# NMR in the
# Life Sciences

# NATO ASI Series

## Advanced Science Institutes Series

*A series presenting the results of activities sponsored by the NATO Science Committee, which aims at the dissemination of advanced scientific and technological knowledge, with a view to strengthening links between scientific communities.*

The series is published by an international board of publishers in conjunction with the NATO Scientific Affairs Division

| | | |
|---|---|---|
| A | **Life Sciences** | Plenum Publishing Corporation |
| B | **Physics** | New York and London |
| C | **Mathematical and Physical Sciences** | D. Reidel Publishing Company Dordrecht, Boston, and Lancaster |
| D | **Behavioral and Social Sciences** | Martinus Nijhoff Publishers |
| E | **Engineering and Materials Sciences** | The Hague, Boston, and Lancaster |
| F | **Computer and Systems Sciences** | Springer-Verlag |
| G | **Ecological Sciences** | Berlin, Heidelberg, New York, and Tokyo |

*Recent Volumes in this Series*

*Series A: Life Sciences*

# NMR in the
# Life Sciences

Edited by

## E. Morton Bradbury

University of California, Davis
Davis, California

and

## Claudio Nicolini

University of Genoa
Genoa, Italy

Plenum Press
New York and London
Published in cooperation with NATO Scientific Affairs Division

Proceedings of a NATO Advanced Study Institute on
NMR in the Life Sciences,
held June 17–29, 1985,
in Erice, Sicily, Italy

Library of Congress Cataloging in Publication Data

NATO Advanced Study Institute on NMR in the Life Sciences (1985: Erice, Sicily)
   NMR in the life sciences.

   (NATO ASI series. Series A, Life sciences; v. 107)
   "Proceedings of a NATO Advanced Study Institute on NMR in the Life
Sciences, held June 17–29, 1985, in Erice, Sicily, Italy"—T.p. verso.
   "Published in cooperation with NATO Scientific Affairs Division."
   Includes bibliographical references and index.
   1. Nuclear magnetic resonance spectroscopy—Congresses. 2. Biomolecules
—Analysis—Congresses. 3. Magnetic resonance imaging—Congresses. I. Brad-
bury, Edwin Morton. II. Nicolini, Claudio A. III. North Atlantic Treaty Organization.
Scientific Affairs Division. IV. Title. V. Series.
QP519.9.N83N38   1985              574.19′285             86-9404
ISBN 0-306-42279-4

© 1986 Plenum Press, New York
A Division of Plenum Publishing Corporation
233 Spring Street, New York, N.Y. 10013

Printed in the United States of America

# PREFACE

This NATO Double Jump Program, held at Erice, Italy, on NMR in the Life Sciences was supported in part by contributions from Oxford Research Systems, Philips International, Technicare Corporation, Varian Instruments, Sciemens Medical, and ESA Control. This program brought together three major research activities in biomedical applications of NMR: high resolution NMR studies of proteins and nucleic acids, in vivo studies of animals, and NMR imaging. Whereas in the development of in vivo NMR and NMR imaging the major technological advances came initially from high resolution NMR spectroscopy, this is no longer the situation. The importance of in vivo NMR and NMR imaging in biomedical science and medical diagnosis has resulted in an explosion of growth in these areas involving schools of medicine, hospitals and instrument manufacturers. Major advances in NMR technology now come from biomedical applications of NMR as well as from high resolution NMR.

Applications of high resolution NMR to the solutions structures of proteins and nucleic acids have been revolutionized by the development of two dimensional NMR Fourier transform techniques and the techniques of biotechnology. Now it is possible, with small proteins up to 10,000-12,000 daltons, by 2D FT NMR techniques to follow the path of the polypeptide backbone through the molecule. The combination of 2D FT NMR techniques with genetically engineered proteins provides one of the most powerful approaches to understanding the principles of protein folding, protein stucture and enzyme catalysis. By site-directed mutagenesis single amino acids in a known protein sequence can be replaced by other amino acids and the effects of those changes assessed on the structure and function of the protein. Major applications of high resolution NMR techniques have been to study the dynamics of proteins and the interactions of ligands with proteins. These have considerably extended our understanding of protein behaviors based on the largely static structures from X-ray crystallography. Major advances have been made in our understanding of the structures and dynamics of nucleic acids in solution by the development of oligonucleotide synthetic techniques. Now it is possible to synthesize oligonucleotides with known sequences and specific substitutions for 2D FT NMR studies of their conformations and conformational behaviors. Strategies have been developed for the assignments of resonances in both small proteins and oligonucleotides. Major questions concerning the functions of nucleic acids which involve the effects of sequence on structure and how specific sequences are recognized by regulatory proteins can now be addressed by the techniques of 2D FT NMR and biotechnology.

In vivo NMR studies of cells in suspension and of organs and tissues are an extension of high resolution NMR techniques but applied to more complex systems. NMR signals derive from the more abundant small molecule metabolites. Determinations of the relative levels of these metabolities provide information on normal and abnormal states of tissues and organs.

Technological questions are concerned with the precise location and spatial resolution of the region in the animal which gives rise to the in vivo spectrum. A major goal is to define the metabolite "profile" of any organ in an animal. In vivo $^{31}$P NMR has been widely used for metabolic studies in a wide range of cells and tissues and organs in small animals. Although very useful, these are restricted by relatively small numbers of phosphate metabolites which can be identified. Major efforts are now being made to extend in vivo NMR by using $^{13}$C and $^{19}$F labelled molecules to answer specific questions concerning metabolic pathways.

NMR imaging is now established as a major technique in medicine for the imaging of soft tissues in normal and diseased states. Major objectives are the development of more inexpensive imagers at lower magnetic fields, the development of real time sequences of images of the beating heart and of blood flow and the coupling of NMR imaging with in vivo NMR so that the regions giving rise to the in vivo spectra can be identified in the NMR image. Major steps have been taken in reaching these objectives.

Many of the objectives outlined above were discussed in detail at the NATO Double Jump Program on NMR in the Life Sciences.

E. M. Bradbury, Professor and Chair, Department of Biological Chemistry, School of Medicine, University of California, Davis, California.

C. Nicolini, Professor and Chair of Biophysics and Institute of Pharmacology, University of Genova School of Medicine, Genova, Italy.

ACKNOWLEDGEMENT: We wish to express our appreciation to Kathleen Martinez and Dorothy Derania for their excellent secretarial assistance in the preparation of this book.

# CONTENTS

# SPECIAL PROBLEMS OF NMR IN $H_2O$ SOLUTION

A. G. Redfield

Department of Biochemistry
Brandeis University
Waltham, MA 02254 U.S.A.

## INTRODUCTION

Most biochemical NMR is performed in aqueous solutions, most often in $D_2O$ containing typically 1% proton impurity as HDO, but also quite often in 80-100% $H_2O$. The latter is necessary if you want to observe exchangeable protons in a macromolecule, or if for some reason replacement of $H_2O$ by $D_2O$ is impractical. The large narrow HDO or $H_2O$ signal, equivalent to up to 100 molar proton concentration, presents various problems which will be outlined here, together with partial solutions.

We have already published several articles on this and related topics,[1,2,3] and in the present article we will avoid repeating the contents of these papers as far as possible. Furthermore, the emphasis will be on techniques that we have used in our own laboratory.

The problem is often presented in terms of the ratios of $H_2O$ molarity to typical solute molarity. This is incorrect since solute signals are often masked by thermal noise in a single free induction decay (FID). The more appropriate comparison is the proton signal-to-thermal-noise amplitude ratio for a typical proton bandwidth into the digitizer of 5 kHz (or 10 ppm at 500 MHz). This ratio is around $2 \times 10^5$ for a 0.2 ml sample at 500 MHz. The digitizer must have dynamic range greater than this, but even a 16 bit digitizer has a signal-to-digitization error of the sixteenth power of two, or $6 \times 10^4$.

Furthermore, another problem arises for macromolecules of size more than about 15 kDalton in $H_2O$. If $H_2O$ is saturated most of the time, either intentionally as in solvent saturation methods (see below) or because the fast repetition of pulses keeps its magnetization well below normal, this saturation can be transferred to the macromolecule and spin-diffuses through it, causing a costly loss in macromolecule NMR signal.[4] Therefore, any method that perturbs the $H_2O$ signal requires a low pulse rate, at a rate less than $T_1^{-1}$ for $H_2O$, or about once every two seconds.

## ENGINEERING AND RELATED ASPECTS

Sixteen bit A/D Converters have sometimes been promoted by instrument makers as a solution to this problem and a necessity for work with $H_2O$, as compared to 12 bit converters. However, it is clear from the last two

1

paragraphs that this is not a complete solution to the problem. There is no question that this and other engineering improvements that will improve the performance of instruments should be encouraged. However, improving linearity and dynamic range of the entire amplifier system to take advantage of the 16 bit A/D may be difficult, and the improvement in actual performance should be evaluated as carefully as possible. Probably there is some advantage to having a 16 bit converter, but not as much as the expected 16-fold improvement over a 12 bit system.

Analog filtering of the signal before A/D conversion to reduce the $H_2O$ signal before conversion is almost always desirable. We have described one carefully thought-out methodology for doing this including computer correction for filter amplitude, as well as phase, varation.[1,2] While first-order phase rotation is generally adequate for this correction, amplitude correction is better because NMR lines close to the filter cut-off can be displayed undistorted. The effect of an analog filter (unlike that of semiselective pulses, described later) can be fully corrected by subsequent data processing. The only disadvantage is loss of dynamic range for peaks close to the cutoff. For selective pulses that discriminate against zero frequency (i.e. the J-R pulse, described later), a dual high pass filter could be used, but this has not been done as far as we know.

Radio and low frequency amplifiers must be arranged with flexibility. Generally the noise level of an amplifier should be about 1/10 the level of the amplified input noise in order to contribute negligible noise power (<1%) while retaining high signal capability. We believe it advantageous to convert a low center frequency (100 kHz in our case) before final (quadrature) conversion to audio frequency because, though more complicated, this allows us to use highly precise analog FET switch conversion in the last stage, to reduce nonlinearity and consequent intermodulation signals (at sums and differences of strong lines). We use triple conversion, to 110 MHz, 6.15, and 100 kHz in the receiver system, and double conversion, from 116.15 MHz, to 110 MHz, and then to 500 MHz in the receiver system. This permits excellent gating by use of multiple gating before mixing, and inexpensive phase shifting of pulses at 6.15 MHz using digital electronics. However, there are workers who believe that multiple down-conversion and low-frequency final conversion is unnecessary and could lead to spurious responses. We also have a fully-linear transmitter system after the 110 MHz level to facilitate precise control of pulse level, including shaped pulses in the future. Instead of the usual non-linear diode arrays we use a Hoult-Richards switch[5] preceeded, in the transmitter line, by a PIN diode switch of standard design (S. Kunz, unpublished), to completely eliminate noise originating in the linear output pulse amplifier.

Software methods[6] to reduce the amplitude of the stored solvent signal serve only a cosmetic purpose in our opinion, except that they do increase the dynamic range of the Fourier Transform (FT) program. However, if the FT program is written in floating point numbers, and/or attention is paid to shift out accumulated roundoff errors in its, dynamic range should not be a problem. These methods should still be useful for compression of 2D data from 32 bit to 16 bit integers, to save storage space and time. We have generalized these methods for arbitrary solvent frequency, and also remove the distortion they produce by post-FT correction (unpublished), for use with a 16-bit FT program; but with a modern (8086-8087 based) computer we no longer need this method of data compression for one-D NMR.

Zero-filling of NMR data is more than a method of interpolation of an N-point spectrum to produce a better looking 2N-point spectra. Rather, it uses the information in the imaginary part of the data set to produce a better value of odd spectral data points (the even points are identical to the points of the N-point FT without zerofilling). However, the sharp end of a long-lasting signal like that of $H_2O$ (See Figure 1 at time T) will produce annoying displacement of the odd points unless the stored data is apodized. We do this, after multiplying the data set by an upward or downward tiling trapezoid ($F_1(t)$ in Fig. 1) which serves to eliminate unwanted data at the end of the FID while approximating resolution

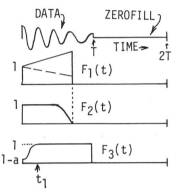

Figure 1. Zerofilled data, and weighting functions described in the text. In $F_1$, the slope can be varied from positive (solid) to negative, as can the cutoff time, under user control. Likewise the parameters a and $t_1$ can be varied. In our system $F_2$ is always goes to zero at the same time as $F_1$, and its cosine cutoff always has the same width of T/4, where T is one fourth the aquisition time.

enhancement or line broadening. The data are then multiplied by an apodization function $F_2(t)$ which effectively multiplies the remaining data by the first quarter of a cosine function. Finally the data are multiplied by a function $F_3$ which reduces or removes the first part of the FID. It is actually the function $F_3 = 1-a[1/2 + 1/2 \cos(t/t_1)]^2$ for $t < \pi t_1$ and $F_2 = 1$ otherwise, where $a<1$ and often $a=1$, and $\pi t_1$ is short compared to the acquisition time. This weighting function gives an approximation to a Gausian convolution-difference spectrum. We believe that Gaussian, rather than Lorenzian (exponential, in the time domain) convolution, is desirable because in theory it produces less far-reaching sag of the baseline away from a strong line. However, Gaussian convolution is the only kind with which we have experience. We use simple cosines, and squares thereof, to speed computation of the weighting function. Actually, these three functions are first computed, then multiplied together, and stored in memory as a single function, and the FID is routinely multiplied by this product function. This weighting is part of the initial subroutine of the FT routine which also includes shuffling of the data according to bit-reversed addresses, a two fold zerofill of the data, and the first set of "butterflies" of the FT. Incidentally, this FT routine is as fast as any we know of for a microcomputer lacking an array processor (1K complex points, 2K total, in about one sec: 8K/16K in ~10 sec). Multiplications are floating point (8087) but additions are time shared 32 bit integer (8086) and butterfly execution is ordered to group together butterflies that use the same sine/cosine values. The 8086/8087 are clocked at 8 MHz.

Details of handling data conversion <u>timing</u> may, or may not, be important. The first pair of complex data points are stored, in analog form, for subsequent conversion within microseconds, exactly $\tau_d$ after the end of the observation pulse, and subsequent samples were taken in intervals $\tau_d$ later, where $\tau_d$ is the dwell time. However, the first conversion pair at time $\tau_d$ is stored as the <u>second</u> point of the FID, while zero is stored as the first point. This is done because the analog filter would certainly put out zero signal at the zero since finite time is required for its output to respond to its input. The receiver system is also gated off for about 50 microsec after the end of the RF pulse, to block the probe tuned circuit ringing from the transmitter pulse.

The <u>NMR tube</u> and <u>shimming</u> can influence the results, and ease of obtaining them, in $H_2O$ solvent. Samples in typical 5 mm NMR tubes having traditional volumes of 0.5 ml or more often give poor baselines because an appreciable part of the sample is in a "bad" part of the field, away from the sensitive region of the probe, but still in region where fringing radio frequency field of the probe will excite $H_2O$, and the probe will pick up the resulting weak signal. The obvious solution is to improve the shimming or get a larger magnet. However, it may be easier to "cheat" on the shimming if one is only interested in, or observing, either only upfield or only downfield of the water resonance: the $z^2$ and $z^4$ shims can often be displaced somewhat to give good lineshape, yet move the field above and below the sample to a lower value, for example, lower value if one is observing downfield of water, thus moving the bad baseline to the upfield side of water where one is not interested. The NMR tube can also be chosen to reduce this problem, by using a semimicro type (Wilmad 510 cp) which confines the sample to the sensitive region of the probe only, and thus eliminates the problem of poor magnet line shape. We generally use a 5 mm tube with 10 mm sample length (volume 0.2 ml). This also optimises sensitivity for a given number of mg of sample, and is a safer way to store samples than is an open 5 mm NMR tube. The disadvantage is that the glass-to-$H_2O$ static magnetic susceptibility mismatch produces line broadening which may be as large as 5 Hz at 500 MHz. We have attempted to replace these tubes with 5 mm tubes having plastic end-filters to continue the sample but with less susceptibility mismatch, without success.

<u>Preirradiation</u> of lines in the proton spectrum for NOE, $T_1$, or exchange rate studies presents problems in $H_2O$ because it stimulates a signal from the water which can be larger than the signal from the observation pulse. This produces baseline curvature in short runs and, more important, it requires running at reduced gain. This problem can be reduced by using a homogeneity <u>spoil</u> pulse, but in our 500 MHz magnet the spoil pulse applied through the shim system must be several msec long, and we have to wait ~10 msec after the spoil to let the eddy currents produced by it to die away. So we asked to the maker of our 500 MHz probes (Cryomagnetic Systems, Indianapolis) to put a spoil coil in our probe, and it works very well. It consists of many turns of fine wire wound on a bobbin on the outside of the glass dewar. This is desirable if you want to

measure short $T_1$'s. A homogeneity spoil pulse interferes with the deuteron lock and to avoid side effects from this interference we turn off the lock system during the time from the start of the spoil pulse to the end of aquisition. During this time the lock field offset is effectively frozen in the equivalent of a track-and-hold circuit.

## SOLVENT SUPPRESSION

So far we have outlined various technical strategies to permit a spectrometer to cope better with a strong solvent or other signal without degraded performance. As indicated at the beginning, these methods are doomed to be inadequate in a modern spectrometer, and we now turn to methods that seek also to drastically reduce selected strong signals such as solvent before they escape from the sample. These can be grouped into three main classes: chemical, which means primarily use of deuterated solvents and, sometimes, other buffer components; solvent saturation methods that seek to reduce the solvent proton signal, or other strong signals, by selectively destroying their magnetization just before pulse excitation; and semiselective pulses that seek not to excite water while appreciably exciting other interesting signals.

### Chemical methods

These have been discussed elsewhere[3] in slight detail. There is not much to say except that the method cannot be used to observe protons that exchange with solvent in a time that is not long compared to the time needed to change solvent and do an experiment, whatever that may be. This precludes its use for most nucleic acid nitrogen protons, and for proton amide protons close to or on the protein surface.

### Solvent saturation

Strategies for solvent saturation can be grouped into two categories. First are more or less continuous wave (CW) methods which use long ($>\sim 0.1$ sec) monochromatic pulses to saturate water during some section of the pulse cycle, generally just after acquisition during the time needed for other spins to recover equilibrium. Doing so is usually possible on modern spectrometers, and, if the power can be suitably reduced, can be very selective and reduce water spinning sidebands as well as the main water signal. This method is most useful as a simple way to selectively eliminate the HDO signal in nominal $D_2O$, to eliminate signals from high concentration protonated buffer components other than $H_2O$, in conjunction with selective pulses to eliminate $H_2O$; and for $\sim$ small macromolecules (MW $< 15,000$) where spin-diffusion from solvated $H_2O$ will not occur rapidly enough to wipe out the spectrum. Saturation methods have the advantage over selective excitation methods (below) that they are more selective than the latter, as lines within only 10-50 Herz of solvent are directly affected; and they are simple. Disadvantages are that they are difficult to use for observation of protons that are rapidly-exchanging with solvent, or for larger macromolecules.

A related second set of pulse preparation techniques use the generally long $T_1$ of $H_2O$ to discriminate and eliminate the $H_2O$ magnetization. We have no experience with these methods; they are rather complicated to set up, are not very selective, and are not widely used.

### Selective excitation

These methods can be grouped into three classes. The first of these includes CW excitation, and correlation or rapid scan NMR which is similar to CW excitation except that rapid frequency sweep excitation is used. In both cases water is largely not excited, by simply stopping the sweep before water is reached. We have discussed these elsewhere.[3] They have largely fallen into disuse probably because they have proven difficult to implement routinely and with high sensitivity.

Soft Pulse Sequences. The remaining selective excitation methods are pulse methods. Long pulse methods[1,2,3] include the plain long (or soft) pulse first introduced long before FT NMR by S. Alexander, and the 214 pulse which is really the composite of an Alexander soft pulse and a 1-1 pulse (below) combined to give a broader region over which the $H_2O$ resonance and its spinning sidebands are selectively unexcited. We have discussed soft pulse methods repeatedly; here we will simply point out relative virtues. The principle advantage is that when well implimented they are easier to use than hard pulse methods and may be more forgiving of some spectrometer defects. These methods do not require excellent rf field inhomogeneity. The principle disadvantages are that they cannot now be implemented on commercial spectrometers without addition of an attenuator in the transmitter line; fine phase control of parts of the pulse is very desirable for the 214 pulse; and pulse amplitude stability (including a lack of pulse-amplitude droop) is required. The latter problem can be circumvented on some spectrometers by eliminating the final amplifier, since less than one watt of power is usually required. Finally, the simple Alexander soft pulse is often forgotten but is still potentially very useful because of its simplicity. At modern high fields radiation damping might prevent a good $H_2O$ null but this could be achieved by appending a short pulse 90° phase-shifted from the long pulse.

Common Problems. A few general comments about selective pulse methods will be inserted here. Most of these methods are unusable for observing both signals very far from solvent, and those close to solvent, in the same run; and many are not suitable for observing both signals upfield from $H_2O$, and downfield, in the same run. Repeated runs with different pulse parameters may then be required. However, this lack of selectivity can be an advantage if uselessly crowded sections of macromolecule spectra can be partly discriminated against, because their signals can also overload the spectrometer, and because the entire set of protons in a macromolecule relax more slowly than do a subset of the protons semiselectively excited, since in the latter case spin diffusion is more effective for the recovery of the excited spins.

The problem of amplitude and phase instability is a serious one that generally requires detailed trouble shooting. The symptom is an unacceptably large variation in solvent signal at the best null point, or a poor null point. In using these sequences it is extremely useful to have a loudspeaker to audibly output the signal and an oscilloscope x-y display to display the two outputs of the quadrature detecter. The excellence of the null is a parameter sometimes given as a figure of merit, and we have heard claims made of a few thousand fold for the reduction of the signal. The best we routinely acheive is about a 200-fold reduction, estimated by comparing the size of the null signal into the A/D computer to the size of the $H_2O$ signal after a 90° pulse. The latter is not measured directly, but is inferred from the signal from a shorter pulse, typically a 1° pulse. A 200-fold null is adequate since it reduces the water signal to within the A/D converter range at a gain setting where the digitizer error is at least one-third the thermal noise.

All selective pulse sequences except the J-R and 1-1 sequences (below) produce serious first order phase distortion of the spectrum. This can be corrected by a first-order correction but this correction produces baseline droop, as discussed elsewhere[2], at the edges of strong lines. Convolution—difference treatment of the data helps cosmetically in some

6

cases, but can distort total intensities of overlapping lines. However, clever successive-approximation, computer correction of the baseline is possible without subjective human intervention.[7] Incidentally, in my opinion this problem is sometimes exaggerated. Delay of the start of data acquisition could produce reported baseline effects called "baseline roll" or "phase roll". We never observe such strong baseline effects (see above, under "timing"), only a very broad curvature due to imperfect $H_2O$ nulling and to the wings of the major aromatic or aliphatic groups of resonances.

Our final general remark concerns the use of phase shifts as well as length adjustment in selective pulses. As described elsewhere we use both fixed and continuously variable phase shifters to get a good $H_2O$ null.[2,3] For a variety of reasons it is desirable to shift the entire phase of selective proton pulses relative to each other, for example in spin-echo or 2D sequences, while maintaining good nulling. It is then by far most flexible and convenient to have completely separate phase shifters for these latter overall shifts. This permits, for example, the use of variable relative phase shifters within a sequence which is very convenient even if not absolutely necessary. And it avoids the necessity of having phase shifts that are precisely 90°, 180°, and 270° as would otherwise be necessary.

HARD PULSE SEQUENCES. We now discuss one class of hard composite pulses. By this we mean composites of short high-power pulses. A large number of these have been demonstrated by now, starting with time-shared versions of Alexander and 214 pulses, and including pulse sequences designed to have broad nulls, narrow nulls, or uniform excitation over a broad band (see, for example, reference 8). We have experience with only one of these which we call a modified J-R pulse, which is essentially the same as sequences called either J-R pulse[7] or 1-1 pulse[9], and limit our discussion to these sequences.

Hard pulse sequences have the advantage that they can be set up and tried (though not necessarily made to work well) on a modern instrument. They are as prone to many of the difficulties outlined above as is the 214 pulse with the possible exception of pulse amplitude droop. Based on our very limited experience, it is somewhat harder to find and optimise the null for hard pulses compared to the soft 214 pulse, and random variations in the null are greater probably because the same nanosecond random variation is bound to be more important for a short high power pulse than for a weak long pulse.

The J-R or 1-1 pulses consist of two theoretically short hard 90° pulses separated by a short time $\tau_p$. The first pulse flips the water magnetization by 90° and the second is suitably phased and timed to return it exactly to the z-axis. This property is independent of whether the two pulses are 90° pulses, or are both some other but equal length, and this is an advantage since the null is rf field independent. More remarkable and useful is that in the case of 90° pulses there is theoretically no first order phase shift in the resulting spectrum although there is an important amplitude distortion. The first pulse puts the entire magnetization in the x-y plane; $\tau_p$ is then picked to allow spins of different frequency to spread apart appreciably in a pizza-shaped distribution in the x-y plane; and the second pulse flips the pizza exactly 90°, so that the $H_2O$ magnetization is back along the z-axis while the other spins all have different z components but their projection is in the same direction. It is this projection which gives the relative phase of different signals and this phase is therefore constant for all sets of protons.

The size of this transverse projection gives the relative sizes of the NMR signals and this is easily shown to be proportional to $\sin (2\pi\Delta f \ \tau_p)$

where $\Delta f$ is the distance in Herz of a line from solvent. Thus $\tau_p$ is set at one half the inverse of the distance in Hertz from the $H_2O$ resonance, of the most interesting part of the spectrum. An added advantage is that the pulse sequence is probably the shortest semiselective sequence available for looking at a given set of lines; a soft pulse or 214 pulse is twice as long.

The J-R pulse[7] is a $90_x-\tau_p-90_{-x}$ sequence and water is jumped down in the first pulse, stays fixed in the rotating frame during $\tau_p$, and returned in an exactly reverse path to the z-axis (J-R stands for "Jump and Return"). The carrier frequency is set equal to the water resonance frequency. The 1-1 pulse[9] is a $90_x-\tau_p-90_x$ sequence and the carrier is placed a distance $2/\tau_p$ in Hertz from water resonance, downfield or upfield of desired part of both water and the desired part of the spectrum. The water magnetization in the rotating frame rotates exactly 180° in the x-y plane during $\tau_p$. The advantage of this variant is that no 180° phase shift is required and it is more straightforward to filter out the computer residual water signal using commercial spectrometers. A disadvantage is that half the storage is wasted though this can easily be fixed by software; also more power is required to see lines on both sides of water. The modified JR sequence that we use[10] is $90_x-\tau_d-90_{\pm y}$. The carrier is placed at the center of a sensitive region of the pulse, $2/\tau_p$ Hertz upfield or downfield of water, and the water magnetization rotates one quarter turn in the x-y plane during $\tau_d$. Whether the second pulse is $90_{+y}$ or $90_{-y}$ depends on whether the carrier frequency is up-or downfield of water. We chose this variant because we do not have much power, and it seemed better to be able to place the carrier at the center of the spectrum. We are generally only interested in the region well downfield of water.

A brief description of our experience with this JR pulse may be useful. Our 3 watt final transmitter provides 50 μsec 90° pulses but for some reason when we use the modified J-R pulse it is much easier to operate with ~35 μsec pulses and it is generally possible to get a flatter baseline after some extensive trial adjustment, with the J-R pulse than with the 214 pulse. Actually, the best J-R baseline sometimes has a linear slope, whereas the best 214 baseline is curved (Fig. 2). Dr. Richard Griffey (unpublished) has programmed our Varian XL-300 to use this modified JR pulse, and found it to work better than the JR or 1-1 pulses on that spectrometer.

The real reason we were interested in the J-R pulse was its lack of a first order phase shift, for use in 2D NMR. In $H_2O$ solutions of larger macromolecules it is obviously highly desirable that all proton pulses be selective against water, to permit higher repetition rates as we described at the beginning. But the first-order phase shifts produced by most such pulses seemed an undesirable complication since we also wished to do pure-phase 2D. The modified J-R pulse has been used successfully by Richard Griffey in our laboratory to obtain 2D NOE (NOESY) spectra of tRNA.

Somewhat surprising was our experience with Hahn spin echoes in $H_2O$ using 90°-180° sequences. What worked best for the 180° pulse was, inelegantly, two modified 90° JR pulses immediately after each other, as compared to a single "180° J-R" pulse in which the spacing is twice that of the composite 90° JR pulse (ie $2\tau_p$). We have not investigated why this is, or worked with other pulses such as a soft 180° pulse.

OTHER AREAS OF NMR

For completeness we mention two related developments. First, remarkable results have recently been obtained in observation of

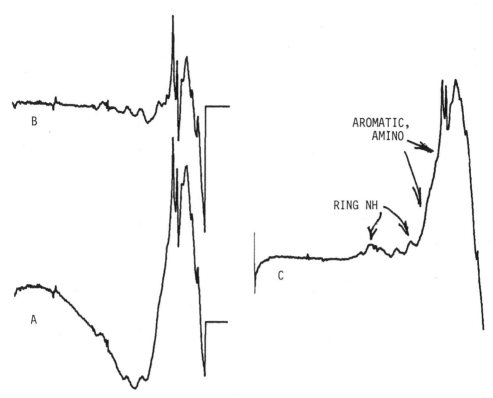

Figure 2. Spectra of approximately one mM tRNA complexed to an equimolar
amount of an enzyme in 90% $H_2O$ buffer. The complex has a
combined molecular weight of about 90 kilodaltons and is
inherently difficult to study for that reason, but it
illustrates the problems connected with such samples. A.
Spectrum obtained with a soft 214 pulse. B. Same data as A,
with a rather severe degree of convolution-difference correction
applied to emphasize sharp lines. C. Spectrum obtained on the
same sample, with less difficulty, using a modified JR pulse as
described in the text.

metabolites in tissues, using a JR pulse[11]. Second, it is my understanding
that frequency-selective pulses are routinely used in NMR imaging, and I
assume that their use is discussed in more detail elsewhere in this
volume.

CONCLUSION

As we stated at the beginning, we have tried not to repeat topics
discussed in our earlier articles, and the reader is referred in particular
to references 2 and 3 as a supplement to the present article. One thing
bears repeating: in biochemical NMR it is worth applying as many of these
techniques as possible at the same time; they are often complementary (for
example in some cases selective pulses and solvent saturation). And the
fact that we may have not emphasized, or not mentioned, certain methods
should not deter you from trying them. Flexibility is the proper approach
to this difficult field.

## ACKNOWLEDGEMENTS

I thank Sara Kunz for help in developing these methods, and all members of my research group over the years for stimulating us to develop them and for their patience while we were working on them. This work was supported by U.S.P.H.S. Grant GM20168. The author is also with the Physics Department and the Rosenstiel Center for Basic Medical Sciences at Brandeis University. This is paper No. 1560 of the Brandeis University Biochemistry Department.

## REFERENCES

1. A. G. Redfield and R. K. Gupta. Adv. Magn. Reson. 5, 81 (1971).
2. A. G. Redfield. NMR: Basic Principles and Progress 13, 152 (1976).
3. A. G. Redfield. Methods Enzymol. 49, 253 (1978).
4. J. D. Stoesz, A. G. Redfield, and D. Malinowski. FEBS Letters 9, 320 (1978).
5. D. I. Hoult and R. E. Richards. J. Magn. Reson. 22, 561 (1976).
6. K. Roth, B. J. Kimber, and J. Feeney. J. Magn. Reson. 41, 302 (1980).
7. P. Plateau, C. Dumas, and M. Gueron. J. Magn. Reson. 54, 46 (1983).
8. P. J. Hore. J. Magn. Reson. 55, 285 (1983).
9. G. M. Clore, B. J. Kimber, and A. M. Gronnenborn. J. Magn. Reson. 54, 170 (1983).
10. A. G. Redfield. Chem. Phys. Lett. 96, 537 (1983).
11. C. Arus, M. Barany, W. M. Westler, and J. L. Markley. J. Magn. Reson. 57, 519 (1984).

# 2D NMR WITH BIOPOLYMERS

Kurt Wüthrich

Institut für Molekularbiologie und Biophysik
Eidgenössische Technische Hochschule
CH-8093 Zürich - Hönggerberg, Switzerland

## INTRODUCTION: 1D AND 2D NMR

With the use of two-dimensional (2D) nuclear magnetic resonance (NMR) experiments (Aue et al., 1976 ; Bax, 1982), the potentialities of NMR for studies of biopolymers can be greatly enhanced. This paper describes 2D NMR experiments which are commonly used for work with proteins and nucleic acids. To familiarize the reader with the subject, 2D NMR is first compared with conventional one-dimensional (1D) experiments.

A normal 1D NMR experiment provides information on the chemical shifts and the spin-spin coupling fine structures of the individual resonances in the spectrum. To obtain additional data on through-bond, scalar connectivities or through-space, dipolar connectivities between individual spins, which provide the basis for resonance assignments and conformational studies in biopolymers (Wüthrich et al., 1982; Wüthrich, 1983), double or multiple irradiation experiments must be used. These rely on selective irradiation of a particular resonance line with a radio frequency (rf) field $\vec{H}_2$ and observation of the resulting effects in the rest of the spectrum. For nuclear Overhauser enhancement (NOE) experiments the selective irradiation is applied prior to the non-selective observation pulse, and for spin decoupling experiments it is applied in a time shared mode during the acquisition of the free induction decay (FID). For work with the complex, crowded spectra of biopolymers (Fig. 1) the use of 1D double irradiation experiments is naturally limited. While the spectral resolution for observation of double irradiation effects in crowded spectral regions has customarily been improved by difference spectroscopy, lack of selectivity for irradiation of individual lines in spectral regions with mutually overlapping resonances is a stringent limitation. Furthermore, since each 1D double resonance experiment usually provides only one (though in favorable cases two to five) connectivities, a very large number of measurements would be required for characterization of the complete network of spin-spin connectivities in a macromolecular structure.

With 2D NMR techniques these natural limitations of 1D experiments can be largely overcome. A 2D NMR experiment uses a two-dimensional laboratory time space in the following sense. Analogous to 1D NMR the FID is recorded during the "detection period", $t_2$, after the observation pulse. However, taking homonuclear correlated spectroscopy (COSY) as an exmaple (Fig. 2D), another non-selective rf-pulse is applied prior to the observation pulse. While no signal is recorded after this first pulse, its influence on the FID, which depends on the length of the "evolution period" $t_1$ between the two pulses, is also recorded during $t_2$. A second laboratory time dimension can thus be created by repeating the same experiment with incrementation of $t_1$. For each value of $t_1$ a FID recorded during $t_2$ is stored, so that a data matrix $s(t_1,t_2)$ is obtained. A 2D Fourier transformation of $s(t_1,t_2)$ then produces the desired 2D frequency spectrum $S(\omega_1,\omega_2)$. In the COSY spectrum of Fig. 3 the chemical shift information is contained in the positions of the peaks along the diagonal from the upper right to the lower left ("diagonal peaks"), and the spin-spin coupling fine structure may also be resolved. In addition, scalar coupling connectivities between individual spins are manifested by "cross peaks" located at the intersections of straight lines parallel to the frequency axes $\omega_1$ and $\omega_2$ through the diagonal peaks. When compared with 1D NMR the most important, fundamental difference for work with biological macromolecules arises because selective connectivities between individual spins are established in experiments which use exclusively non-selective rf-pulses (Fig. 2). In addition, a single COSY experiment can in principle delineate all spin-spin coupling connectivities between protons in a macromolecular structure, and it is thus much more efficient than the use of 1D spin decoupling experiments. Furthermore, because the resonance peaks are spread out in two dimensions, the spectral resolutions is usually substantially improved.

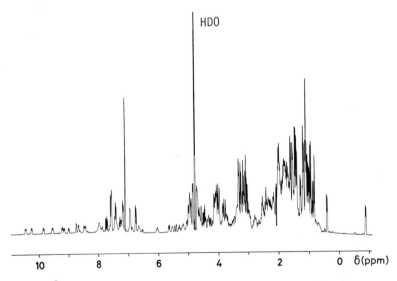

Fig. 1. 1D [1]H NMR spectrum at 360 MHz recorded in a freshly prepared 0.01 M solution of the protease inhibitor K from the venom of the black mamba (Dendroaspis polylepis polylepis), pD = 3.4, T = 25°C.

EXPERIMENTAL SCHEMES FOR 2D NMR SPECTROSCOPY

A general scheme for 2D NMR spectroscopy includes four successive time periods (Fig. 2A). The preparation period usually consists of a long delay time, during which thermal equilibrium is attained, followed by one or several rf-pulses to create coherence. During the evolution period the coherence evolves and at the end of this interval the system assumes a specified state which depends on the elapsed time $t_1$ and the spin Hamilton operator, $\mathcal{H}^{(1)}$, which is effective during $t_1$. The mixing period may include pulses and delay intervals. During the detection period the system evolves further under the effective spin Hamilton operator, $\mathcal{H}^{(2)}$, and the resulting FID is recorded and stored as $s'(t_2)$. The lengths of the preparation, mixing and detection periods are in principle invariant for all the experiments needed to obtain a complete 2D data set, $s(t_1,t_2)$, whereas $t_1$ is incremented between the individual measurements $s'(t_2)$. In the 2D spectrum, $S(\omega_1,\omega_2)$, obtained by 2D Fourier transformation of $s(t_1,t_2)$ (Fig. 3), the precession frequencies during evolution and detection (i.e. under $\mathcal{H}^{(1)}$ and $\mathcal{H}^{(2)}$, respectively) determine the coordinates of the signal peaks. The mixing process determines the frequency pairs, $(\omega_1,\omega_2)$, which produce peaks of non-vanishing intensity. Of the four periods in Fig. 2A, preparation, evolution and detection are mandatory, whereas a mixing period is necessary for certain 2D NMR experiments only.

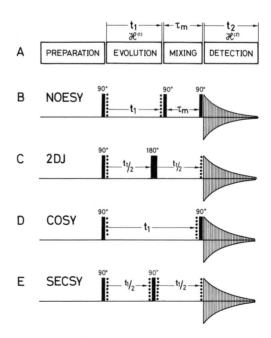

Fig. 2. (A) General experimental scheme for 2D NMR spectroscopy. (B)-(E) Experimental schemes for four homonuclear [1]H 2D NMR experiments. The dotted lines indicate the bounds of the evolution period in the different experiments.

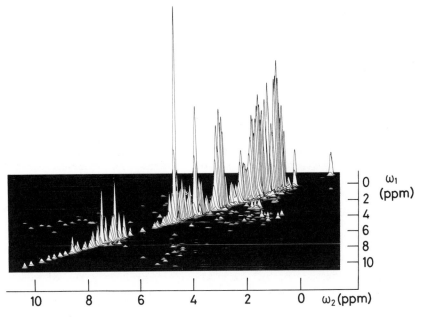

Fig. 3. $^1$H COSY spectrum at 360 MHz of the inhibitor K in $D_2O$
(same sample as Fig. 1).

The four experiments presented in Fig. 2, B-E, have been of central
importance for the early development of $^1$H 2D NMR studies with biopolymers.
In all cases the preparation consists of a delay interval, which can be
adjusted according to $T_1$ of the spins of interest, and a 90$^o$ pulse at the
end, and the detection is also the same for the four measurements. The 2D
nuclear Overhauser enhancement (NOESY) experiment requires an extensive
mixing period separated from the evolution and detection periods by two
90$^o$ pulses (Fig. 2B). In its outlay it thus coincides exactly with the
general scheme of Fig. 2A. NOESY delivers spectra with the appearance of
Fig.3, but in contrast to COSY the cross peaks put into evidence dipole-
dipole coupling between nuclear spins in close spatial proximity, which
gives rise to NOE's (Anil Kumar et al. 1980). The same experiment can be
employed for studies of magnetization transfer by chemical exchange or
physical exchange processes (Meier and Ernst, 1979).

In 2DJ-resolved spectroscopy the evolution period contains a 180$^o$
pulse in the middle, and there is no mixing period (Fig. 2C). At the end
of the evolution a spin echo is produced, which for weakly coupled spin
systems manifests exclusively the spin-spin couplings. 2DJ-spectroscopy
thus affords a separation of spin-spin coupling fine structure and chemical shifts, so that after suitable data manipulation the resonance
multiplets are manifested along the $\omega_1$-axis perpendicular to the chemical
shift axis $\omega_2$ (Aue et al., 1976 ; Nagayama et al. 1977; 1978). Fig. 4
illustrates that the spectral resolution can be greatly improved by the
2DJ technique and that this experiment readily identifies all components
of a given multiplet.

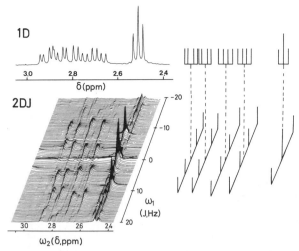

Fig. 4. Improved resolution in 2DJ spectra when compared to 1D NMR.
The [1]H NMR spectrum of a mixture of Ala, Ile, Met, Tyr and
His (0.1 M each, $D_2O$, pD 10.6, 25°C; 360 MHz) between 2.4
and 3.0 ppm contains a triplet and four doublets of doublets
corresponding to $\gamma CH_2$ of Met and $\beta CH_2$ of Tyr and His. The
schemes on the right indicate the arrangements of the multiplets in the experimental spectra. (From Wüthrich et al., 1979).

In COSY the mixing is obtained by the 90° pulse separating evolution
and detection (Fig. 2D). COSY produces correlation maps which display the
connectivity of nuclei by scalar spin-spin coupling (Fig. 3) and thus
provides information on proximity of nuclei along the chemical bonds
(Aue et al., 1976; Nagayama et al., 1980; Bax and Freeman, 1981).

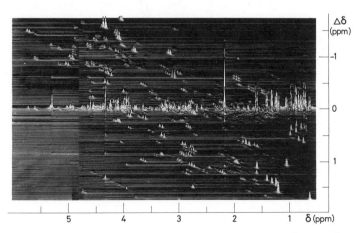

Fig. 5. 360 MHz SECSY spectrum of a 0.01 M solution of BPTI in $D_2O$,
pD 7.0, 68°C. Except for the aromatic region, the complete
spectrum of the non-labile protons is shown. (From Nagayama
et al., 1980).

Spin echo correlated spectroscopy (SECSY) (Fig. 2E) is a variant of COSY using delayed detection (Nagayama et al., 1979; 1980). Formally it resembles the 2DJ experiment, from which it can be derived by replacing the 180$^O$ spin echo pulse by a 90$^O$ mixing pulse. Delayed acquisition results in a different outlay of the correlation map (Fig.5). SECSY peaks corresponding to the diagonal peaks in COSY are on a horizontal line through the center of the spectrum, and the pairs of cross peaks in symmetrical positions relative to the diagonal in COSY lie on straight lines at an angle of 45$^O$ relative to the horizontal axis. Compared to COSY, a SECSY spectrum occupies less memory space along $\omega_1$. Another important difference between the two experiments arises because in spectra recorded with delayed acquisition the absorption and dispersion mode components cannot routinely be separated (Wider et al., 1984).

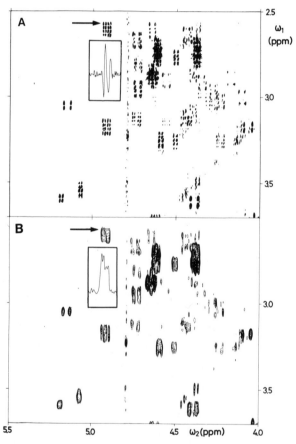

Fig. 6. Improved resolution in phase sensitive COSY. The same time domain data set recorded for rabbit liver metallothionein-2 (0.005 M, in $D_2O$, pD 7.0, 24$^O$C at 500 MHz was transformed (A) in the phase sensitive mode, (B) in the absolute value mode. Otherwise identical data handling was applied for the two spectra. A region containing αH-βH cross peaks is shown. The insets contain cross sections along $\omega_2$ through the higher field αH-βH cross-peak of Asp 2 taken at the $\omega_1$-position indicated by the arrow. In the contour plots positive and negative levels are not distinguished.

## ABSOLUTE VALUE AND PHASE SENSITIVE MODE

The 2D Fourier transformation of the time domain data set $s(t_1,t_2)$ can be considered as consisting of two subsequent 1D transformations, usually first with respect to $t_2$ and then with respect to $t_1$. This yields a complex frequency domain data matrix

$$S(\omega_1,\omega_2) = R(\omega_1,\omega_2)+iI(\omega_1,\omega_2), \tag{1}$$

where both $R(\omega_1,\omega_2)$ and $I(\omega_1,\omega_2)$ can contain a mixture of absorptive and dispersive signals. Until 1983 the spectra of biopolymers were presented in the absolute value mode

$$|S(\omega_1,\omega_2)| = [R^2(\omega_1,\omega_2)+I^2(\omega_1,\omega_2)]^{1/2}. \tag{2}$$

Two different procedures for obtaining pure 2D absorption spectra were then implemented for use with large data matrices (States et al. 1982; Marion and Wüthrich, 1983), and presently the phase sensitive mode is used almost exclusively. The main advantages of absorption spectra are the higher resolution and the possibility of distinguishing between positive and negative intensities.

Fig. 6 illustrates the improvement of the spectral resolution which can be achieved with otherwise identical data recording and manipulation by the phase sensitive mode when compared to the absolute value mode. In the absolute value spectrum one recognizes outlines of the cross peaks with only partly resolved multiplet fine structure along $\omega_2$. The pure absorption mode cross peaks show well resolved multiplet fine structure in both frequency dimensions. The improved resolution is a consequence both of the narrower absorption lines and the antiphase intensity distribution in the absorption mode multiplets. In practice the antiphase fine structure patterns often enable unambiguous identification of cross-peaks in difficult situations, for example in noisy regions, near the diagonal, or in areas crowded with mutually overlapping cross-peaks.


## SUPPRESSION OF THE SOLVENT RESONANCE

Both resonance assignments and structure determination in biopolymers by NMR depend critically on observation of potentially labile protons, for example the backbone amide protons in proteins or the hydrogen bonded imino protons in the Watson-Crick base pairs of nucleic acids. 2D spectra must therefore often be recorded in $H_2O$ solution, so as to prevent loss of cross peaks with labile protons. The spectroscopist then faces serious experimental problems, since the weak solute signals (typical concentration range 0.001 to 0.01 M) have to be detected in the presence of the huge signal from the water protons (concentration 110 M). To work under these conditions, different 2D NMR procedures are employed for experiments with slowly exchanging interior amide protons in proteins, the more rapidly exchanging solvent accessible amide protons in proteins at slightly acidic pH, or the highly labile protons in nucleic acids or in polypeptides at high pH.

Interior amide protons in proteins can often be observed in $D_2O$, so that no special precautions are needed for suppression of the solvent line (Wagner et al., 1981). Even when dealing with more rapidly exchanging amide protons in $H_2O$ solutions of proteins, these can usually be studied using selective saturation of the solvent line (Wider et al., 1984).

Four experimental schemes, which have all been used in practice for both COSY and NOESY, are shown in Fig. 7. In these schemes, time shared irradiation during $t_2$ (A and C) tends to produce spurious signals in the spectra, and continuous irradiation during $t_1$ (B and C) can cause Bloch-Siegert shifts for resonance lines near the solvent (Wider et al., 1983). However, since the $t_1$-values employed for work with biological macromolecules are relatively short, satisfactory suppression can be achieved with the experiment of Fig. 7 D, which therefore is in most cases the best choice. Fig. 8 shows a representative spectrum recorded with this technique. The major residual perturbation, i.e. a band of $t_1$-noise at the $\omega_2$-position of the solvent line, was in this example removed by symmetrization (Baumann et al., 1981). Furthermore, the cross peaks with $\alpha$-protons which overlap with the solvent line are "bleached out" (Anil Kumar et al., 1980), so that a narrow spectral region of approximately $\pm$ 0.05 ppm about the solvent position is "empty". Typically, up to five cross peaks are thus lost in the COSY "fingerprint" (Wagner and Wüthrich, 1982) of a small protein. A complete data set can usually be obtained by combination of measurements at two different temperatures.

Solvent suppression in $H_2O$ solutions of nucleic acids, or polypeptides under conditions of rapid exchange, can be achieved by use of semi-selective pulses in the 2D NMR experimental schemes (Redfield and Kunz, 1979). For example with the use of a time shared long pulse as the observation pulse in the NOESY scheme, the solvent resonance can be suppressed by a factor of 200 to 500 (Haasnoot and Hilbers, 1983). Further suppression of the water peak by a factor 50 to 200 can then be achieved by digital shift accumulation, so that overall a suppression by a factor $1x10^4$ to $1x10^5$ can be obtained.

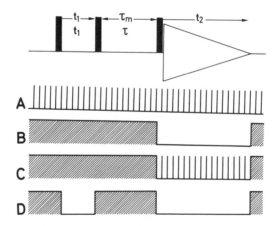

Fig. 7. Solvent suppression by saturation in $H_2O$ solutions
of proteins. The traces A to D show four different
switching cycles for the selective irradiation of the
water resonance during a NOESY experiment (top trace).
A shaded bar indicates continuous irradiation, vertical lines represent time shared irradiation, and empty
spaces indicate that the decoupler was turned off.
(From Wider et al., 1983).

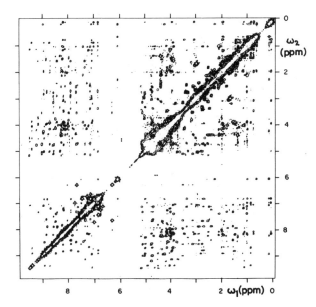

Fig. 8. $^1$H NOESY spectrum of the protein bull seminal
inhibitor (BUSI IIA) in $H_2O$ (0.016 M solution,
pH 4.9, 45$^\circ$C) recorded at 500 MHz. Residual
perturbations from the water suppression by
selective saturation (Fig. 7) were removed
by symmetrization. (From Strop et al., 1983).

DATA PROCESSING

The appearence of 2D NMR spectra obtained from recordings with a
given set of performance parameters can be improved by multiplication
of the time domain data set $s(t_1,t_2)$ with suitable weighting functions
$h_2(t_2)$ and $h_1(t_1)$. Base line correction and resolution enhancement are
routinely applied. Much work has been invested for optimizing weighting
functions for resolution enhancement in spectra of proteins or nucleic
acids (e.g. Campbell et al., 1973). For 2D work with biopolymers the sine
bell (DeMarco and Wüthrich, 1976), or in improved versions a shifted sine
bell (Wagner et al., 1978) or a squared sine bell are very easily generated and applied. Rather strong resolution enhancement is indispensable
for the presentation of absolute value 2D NMR spectra of macromolecules.
As an illustration of the effects which one can expect from the application of a suitable weighting function selected from the wide variety
of different resolution enhancement routines, Fig. 9 presents data obtained with micelle-bound glucagon (Wider et al., 1982; 1984). After
multiplication with a cosine function, which produces no resolution
enhancement, the broad tails of the absolute value peaks in the spectrum
of Fig. 9A mask the information content of the spectrum, whereas
numerous cross peaks were resolved after multiplication with a squared
sine bell (Fig. 9B).

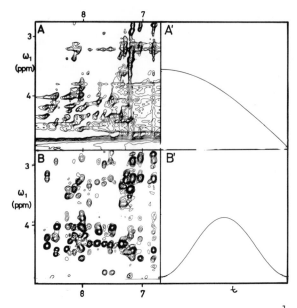

Fig. 9. Improvement of an absolute value 2D [1]H NMR spectrum by different resolution enhancement functions. A region from a 500 MHz [1]H NOESY spectrum of a sample of the polypeptide hormone glucagon bound to perdeuterated dodecylphosphocholine micelles is shown as obtained after digital filtering in both dimensions with (A) the cosine function A', (B) the sine squared function B'. (From Wider et al., 1984).

ACKNOWLEDGEMENTS

My thanks go to the many colleagues mentioned in the references who worked with enthusiasm on the development of these experiments, and to Mrs. E. Huber and Mrs. E.H. Hunziker for the careful preparation of the manuscript and the figures. Financial support for this work was over the years obtained from the Schweizerischer Nationalfonds and from the Kommission zur Förderung der Wissenschaftlichen Forschung.

REFERENCES

Anil Kumar, Ernst, R.R., and Wüthrich, K., 1980, A Two-Dimensional Nuclear Overhauser Enhancement (2D NOE) Experiment for the Elucidation of Complete Proton-Proton Cross-Relaxation Networks in Biological Macromolecules, Biochem. Biophys. Res. Comm., 95:1.

Anil Kumar, Wagner, G., Ernst, R.R., and Wüthrich, K., 1980, Studies of J-Connectivities and Selective [1]H-[1]H Overhauser Effects in $H_2O$ Solutions of Biological Macromolecules by Two-Dimensional NMR Experiments, Biochem. Biophys. Res. Comm., 96:1156.

Aue, W.P., Bartholdi, E., and Ernst, R.R., 1976, Two-Dimensional
    Spectroscopy. Application to NMR. J. Chem. Phys., 44:2229.
Aue, W.P., Karhan, J., and Ernst, R.R., 1976, Homonuclear Broad Band
    Decoupling and Two-Dimensional J-Resolved NMR Spectroscopy,
    J. Chem. Phys., 64:4226.
Baumann, R., Wider, G., Ernst, R.R., and Wüthrich, K., 1981, Improvement
    of 2D NOE and 2D Correlated Spectra by Symmetrization, J. Magn.
    Reson., 44:402.
Bax, A., 1982, "Two-Dimensional Nuclear Magnetic Resonance in Liquids,"
    Reidel, London.
Bax, A., and Freeman, R., 1981, Investigation of Complex Networks of
    Spin-Spin Coupling by Two-Dimensional NMR, J. Magn. Reson., 44:542.
Campbell, I.D., Dobson, C.M., Williams, R.J.P., and Xavier, A.V., 1973,
    Resolution Enhancement of Protein PMR Spectra Using the Difference
    between a Broadened and a Normal Spectrum, J. Magn. Reson., 11:172.
DeMarco, A., and Wüthrich, K., 1976, Digital Filtering with a Sinusiodal
    Window Function: An Alternative Technique for Resolution Enhancement
    in FT NMR, J. Magn. Reson., 24:201.
Haasnoot, C.A.G., and Hilbers, C.W., 1983, Effective Water Resonance
    Suppression in 1D- and 2D-FT-[1]H NMR Spectroscopy of Biopolymers
    in Aqueous Solution, Biopolymers, 22:1259.
Marion, D., and Wüthrich, K., 1983, Applications of Phase Sensitive Two-
    Dimensional Correlated Spectroscopy (COSY) for Measurements of
    [1]H-[1]H Spin-Spin Coupling Constants in Proteins, Biochem. Biophys.
    Res. Comm., 113:967.
Meier, B.H., and Ernst, R.R., 1979, Elucidation of Chemical Exchange
    Networks by Two-Dimensional NMR Spectroscopy: The Heptamethyl-
    benzenonium Ion, J. Am. Chem. Soc., 101:6441.
Nagayama, K., Anil Kumar, Wüthrich, K., and Ernst, R.R., 1980, Experi-
    mental Techniques of Two-Dimensional Correlated Spectroscopy,
    J. Magn. Reson., 40:321.
Nagayama, K., Bachmann, P., Wüthrich, K., and Ernst, R.R., 1978, The Use
    of Cross-Sections and of Projections in Two-Dimensional NMR
    .Spectroscopy, J. Magn. Reson., 31:133.
Nagayama, K., Wüthrich, K., Bachmann, P., and Ernst, R.R., 1977, Two-
    Dimensional J-Resolved [1]H n.m.r. Spectroscopy of Biological
    Macromolecules, Biochem. Biophys. Res. Comm., 78:99.
Nagayama, K., Wüthrich, K., and Ernst, R.R., 1979, Two-Dimensional Spin
    Echo Correlated Spectroscopy (SECSY) for [1]H NMR Studies of Bio-
    logical Macromolecules, Biochem. Biophys. Res. Comm., 90:305.
Redfield, A.G., and Kunz, S.D., 1979, Proton Resonance Spectrometer for
    Biochemical Application, in "NMR and Biochemistry", S.J. Opella
    and P. Lu, eds., Dekker, New York.
States, D.J., Haberkorn, R.A., and Ruben, D.J., 1982, A Two-Dimensional
    Nuclear Overhauser Experiment with Pure Absorption Phase in
    Four Quadrants, J. Magn. Reson., 48:286.
Strop, P., Wider, G., and Wüthrich, K., 1983, Assignment of the [1]H
    Nuclear Magnetic Resonance Spectrum of the Proteinase Inhibitor
    IIA from Bull Seminal Plasma by Two-Dimensional Nuclear Magnetic
    Resonance at 500 MHz, J. Mol. Biol., 166:641.
Wagner, G., Anil Kumar, and Wüthrich., 1981, Systematic Application of
    Two-Dimensional [1]H Nuclear-Magnetic-Resonance Techniques for Studies
    of Proteins. 2. Combined Use of Correlated Spectroscopy and Nuclear
    Overhauser Spectroscopy for Sequential Assignments of Backbone Re-
    sonances and Elucidation of Polypeptide Secondary Structures, Eur.
    J. Biochem., 114:375.

Wagner, G., and Wüthrich, K., 1982, Sequential Resonance Assignments in Protein $^1$H Nuclear Magnetic Resonance Spectra. Basic Pancreatic Trypsin Inhibitor, J. Mol. Biol., 155:347.

Wagner, G., Wüthrich, K., Tschesche, H., 1978, A $^1$H Nuclear-Magnetic-Resonance Study of the Solution Conformation of the Isoinhibitor K from Helix pomatia, Eur. J. Biochem., 89:367.

Wider, G., Hosur, R.V., Wüthrich, K., 1983, Suppression of the Solvent Resonance in 2D NMR Spectra of Proteins in $H_2O$ Solution, J. Magn. Reson., 52:130.

Wider, G., Lee, K.H., and Wüthrich, K., 1982, Sequential Resonance Assignments in Protein $^1$H Nuclear Magnetic Resonance Spectra. Glucagon Bound to Perdeuterated Dodecylphosphocholine Micelles, J. Mol. Biol., 155:367.

Wider, G., Macura, S., Anil Kumar, Ernst, R.R., and Wüthrich, K., 1984, Homonuclear Two-Dimensional $^1$H NMR of Proteins. Experimental Procedures, J. Magn. Reson., 56:207.

Wüthrich, K., 1983, Sequential Individual Resonance Assignments in the $^1$H NMR Spectra of Polypeptides and Proteins, Biopolymers, 22:131.

Wüthrich, K., Nagayama, K., and Ernst, R.R., 1979, Two-Dimensional NMR Spectroscopy, Trends in Biochemical Sciences, 4:N178.

Wüthrich, K., Wider, G., Wagner, G., and Braun, W., 1982, Sequential Resonance Assignments as a Basis for Determination of Spatial Protein Structures by High Resolution Proton Nuclear Magnetic Resonance, J. Mol. Biol., 155:311.

# PROTON ASSIGNMENT STRATEGIES IN NUCLEIC ACID NMR STUDIES

Brian R. Reid

Chemistry and Biochemistry Departments,
University of Washington, Seattle, WA 98195

The last few years have seen a rapid expansion in our ability to study nucleic acids and proteins of increasing size and spectral complexity by high-resolution NMR spectroscopy (see Kearns, 1984, and Wemmer & Reid, 1985, for recent reviews). An important factor in our ability to study biopolymers in the 8,000 - 16,000 mol. wt. range is the sensitivity and resolution of modern NMR spectrometers with magnetic field strengths in the 11-12 Tesla range (ca. 500 MHz). Even at such frequencies, the NMR spectra of 10,000 dalton biopolymers are very crowded, with many overlapping resonances, and the introduction of two-dimensional NMR spectroscopy (2DNMR) has been an equally important development. As in all forms of spectroscopy, the ability to specifically assign the majority of resonance peaks is the first crucial step in any detailed study and 2DNMR has facilitated the ease and speed of assigning relatively complicated spectra. In this paper I shall present the techniques and strategies for assigning nucleic acid NMR spectra, with particular emphasis on short DNA molecules containing 10-20 base pairs. In presenting these assignment methods I shall draw on examples taken from the work of several members of my laboratory to whom I am grateful, particularly Dennis Hare, David Wemmer and Shan-Ho Chou.

## TYPES OF PROTONS IN DNA

DNA consists of deoxynucleoside units containing a deoxyribose sugar to which one of the four common heterocyclic bases adenine (A), guanine (G), cytosine (C) or thymine (T) is linked - as shown in Figure 1. In terms of through-bond (scalar) J-coupling, each deoxyribose consists of a seven proton coupled spin system, i.e. the 1', 2', 2", 3', 4', 5' and 5" protons, that are expected to exhibit spin-spin splitting. The bases A, T, G, and C constitute four independent spin systems that are not J-coupled to the sugar protons. It is worth

23

noting that cytidine is the only base containing vicinal protons on adjacent carbons; the cytidine H5 and H6 protons should be split into doublets whereas the remaining non-exchangeable aromatic protons (T-H5, G-H8, A-H8 and A-H2) should appear as singlets. Thus, including the deoxyribose rings, there are only 5 types of spin systems found in DNA. From NMR spectra of the four mononucleosides, there are six major spectral regions in which DNA protons generally resonate. They are as follows:

1) 7 to 8 ppm - C8H of A and G, C2H of A, C6H of T and C.
2) 5.2 to 6.2 ppm - C5H of C, deoxyribose 1'H.
3) 4.6 to 5.1 ppm - deoxyribose 3'H.
4) 3.6 to 4.6 ppm - deoxyribose 4'H, 5'H and 5"H.
5) 1.7 to 3.0 ppm - deoxyribose 2'H and 2"H.
6) 1.0 to 1.7 ppm - methyl of T.

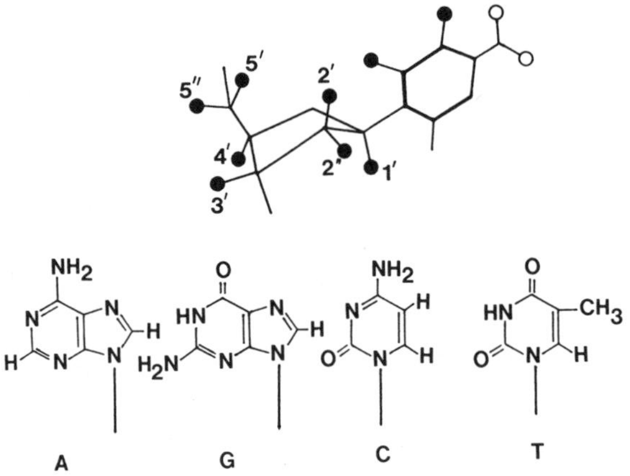

Figure 1. A typical deoxynucleoside (deoxycytidine) in the B-DNA conformation. Non-exchangeable protons are shown as filled circles; the exchangeable amino protons are shown as open circles. Note the proximity of the base H6 to its own 2' and 1' protons.

Figure 2 shows the NMR spectra of a short relatively simple DNA duplex and a larger more complicated DNA sequence. The simpler upper spectrum is of the Eco RI DNA sequence d(CGCGAATTCGCG)$_2$ which, because of the two-fold symmetry

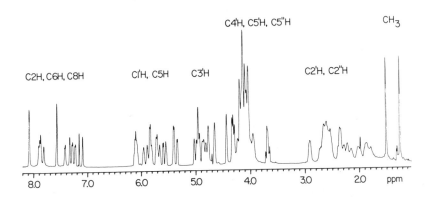

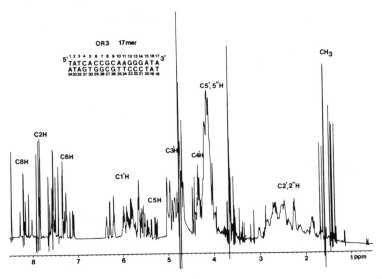

Figure 2. The NMR spectra of CGCGAATTCGCG (upper) and OR3 operator DNA (lower). Resonances occur in six discrete chemical shift regions as described in the text.

of the duplex. contains only six unique base pairs i.e. the protons from twelve nucleotides. The resolution is such that the cytidine doublets in the aromatic region can be identified by visual inspection. The more complicated lower spectrum is of the 17 base pair bacteriophage lambda OR3 operator. It contains resonances from 34 unique nucleotides (about 300 protons) but. despite the spectral crowding. the six major spectral regions are still discernible and any given resonance can usually be assigned to a specific proton type by its chemical shift. I shall now discuss specific assignments and how they are made.

25

## 2DNMR ASSIGNMENT METHODS

An important goal in assigning spectra is the determination of vicinal proton spin systems that are coupled through three covalent bonds, and dipolar coupled spins that reside close to each other in space. Although a relatively simple DNA spectrum such as the upper spectrum in Figure 2 could, in theory, be assigned by a series of one-dimensional decoupling and selective saturation experiments, this would be extremely laborious and time-consuming; the advantage of 2DNMR is that the equivalent information can be obtained in a single experiment. The COSY experiment (Wagner & Wuthrich 1982) is the two-dimensional analog of one-dimensional decoupling and reveals all J-coupled proton pairs simultaneously. Using a $90°-t_1-90°-t_2$ pulse sequence with several hundred incremented $t_1$ values, the resulting data matrix $S(t_1, t_2)$ is Fourier transformed with respect to $t_1$ and $t_2$ to generate the two-dimensional spectrum $S(w_1, w_2)$, usually presented as a contour plot. The one-dimensional spectrum appears on the diagonal $(w_1 = w_2)$ but coherence transfer between J-coupled proton pairs leads to off-diagonal cross peaks at the intercept of the two corresponding frequencies. Thus the 1'-2', 1'-2", 3'-2', 3'-2" and 3'-4' couplings for each sugar are easily detected and the majority of the sugar protons can be segregated into individual deoxyribose spin systems. Furthermore the cytidine H5-H6 couplings are obvious in the 1) - 2) spectral region and, with care, even the weak (1Hz) four-bond thymine H6-Me couplings can be seen in the 1) - 6) region. At this stage the purine protons in region 1) can be identified by elimination. The COSY spectrum corresponding to the d(CGCGAATTCGCG)$_2$ spectrum shown in the upper portion of Figure 2 can be found in Hare et al (1983).

After identifying the coupled spin systems, the NOESY spectrum is required to specifically assign a given resonance to a particular residue in the DNA sequence. The NOESY pulse sequence, $90° - t_1 - 90° - \tau_m - 90° - t_2$, includes an additional pulse and a mixing time, $\tau_m$ of ca. 0.3 sec during which dipolar cross-relaxation between proximal protons is allowed to occur. Since the cross-saturation phenomenon falls off as $r^6$, only very close (<5 Å) proton pairs will show cross-peaks and the NOESY spectrum therefore reveals through-space proximities within the molecule. Usually the mixing time is also randomly jittered about the mean value to cancel zero quantum through-bond coherence transfer.

The NOESY spectrum of d(CGCGAATTCGCG)$_2$, from which specific assignments can be made, is shown in Figure 3. From the multitude of cross peaks, there are obviously extensive networks of proximal protons throughout the DNA molecule, i.e. the nuclear Overhauser effect (NOE) from region 1 (aromatic base protons) is particularly strong to protons in region 2 (1'H), region 3 (3'H), region·5 (2'H and 2"H) and region 6 (methyl) indicating efficient dipolar coupling (close proximity) between these proton sets. The four very intense cross peaks between regions 1 and 2 also appear in the COSY spectrum and are therefore the H5-H6 pairs of the cytidine residues. One can begin assignments either by identifying the 5'- and 3'-terminal residues in the chain (see below) or by

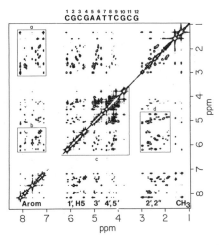

Figure 3. The NOESY spectrum of CGCGAATTCGCG. THe off-diagonal cross peaks represent NOE contacts between various types of protons.

identifying specific unique internal residues. For instance the two methyl resonances at 1.24 and 1.51 ppm obviously belong to T7 and T8. The 1.24 ppm methyl shows a COSY and NOESY cross peak at 7.11 ppm (its own H6) and a cross peak to a purine resonance at 8.09. From the internal sequence A6-T7-T8-C9, T8 has pyrimidines on either side and the 1.24 ppm methyl must belong to T7 rather than T8; the T7-Me to A6-H8 NOE corroborates the right-handedness of the DNA helix. Thus, by elimination, the 1.51 ppm and 7.35 ppm resonances, which show a weak 1 Hz four-bond coupling in the COSY spectrum (Hare et al., 1983), must belong to the methyl and H6 protons respectively of T8. Now that the most upfield aromatic proton at 7.11 ppm is established as the H6 of T7, the horizontal row along this frequency reveals the family of resonances within 5 Å of this proton. The 1.51 ppm to 7.11 ppm cross peak establishes that the methyl group of T8 is close to the H6 of T7 i.e. there are NOE connectivities between the base "side chains". Furthermore, in the 1-2 region, the 7.11 ppm H6 of T7 shows NOEs to two different sugar 1' protons. Regardless of the glycosidic dihedral angle, a pyrimidine H6 (or a purine H8) cannot be more than 4.5 Å from

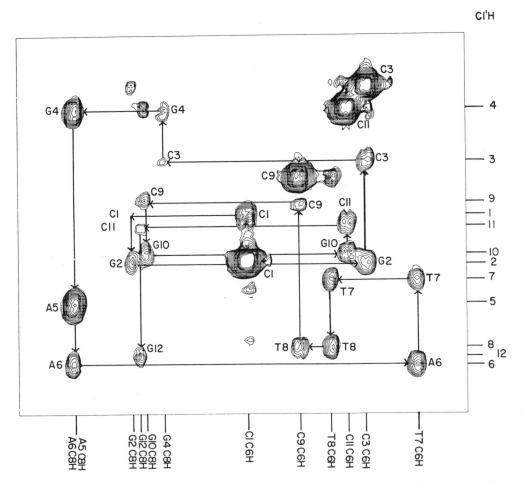

Figure 4. Expanded view of the aromatic-1'H cross peaks from box b in Figure 3. The sequential inter-residue connectivity from C1 to G12 is traced by arrows.

its own 1'H, so one of these cross peaks must be the 1'H of T7. The fact that there is an additional cross peak to a neighboring 1'H constitutes another network of inter-residue NOE connectivities between base protons and backbone protons of a neighboring deoxyribose. From the right-handedness of the helix, the additional 1'H NOE must be to the preceding (5'-side) sugar; in idealized B-DNA (Arnott & Chandrasekaran, 1984) the distance from a given H6 to the (n-1) 1'H is 3.52 Å, whereas the distance to the (n+1) 1'H is 7.5 Å. The fact that each aromatic H6 or H8 has NOEs to two 1'H peaks, and vice-versa, means that there should be a zig-zag path of aromatic -1'H connectivities along the entire DNA chain. This region of cross peaks from Figure 3 is shown in expanded form in Figure 4. As expected, one can easily trace a sequential path of inter-residue connectivities from

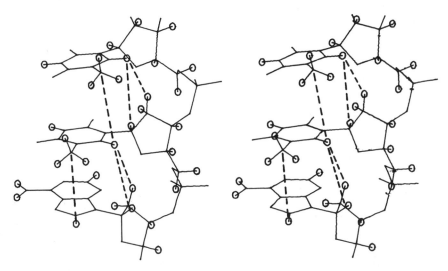

Figure 5. Stereo view of the A6-T7-T8 region in an idealized B-DNA sequence. Note the inter-residue connectivities from the methyl and H6 proton of T7.

one end of the DNA chain to the other, thus specifically assigning each 1'H to its corresponding residue in the sequence. Since each 1'H was previously associated with the other protons of that deoxyribose spin system by J-coupling via the COSY spectrum, one has, in principle, now assigned all the sugar protons and all the base H8 or H6 protons. However, there is an additional connectivity network throughout the molecule by which one can independently check the resulting assignments i.e. there is redundancy in the NOESY spectrum. In the bottom right corner of Figure 3 one observes at least three cross peaks in the 2-3 ppm region for each aromatic proton. These are NOEs from each H8 or H6 to its own 2' and 2" protons and to the 2"H of the preceding residue (located 2.2-2.3 Å away in idealized DNA). Thus there is an independent network of aromatic -2"H connectivities along the DNA chain from which sequential assignments can equally well be made. These methods of seqential assignment from two-dimensional NOESY spectra were first applied to DNA spectra in 1983 (Hare et al. 1983; Scheek et al. 1983, 1984). A molecular graphics picture of a DNA chain showing the major inter-residue NOEs in the NOESY map is shown in Figure 5.

## INTERATOMIC DISTANCES AND LIMITS OF THE METHOD

The fact that, in biopolymers of this size, the NOE between two protons is a result of cross-relaxation, which in turn depends on the distance between the protons, suggests that distance information can somehow be extracted from the NOESY spectrum. However, one must exercise some caution in deriving distances because more distant protons can produce apparent NOEs that exaggerate their proximity via a process termed spin-diffusion (Kalk & Berendsen, 1976). Nevertheless at sufficiently short mixing times, or by measuring the time-dependence of the cross-peak build-up, one can indeed extract relatively accurate distance information. In the absence of local motion, for a sufficiently large polymer such that $\omega\tau_c \gg 1$, the cross-relaxation rate is given by:

$$R_1 = \frac{\gamma^4 h^2}{10} \frac{\tau c}{r^6}$$

Thus one can evaluate the distance, r, by measuring the amount of cross-relaxation if the rotational correlation time, $\tau_c$, is known. Even without determining $\tau_c$, one can determine interproton distances by relating NOE intensities to the corresponding intensities for known proton pairs at a known fixed distance. Figure 6 shows the NOESY cross peaks at a short mixing time between aromatic and 1' protons and between aromatic and 2'2" protons. Thus each horizontal row contains distance information from each purine H8 or pyrimidine H6 to five or six proximal protons (three of its own protons and two or three protons of the 5'-neighbor). However the left spectrum also contains four strong cross peaks from H5-H6 protons of the four cytidine residues; the H5-H6 distance in cytidine is fixed at 2.45 Å and hence these cross peaks serve as internal "yardsticks" to which other distances can be scaled and evaluated. In determining distances this way one must evaluate the volume integral of the cross peaks since different peaks have different lineshapes. It is also worth noting that the four cytidine H5-H6 cross peaks have identical intensities indicating that there is no differential local motion between positions 1, 3, 9 and 11 in the sequence. When the base-sugar distances evaluated in this way are compared to the corresponding distances in the crystal structure of this DNA sequence (Dickerson & Drew 1981), they agree to better than 0.4 Å, establishing that NOESY maps are indeed a reliable source of interatomic distance information in a DNA molecule. Thus the entire NOESY map in Figure 3 actually contains hundreds of proton-proton distances; these spatial constraints effectively define the three-dimensional structure of the molecule in distance space. However, deriving the structure from this distance matrix is a non-trivial operation requiring computerized matrix methods (Crippen, 1981).

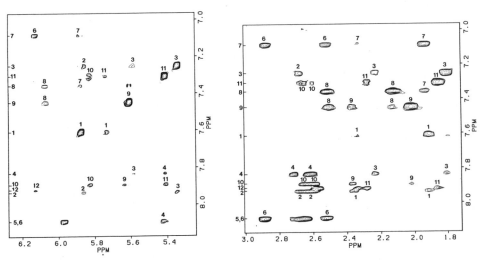

Figure 6. NOESY cross peaks to 1' protons (left) and to 2' and 2" protons (right) from the twelve H6/H8 aromatic protons of CGCGAATTCGCG. These data were obtained with a 0.1 sec mixing time.

The ability of the COSY/NOESY methods described above to assign the spectra of larger DNA molecules is limited only by spectral resolution of the off-diagonal cross peaks. The spectra of Pribnow box promoter sequences (24 unique residues) have been assigned by these methods (Wemmer et al. 1984a) as have operator sequences containing 34 residues (Wemmer et al., 1984b). In these non-symmetrical DNA sequences the sequential connectivities down each strand must be traced separately. With a 500 MHz spectrometer using phase-sensitive pure absorption data manipulation (States et al., 1982), one can assign DNA duplexes containing up to 50-60 unique nucleotides with these techniques i.e. 25-30 base pairs with no symmetry or 50-60 base pairs of DNA duplex with two-fold symmetrical sequences. When field strengths above 11.7 Tesla become available there is no reason why even longer DNA molecules cannot be assigned by 2DNMR.

# ALTERNATE CONFORMATIONS - REAL STRUCTURES

The above-described inter-residue connectivities lead to sequential assignments for DNA duplexes only if they have a conformation that is close to B-form DNA. For atypical alternate conformations of DNA this approach will not work and one obviously has to use different assignment strategies. An interesting example of an alternate DNA conformation is the hairpin structure adopted by d(CGCGTATACGCG)$_2$ under conditions of low ionic strength, low concentration or high temperature. At 40°C in 10 m$\underline{M}$ phosphate at a concentration of 3-4 mM, the duplex and hairpin conformations exist in equilibrium with forward and reverse rate constants that are conveniently measurable by NMR. Thus the NOESY spectrum contains a set of cross peaks due to B-DNA from which the protons in the duplex conformer can be assigned by the standard procedures described above. However, the two-dimensional spectrum also contains more intense cross peaks due to chemical exchange between duplex and hairpin forms. These exchange cross peaks between the hairpin and duplex conformations allow the assignments of known protons in the duplex conformer to be carried over to the hairpin conformer. Thus the hairpin form can be assigned by exchange transfer from the duplex, obviating the need for reassigning this new conformation from scratch (Wemmer et al. 1985).

We have also studied fixed non-complementary hairpin sequences of the type d-CGCGTTTTCGCG (Hare & Reid, 1985). In such sequences the first four residues and the last four residues form a base paired unimolecular duplex with each other that can be assigned by standard sequential methods. However, the central four T residues in the loop must adopt an atypical conformation in order to trace a 180° backbone turn. This is revealed by the absence of "standard" inter-residue connectivities and the appearance of new "unexpected" cross peaks in the NOESY map. For instance the 1'H of T6 is no longer within NOE distance of the H6 of T7. However, the methyl group of T7 has now moved close to the H6 and the 1'H of T5 (the next-nearest linear neighbor) resulting in two new cross peaks. Such atypical proximities represent extremely informative clues about the three-dimensional folding of the loop. By converting these NOEs into quantitative distances and embedding this distance matrix in three-dimensional space followed by refinement against the experimental distances, Dennis Hare has been able to produce a computer-generated structure that satisfies all of the experimental distance constraints (Hare & Reid, 1985). Thus, far from being an awkward complication, these "anomalous" NOEs can be used to derive the three-dimensional structure of interesting alternate conformations of DNA.

# EXCHANGEABLE PROTONS - HELIX DYNAMICS

Up to this point I have restricted my discussion to non-exchangeable carbon-bound protons in DNA. However, the hydrogen bonded amino and imino protons that hold the complementary base pairs together constitute an entirely different

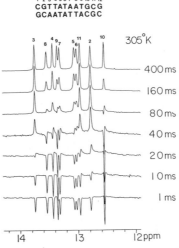

Figure 7. Inversion recovery data on the ten internal imino protons of a -10 promoter sequence. Note the much faster recovery of TA3 (due to solvent exchange) compared to GC10.

class of protons from which dynamic information can be extracted. The imino or ring NH proton of G and T is extremely deshielded, resonating in the 10-11 ppm region of the spectrum. In single-stranded random coil polynucleotides the imino protons exchange extremely rapidly with solvent and are thus not detectable in

$D_2O$ solution. In $H_2O$ solution the presence of narrow resolved imino proton resonances in the 12-14 ppm region of DNA NMR spectra indicates that, on the NMR timescale, the Watson-Crick base pairs have long lifetimes in the hydrogen bonded state in the interior of the double helix. However, the fact that such resonances are not detectable in freshly dissolved $D_2O$ solutions, even in native double-helical DNA, indicates that transient helix opening and solvent exchange must occur on the seconds-to-minutes timescale. Thus when an imino proton resonance is selectively saturated or inverted, in addition to the physical process of spin-lattice relaxation and cross-relaxation, these resonances will also contain a significant contribution from solvent exchange in their rate of z-magnetization recovery if the rate of base pair opening equals or exceeds the rate of $T_1$ relaxation. This fact allows us to measure helix-coil dynamic processes at different positions in a native DNA sequence.

The top spectrum in Figure 7 shows the fully relaxed imino proton resonances of a twelve base pair DNA duplex containing the -10 Pribnow promoter sequence TTATAATG. The various peaks have been assigned to their respective base pairs by sequential imino proton NOEs (Chou et al. 1984) and are labelled with their base pair number. Upon inverting only the imino protons, the rate of recovery of each resonance can be monitored by sampling the spectrum at various time intervals. The rapid recovery of base pairs 2 and 11 at over 20 $sec^{-1}$ is indicative of rapid solvent exchange due to end-fraying of the duplex (base pairs 1 and 12 have completely exchanged out of the spectrum at 32°C). One step further into the helix, base pair 10 recovers at only 5 $sec^{-1}$ due entirely to $T_1$ relaxation only, whereas base pair 3 recovers at 17 $sec^{-1}$ which is predominantly solvent exchange. Thus by subtracting out the $T_1$ contribution to recovery, we can conclude that the third base pair from the left is opening at at least 14 $sec^{-1}$ while the third base pair from the right opens no faster than 1 $sec^{-1}$. Similarly base pairs 4 and 5 exchange more frequently than do 8 and 9, leading to the conclusion that the left end of the promoter sequence is more labile than the right end. This may be physiologically relevant since this region of the promoter is involved in forming the non-paired "open complex" with RNA polymerase and the direction of initiation and elongation is from left to right as the sequence is written. The ability to measure helix opening rates at each position in the DNA allows one to estimate the activation energy for the helix-coil transition for each base pair by means of temperature-dependent studies (Chou et al. 1984). The experimentally observed recovery rates ($k_{op} + 1/T_1$) as a function of temperature are shown as Arrhenius plots in Figure 8. When the magnetic contribution from cross-relaxation is subtracted from these slopes, one obtains helix-coil activation energies of only 23 kcal/mol for the central base pairs AT5 and TA6. Such low values, which are

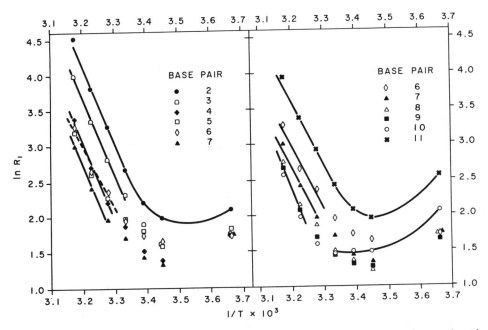

Figure 8. Arrhenius plots of the recovery rate versus inverse temperature for the ten imino protons of the promoter sequence in Figure 7. In the low temperature (no opening) region the recovery rate slows down with increasing temperature due to more rapid molecular tumbling. After subtracting this cross-relaxation component, the activation energy for base pair opening can be obtained from the temperature dependence of the exchange rate.

actually lower than the exchange activation energies for TA4 and AT7, argue strongly for independent non-cooperative opening of the interior base pairs in this promoter sequence. Thus kinetic studies on exchangeable protons in DNA contribute a quite different and extremely valuable type of information that can be combined with the structural data obtained by 2DNMR of non-exchangeable protons.

Acknowledgements: The majority of the research described in this article was supported by a National Institutes of Health Program Project Grant, PO1 GM32681. An instrumentation grant from the Murdock Foundation is gratefully acknowledged.

## References

Arnott, S. & Chandrasekaran, R. (1984) - private communication.

Chou, S.H., Wemmer, D.E., Hare, D.R. & Reid, B.R. (1984) Biochemistry, 23, 2257.

Crippen, G.M. (1981) Distance Geometry and Conformational Calculations, Research Studies Press/Wiley, Chichester.

Dickerson, R.E. & Drew, H.R. (1981) J. Mol. Biol., 149, 761.

Hare, D.R., Wemmer, D.E., Chou, S.H., Drobny, G. & Reid, B.R. (1983) J. Mol. Biol., 171, 319.

Hare, D.R. & Reid, B.R. (1985) Biochemistry, submitted.

Kearns, D.R. (1984) CRC Crit. Rev. Biochem., 15, 237.

Scheek, R.M., Russo, N., Boelens, R. & Kaptein, R. (1983) J. Am. Chem. Soc., 105, 2914.

Scheek, R.M., Boelens, R., Russo, N., van Boom, J.H. & Kaptein, R. (1984) Biochemistry, 23, 1371.

States, D.J., Haberkorn, R.A. & Ruben, D.J. (1982) J. Magn. Reson., 48, 286.

Wagner, G. & Wuthrich, K. (1982) J. Mol. Biol., 155, 347.

Wemmer, D.E., Chou, S.H., Hare, D.R. & Reid, B.R. (1984 a) Biochemistry, 23, 2262.

Wemmer, D.E., Chou, S.H. & Reid, B.R. (1984 b) J. Mol. Biol., 180, 41.

Wemmer, D.E. & Reid, B.R. (1985) Ann. Rev. Phys. Chem., 36, 105.

Wemmer, D.E., Chou, S.H., Hare, D.R. & Reid, B.R. (1985) Nucl. Acids Res., 13, 3755.

# GENETIC METHODS IN HIGH-RESOLUTION NMR STUDIES OF PROTEINS

Michael A. Weiss, Anna Jeitler-Nilsson*, Nancy J. Fischbein,
Martin Karplus, and Robert T. Sauer*

Department of Chemistry
Harvard University
Cambridge, Massachusetts 02138

*Department of Biology
Massachusetts Institute of Technology
Cambridge, Massachusetts 02139

## INTRODUCTION

Many biomolecules have long rotational correlation times and thus give rise to broad NMR resonances in solution. A variety of strategies have been devised to overcome this limitation. Resolution enhancement algorithms have permitted the study of flexible regions of structures as large as Tobacco Mosaic Virus (1-3); one-dimensional and two-dimensional pulse sequences may also be used to selectively observe flexible spin systems (4,5). In addition, the introduction of nuclear spin labels has facilitated the identification of individual residues (6-9). In this paper we describe how the techniques of molecular biology may be employed to facilitate the NMR study of large proteins. Illustrative examples will be taken from our studies of the bacteriophage $\lambda$ repressor (10-12).

Bacteriophage $\lambda$ repressor contains two structural domains: an N-terminal domain that mediates sequence-specific DNA binding, and a C-terminal domain that mediates oligomerization (13,14). The crystal structure of the N-terminal domain has been determined and has been used to model the interaction of repressor with operator DNA (15,16). The gene encoding the $\lambda$ repressor has been cloned into overexpression plasmids (17,18), and has been subject to extensive genetic analysis (19,20). Thus, large quantities of wild-type, genetically altered, or isotopically enriched protein may be conveniently purified for NMR study.

## An Overexpression System

An overexpression system for $\lambda$ repressor was constructed by Amann et al. (18), using the strong promoter tac, first described by DeBoer et al. (21). This promoter, which contains the -10 region of the lacUV5 promoter and the -35 region of the trp promoter, can direct the expression of $\lambda$ repressor in E. coli to levels as high as thirty percent of total cellular protein. Its bipartite structure is shown in Figure 1 (lower left). Plasmid pEA301, shown in Panel A of Figure 1, contains only the -35 region of the trp promoter adjacent to a unique ClaI restriction site. Wild-type or genetic-

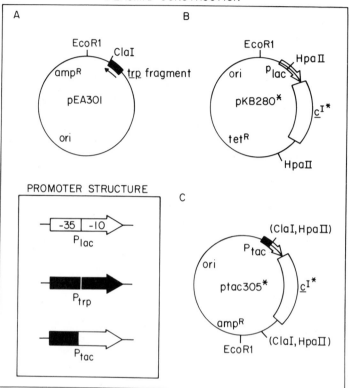

PLASMID CONSTRUCTION

Figure 1. Overexpression system for bacteriophage λ repressor developed by Amann et al. (18) using the hybrid tac promoter (21). As shown in the box inset in the lower left-hand corner, the tac promoter contains the -35 region of the trp promoter and the -10 region of the lac promoter. Under the control of this strong promoter in E. coli, λ repressor can constitute up to 30% of total cellular protein, thus facilitating the biosynthetic incorporation of spin labels. (A) Plasmid pEA301 contains only the -35 region of the trp promoter adjacent to a unique ClaI site, into which wild-type or genetically altered repressor genes (cI) can be subcloned. (B) Plasmid pKB280, which expresses repressor under the control of the lac promoter (17), has been subject to extensive genetic analysis (19,20). A HpaII restriction fragment containing mutant repressor genes (cI*) and the -10 region of the lac promoter can be recloned into the ClaI site of pEA301, to generate plasmid ptac305 (C). This construction, which results in formation of the hybrid tac promoter, enables large quantities of mutant proteins to be purified (10,11, 19,20).

altered repressor genes may be inserted into this site to generate over-expression plasmids. For example, Nelson et al. (19) and Hecht et al. (20) have isolated and sequenced an extensive collection of mutant λ repressor alleles under the control of a lac promoter in plasmid pKB280 (17), as shown in Panel B of Figure 1. A HpaII restriction fragment containing the mutant allele and the -10 region of the lac promoter may be subcloned into pEA301 to create plasmid ptac305. In this construction the tac promoter is regenerated, as shown in Panel C of Figure 1.

Such an overexpression system has several convenient features for bio-physical studies. First, the large degree of overproduction expedites purification of the protein. Smaller scale fermentation and fewer purifica-tion steps may be required. In addition, even in the early stages of purifi-cation, the desired product may be identified by gel electrophoresis rather than more laborious functional assays. Second, inducibility of the desired gene (for example, by inhibition of lac repressor control of the tac promoter) makes biosynthetic incorporation of isotopically enriched substrates more efficient. Label may be incorporated into the protein of interest following induction, with less "wasted" in the mass of cellular proteins. Finally, a portable promoter system enables wild-type and genetically altered alleles to be interchanged, permitting any suitably cloned mutant to be overproduced, purified and characterized.

## Example: Deuterium Labeling

The N-terminal domain of λ repressor, which mediates recognition of operator DNA, may be isolated as a fragment of 102 residues (12). This species forms a dimer in solution of molecular weight 22 kd. The aliphatic region of its proton NMR spectrum at 500 Megahertz is shown in Panel A of Figure 2. The resonances are in general broad, consistent with the size of the protein. Three methyl resonances are resolved in the upfield region of the spectrum between +/- 0.5 ppm. On the basis of two-dimensional methods (22), they may be assigned to either leucine or valine spin systems. The two are difficult to distinguish in a protein of this size because connectivities through their respective methylenes are difficult to trace.

Leucine and valine resonances may be rigorously distinguished by selective deuterium labeling. The aliphatic spectrum of an N-terminal fragment containing perdeuterated leucine is shown in Panel B of Figure 2. The methyl resonance near -0.2 ppm (indicated by asterisk in Figure 2) is virtually absent; it is thus assigned to a leucine. In contrast, the methyl resonance near +0.2 ppm, assigned to Val47, is unaffected by the leucine label.

## STRUCTURE-FUNCTION RELATIONSHIPS IN λ REPRESSOR

Intact λ repressor, in contrast to its proteolytic fragments, has not been crystallized, and there is little direct evidence concerning its struc-ture. Solution NMR studies are limited by the broad spectrum resulting from repressor aggregation. At the millimolar concentrations used for NMR, λ repressor has an apparent molecular weight in excess of one million daltons (23). Nevertheless, valuable information may be obtained from NMR data through the application of genetic techniques. In the following sections we will review two structural and dynamic features of the protein: the relationship between the N-terminal and C-terminal domains, and the dynamics of the N-terminal arm. These studies are described in detail elsewhere (10-12).

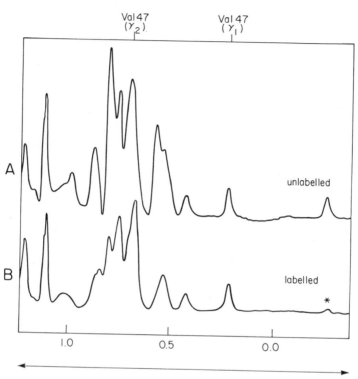

Figure 2. Aliphatic region of the [1]H-NMR spectrum of the N-terminal domain of
λ repressor at 500 Megahertz and 30°C (Francis Bitter National
Magnet Laboratory): (A) unlabelled, and (B) perdeuterated leucine
has been biosynthetically incorporated. In both spectra resolution
was enhanced by convolution difference with parameters GM4, EM20,
and subtraction factor 0.9. The protein was made 5 mM (monomer
concentration) in a buffer consisting of 200 mM KC1, 50 mM potassium phosphate (pD 7.4), 1 mM sodium azide and 0.1 mM EDTA in 99.9%
deuterium oxide. Three methyl resonances are shifted upfield,
between +0.5 ppm and -0.5 ppm; such shifts are often due to ring-
current effects from nearby aromatic groups. Val47, for example,
is near Phe51 in the hydrophobic interior of the domain. Valine
and leucine spin systems can be difficult to distinguish by two-
dimensional methods, especially in large proteins. The difficulty
arises from the chemical similarity of these branched-chain aliphatic residues, which differ only in the number of methylenes. Deuterium labeling provides a rigorous method to assign these spin
systems. Almost complete enrichment can be obtained in prototro-
phic strains by feedback inhibition with valine and isoleucine.

## Domain Organization of λ Repressor

λ repressor contains two structurally and functionally distinct domains (13,14). The isolated N-terminal domain retains the regulatory properties of the intact molecule, and protection experiments show that the fragment and intact repressor contact operator DNA in the same way. The C-terminal domain does not bind DNA, but contains strong dimer and higher-order contacts. In this section we will show that the N-terminal domain is only loosely tethered to the C-terminal domain in the intact repressor structure.

In Figure 3 the aliphatic spectrum of intact repressor (bottom panel) is compared with the aliphatic spectra of the isolated N-terminal domain (middle panel) and of the isolated C-terminal domain (top panel). Broad resonances are observed in the intact spectrum that correspond to the upfield-shifted methyl resonances of the N-terminal domain, but not to the upfield-shifted resonances of the C-terminal domain. It appears that the C-terminal resonances do not appear in the spectrum of the intact repressor. If these correspondences are meaningful (i.e., the broad resonances in the intact spectrum can be rigorously assigned to protons in the N-terminal domain),

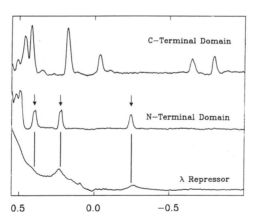

Figure 3. (Bottom Spectrum) Aliphatic [1]H-NMR spectrum of intact λ repressor at 500 Megahertz and 30°C as described in the legend to Figure 2. A convolution difference with parameters GM6, EM30, 0.9 was applied. (Middle) Aliphatic spectrum of the isolated N-terminal domain as a fragment of 90 residues. A convolution difference with parameters GM4, EM20, 0.1 was applied. (Top) Aliphatic spectrum of a C-terminal fragment; a convolution difference with parameters GM4, EM20, 0.9 was applied.

then this implies that at high repressor concentrations the N-terminal domain tumbles more quickly than the C-terminal domain. However, since the two domains are covalently connected, they must be only loosely tethered to each other. Although the extreme line broadening that underlies the loss of C-terminal resonances is a consequence of aggregation at high repressor concentrations, the independent mobility of the two domains is an inherent dynamical property of repressor.

In order to verify that the correspondences of chemical shifts observed in Figure 3 are meaningful, an assignment technique is required. Since the broad resonances of intact repressor are not amenable to standard double resonance and two-dimensional NMR methods, an alternative technique for assignment is needed.

In the course of studying mutant repressors (19,20) we observed that substitution of tyrosine for glutamine at residue 44 selectively shifts resonances in the N-terminal domain. These site-specific perturbations may be conveniently observed in the aromatic region of the NMR spectrum, whose resonances provide sensitive markers for tertiary structure (10-12). The N-terminal domain contains four tyrosines, two phenylalanines and no histidine or tryptophan (13,23). Resonances arising from aromatic protons in the isolated domain (residues 1-90) are shown in Panel A of Figure 4. Three of the tyrosines (not labeled in the figure) have chemical shifts near that of free tyrosine, whereas the fourth is shifted upfield. The latter spin system has been assigned to Tyr22, the sole buried tyrosine in the N-terminal domain monomer (15). Both pheylalanines are buried in the crystal structure; their assignments are given in Figure 4. Tyr22, Phe51 and Phe76 form a major part of the hydrophobic core of the N-terminal domain. As illustrated in Panel A of Figure 5, Tyr22 and Phe51 are neighbors and their aromatic rings are partially stacked. Phe76 is not stacked against either of the other internal aromatics, but it still quite close to them. The relative proximity of Tyr22, Phe51 and Phe76 give rise to distinctive magnetic environments; the large chemical shift dispersion observed in their NMR resonances reflects the native structure of the N-terminal domain.

The aromatic NMR spectrum of the Tyr44 mutant N-terminal domain (as a fragment of 90 residues) is shown in Panel C of Figure 4. The resonances from Tyr22 and Phe51 are shifted a small amount upfield, whereas those from Phe76 are not affected. As shown in Panel A of Figure 5, Tyr22 and Phe51 are closer to the site of the mutation. The overall pattern of resonances for the Gln44 (wild-type) and Tyr44 (mutant) fragments is, however, similar. The one exception is the newly introduced Tyr44 spin system, which is well resolved in the two-dimensional correlated spectrum shown in Panel B of Figure 5. The similarity between the spectra of the wild-type and mutant spectra suggests that the mutant domain retains a native conformation. The differences between the spectra suggest that the Tyr44 substitution causes a small perturbation, either structural or inductive, that selectively shifts the Tyr22 and Phe51 resonances. These selective shifts provide a means of correlating resonances present in both intact repressor and the isolated N-terminal domain.

The aromatic spectrum of intact wild-type repressor is shown in Panel B of Figure 4. Just as was observed for the aliphatic resonances in Figure 3, broad resonances appear in the intact spectrum that correspond to peaks in the spectrum of the isolated N-terminal domain. In Panel D of Figure 4, the aromatic spectrum of the intact mutant repressor is shown. Broad resonances corresponding to Tyr22 and Phe51 are observed to be shifted relative to their positions in the wild-type spectrum. These shifts are identical to those observed for the wild-type and mutant isolated N-terminal domains. Since Tyr44 causes the same shifts both in intact repressor and in the isolated N-terminal domain, the resonances affected in the two cases must correspond.

This permits the assignment of specific resonances in the spectrum of intact
λ repressor and makes rigorous the conclusion that in the intact structure
the N-terminal domain and C-terminal domain are dynamically independent.

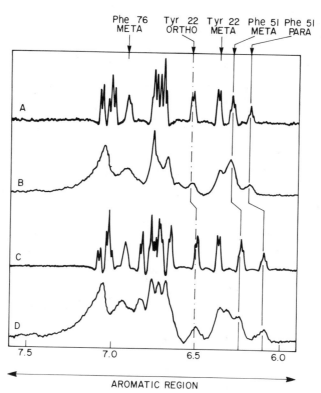

Figure 4. Portion of the aromatic region of the $^1$H-NMR spectra at 500 Megahertz of (A) wild-type N-terminal fragment (residues 1-90); (B)
wild-type intact repressor; (C) Tyr44 mutant N-terminal fragment
(residues 1-90); and (D) Tyr44 mutant intact repressor. Partial
assignments for Tyr22, Phe51 and Phe76 are given. These aromatic
groups are buried in the hydrophobic interior of the N-terminal
domain and provide markers for tertiary structure. The Tyr44 mutation causes selective shifts in the resonances of Tyr22 and Phe51.

A. model                                    B. spectrum

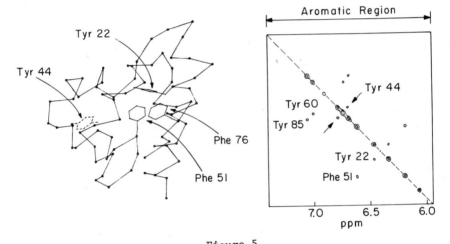

Figure 5.

The N-Terminal Arm of λ Repressor

Many prokaryotic regulatory proteins appear to recognize their DNA binding sites by a common mechanism (for review, see (24)). Such proteins are thought to make sequence-specific contacts by inserting an α helix, the "recognition helix," into the major groove of DNA. In addition to a recognition helix, λ repressor contains an extended N-terminal arm that is proposed to wrap around the DNA ( 5 ,11,15,16,25,26). This model is illustrated in Figure 6.

In the crystal the N-terminal arm consists of the first six residues, Ser1-Thr2-Lys3-Lys4-Lys5-Pro6. No electron density was observed for the first three residues, and the next three extend away from the rest of the protein (15). Repressor fragments with altered arms exhibit reduced operator affinity, as does a point mutation, Lys4 → Gln (19,20,25). In addition, such alterations cause a change in the protection pattern in the major groove on the back of the operator site. Thus, the arms are imagined to reach around the double helix to contact the major groove on the back surface of the DNA. Eliason et al. (26) have recently shown that the N-terminal arm is responsible for determining the effects of operator mutations on the back surface; i.e., the arm "reads" the DNA sequence at these positions.

In order to study the structure, dynamics and interactions of the N-terminal arm in solution, it is necessary as a first step to assign resonances from the N-terminal residues. Since the spectrum of the intact λ

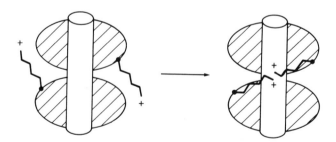

BACK OF OPERATOR SITE

Figure 6.  Schematic representation of the proposed role of the N-terminal Arm in the λ repressor-operator complex. The arms are assumed to be flexible in solution and to wrap around the operator DNA (cylinder). Most of the protein (hatched dimer) contacts the front surface of the DNA, where the recognition helix contacts the major groove. The N-terminal arm is thought to contact the back surface of the DNA. Although N-terminal arms may be an unusual feature among the helix-turn-helix class of regulatory proteins, the use of flexible regions in protein-nucleic acid interactions may be a general motif. λ Cro repressor appears to have flexible C-terminal residues properly positioned to contact the phosphate backbone (24).

45

repressor is not amenable to standard NMR techniques, as above an alternate method of assignment is required.

Eliason et al. (5, 26) have constructed by recombinant DNA techniques a series of mutant repressors containing successive N-terminal deletions. These genetically altered proteins exhibit a progressive loss of operator affinity and demonstrate the importance of the N-terminal arm in operator recognition. In addition, they provide a means of assigning NMR resonances from the N-terminal residues. Since the removal of these residues does not perturb the global structure of the domain (12), resonances that are absent in the mutant spectra may be assigned to the N-terminal arm.

A portion of the aliphatic region of the intact wild-type repressor spectrum is shown in Panel A of Figure 7. An envelope of broad resonances is observed, assigned to the N-terminal domain in the previous section. In addition, a sharp methyl doublet is observed near 1.1 ppm. This sharp feature may be rigorously assigned to Thr2 in the N-terminal arm by comparing the wild-type spectrum to a spectrum of a deletion mutant lacking Ser1-Thr2-Lys3. Although the broad envelope of resonances is essentially unperturbed by the absence of the first three residues, the sharp doublet near 1.1 ppm does not appear. Thus, this methyl resonance comes from Thr2; its linewidth (or spin-spin relaxation time) suggests that the N-terminal residues are reorienting independently of overall macromolecular tumbling. From this we conclude that the arm is flexible in solution, an essential feature of the current model of the λ repressor-operator complex.

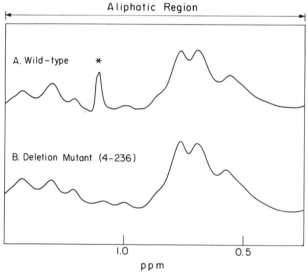

Figure 7. Assignment of Thr2 by recombinant DNA methods (5, 26).

## DISCUSSION

Two-dimensional NMR methods, discussed elsewhere in this volume, have made possible systematic assignment methods for small proteins and oligonucleotides. Sequential assignment strategies, which rely upon the characteristic secondary structures of these biopolymers, underlie efforts to determine three-dimensional structures in solution from NMR data. Despite the promise of these techniques, their application to large biological systems is fundamentally limited by rapid spin-spin relaxation and broad resonances. Nevertheless, NMR spectroscopy can provide valuable information concerning even large systems. Genetic engineering, the ability to clone, overproduce, and mutagenize the gene for a protein of interest, enables site-specific structural or dynamic information to be obtained.

## ACKNOWLEDGEMENTS

We thank Jim Eliason, Hillary Nelson, Michael Hecht, and Kathy Hehir for plasmids and advice regarding repressor genetics; Carl Pabo and Mitch Lewis for the coordinates of the N-terminal domain of $\lambda$ repressor and for helpful discussion; Dinshaw Patel, Ponzy Lu, David States, Rich Griffey, David Ruben, and Alfred Redfield for advice regarding NMR techniques. This work was supported in part by grants from the National Institutes of Health to Professors Robert T. Sauer, Martin Karplus and Mark Ptashne. The 500 MHz spectra were recorded at the High Field NMR Resource of the Francis Bitter National Magnet Laboratory (NIH, RR-00995). Michael A. Weiss was supported in part by a Medical Scientist Training Program at Harvard Medical School (GM-07753).

## REFERENCES

1. N. Wade-Jardetzky, R. P. Bray, W. W. Conover, O. Jardetzky, N. Geisler, and K. Weber, Differential Mobility of the N-Terminal Headpiece in the lac Repressor Protein, J. Mol. Biol. 128:259 (1979).
2. O. Jardetzky, K. Akasaka, R. Vogel, S. Morris, and K. C. Holmes, Unusual Segmental Flexibility in a Region of Tobacco Mosaic Virus Coat Protein, Nature 273:564 (1978).
3. S. Highsmith, K. Akasaka, M. Konrad, R. Goody, K. Holmes, N. Wade-Jardetzky, and O. Jardetzky, Internal Motions in Myosin, Biochemistry 18:4238 (1979).
4. I. D. Cambell, C. M. Dobson, R. J. P. Williams, and P. E. Wright, Pulse Methods for the Simplification of Proton NMR Spectra, FEBS Lett. 57:96 (1975).
5. M. A. Weiss, J. L. Eliason, and D. J. States, Dynamic Filtering by Two-Dimensional NMR with Application to Phage $\lambda$ Repressor, Proc. Natl. Acad. Sci. USA 81:6019 (1984).
6. M. A. C. Jarema, K. T. Arndt, M. Savage, P. Lu, and J. H. Miller, Genetic Insertion of Nuclear Spin Labels in the lac Repressor, J. Biol. Chem. 256:6544 (1981).
7. M. A. C. Jarema, P. Lu, and J. H. Miller, Genetic Assignment of Resonances in the NMR Spectrum of a Protein: lac Repressor, Proc. Natl. Acad. Sci. USA 78:2707 (1981).
8. R. H. Griffey, C. D. Poulter, A. Bax, B. L. Hawkins, Z. Yamaizumi, and S. Nishimura, Multiple Quatum Two-Dimensional 1H-15N NMR Spectroscopy: Chemical Shift Correlation Maps for Exchangable Imino Protons of E. coli tRNAmet in Water, Proc. Natl. Acad. Sci. USA 80:5895 (1983).
9. R. H. Griffey, A. G. Redfield, R. E. Loomis, and F. W. Dahlquist, Nuclear Magnetic Resonance Observation and Dynamics of Specific Amide Protons in T4 Lysozyme, Biochemistry 24:817 (1985).

10. M. A. Weiss, M. Karplus, D. J. Patel, and R. T. Sauer, Solution NMR Studies of Intact λ Repressor, <u>J. Biomol. Struc. Dyn.</u> 1:150 (1983).

11. M. A. Weiss, R. T. Sauer, D. J. Patel, and M. Karplus, The N-Terminal Arm of λ Repressor: a 1H-NMR Study, <u>Biochemistry</u> 23:5090 (1984).

12. M. A. Weiss, M. Karplus, and R. T. Sauer, Complete Assignment of the Aromatic Resonances of λ Repressor, manuscript in preparation.

13. C. O. Pabo, R. T. Sauer, J. M. Sturtevant, and M. Ptashne, The λ Repressor Contains Two Domains, <u>Proc. Natl. Acad. Sci. USA</u> 76:1608 (1979).

14. R. T. Sauer, C. O. Pabo, B. J. Meyer, M. Ptashne, and K. C. Backman, Regulatory Functions of the λ Repressor Reside in the Amino Terminal Domain, <u>Nature</u> 279:396 (1979).

15. C. O. Pabo and M. Lewis, The Operator-Binding Domain of λ Repressor: Structure and DNA Recognition, <u>Nature</u> 298:443 (1982).

16. M. Lewis, A. Jeffrey, J. Wang, R. Ladner, M. Ptashne, and C. O. Pabo, Structure of the Operator-Binding Domain of Bacteriophage λ Repressor: Implications for DNA Recognition and Gene Regulation, <u>Cold Spring Harbor Symp. Quant. Biol.</u> 47:435 (1983).

17. K. Backman, M. Ptashne, and W. Gilbert, Construction of Plasmids Carrying the <u>cI</u> Gene of Bacteriophage Lambda, <u>Proc. Natl. Acad. Sci. USA</u> 73:4174 (1976).

18. E. Amann, J. Brosius, and M. Ptashne, Vectors Bearing a Hybrid <u>trp-lac</u> Promoter Useful for Regulated Expression of Cloned Genes in <u>E. coli</u>, <u>Gene</u> 25:167 (1983).

19. H. C. M. Nelson, M. Hecht, and R. T. Sauer, Mutations Defining the Operator-Binding Sites of Bacteriophage λ Repressor, <u>Cold Spring Harbor Symp. Quant. Biol.</u> 47:441 (1983).

20. M. Hecht, H. C. M. Nelson, and R. T. Sauer, Mutations in λ Repressor's Amino-Terminal Domain: Implications for Protein Stability and DNA Binding, <u>Proc. Natl. Acad. Sci. USA</u> 80:2676 (1983).

21. H. A. deBoer, L. J. Comstock, and M. Vasser, The <u>tac</u> promoter: a Functional Hybrid Derived from <u>trp</u> and <u>lac</u> Promoters, <u>Proc. Natl. Acad. Sci. USA</u> 80:21 (1983).

22. E. R. Zuiderweg, R. Kaptein, and K. Wuthrich, Secondary Structure of the <u>lac</u> Repressor DNA-Binding Domain by Two-Dimensional 1H Nuclear Magnetic Resonance in Solution, <u>Proc. Natl. Acad. Sci. USA</u> 80:5837 (1983).

23. R. T. Sauer and R. Anderegg, Primary Structure of the λ Repressor, <u>Biochemistry</u> 17:1092 (1978).

24. C. O. Pabo and R. T. Sauer, Protein-DNA Recognition, <u>Ann. Rev. Biochem.</u> 53:293 (1984).

25. C. O. Pabo, W. Krovatin, A. Jeffrey, and R. T. Sauer, N-Terminal Arms of λ Repressor Wrap around the Operator DNA, <u>Nature</u> 298:441 (1982).

26. J. L. Eliason, M. A. Weiss, and M. Ptashne, NH2-Terminal Arm of Phage λ Repressor Contributes Energy and Specificity to Repressor Binding and Determines the Effects of Operator Mutations, <u>Proc. Natl. Acad. Sci. USA</u> 82:2339 (1985).

# DETERMINATION OF MACROMOLECULAR STRUCTURE AND DYNAMICS BY NMR

Oleg Jardetzky, Andrew Lane, Jean-Francois Lefevre, and Olivier Lichtarge
Stanford Magnetic Resonance Laboratory

Barbara Hayes-Roth and Bruce Buchanan
Knowledge Systems Laboratory and Department of Computer Science
Stanford University, Stanford, CA 94305, U.S.A.

## INTRODUCTION

The possibility of defining solution structures of proteins and nucleic acids from NMR data has been advanced for many years [1, 2, 3]. In several cases, partial successes have been achieved [4, 5, 6]. However, a closer examination of the lines of argument used in the interpretation of NMR data forces one to conclude that they have not led to the development of an independent, generally applicable method for this purpose. The most successful examples (5, 6) have relied heavily on prior knowledge of the crystal structure - or of very similar crystal structures - and/or on a priori additional constraints, such as the assumption that a single rigid structure exists in solution which can be calculated from the data by minimizing either an error function or the energy of the structure. The danger of such procedures has been discussed elsewhere [8, 9, 10].

At this point techniques for the efficient collection of NMR data useful for structure determinations are readily available and the limiting factors are the techniques of interpretation. The basic problem of interpreting spectroscopic data in structural terms stems from the fact that the measured parameters represent motional (as well as ensemble) averages. For non-rigid systems a unique relationship between measured spectroscopic parameters and structural parameters, such as interatomic distances and coordinates, does not exist, and a straightforward calculation of the structure from experimental data is not possible. Nevertheless, the NMR parameters, being a function of only distances and motional frequencies and amplitudes, have a _relatively_ well defined relationship to interatomic distances. Since both the distances and time factors are unknown, a procedure for deducing structures from NMR data, if it is is to be general, must take the dynamics of the structure explicitly into account. Our aim is to rigorously deduce structures from experimental data - including NMR and other physical measurements - rather than to follow the current practice of inventing plausible structures that on certain assumptions are consistent with the data, but in reality may or may not be correct. The resulting structures can not be expected to have the same precision as the structures derived from X-ray crystallography. They will be structures defined within the limits of uncertainty of the spectroscopic method. The method for obtaining such structures is described here.

The strategy proceeds in four steps and requires prior knowledge of the amino acid sequence. The first step is the definition of secondary structure by COSY-NOESY and relayed NOE methods which have now become standard. The second is the refinement of the localized secondary structure as discussed below. The third is the definition of the topology of the folded structure (for proteins and, if applicable, for a nucleic acid), taking the secondary structure as a given and using long range constraints (e.g. NOEs between remote residues as obtained by 2DFT techniques) as well as information on surface atoms. To carry out this step we have developed an Expert (Artificial Intelligence) System called PROTEAN. Recognizing that at this level the problem is undetermined for a precise structure calculation, the Artificial Intelligence Program defines the entire family of structures compatible with the experimentally available set of constraints. The fourth step of the strategy is a refinement of the tertiary structure. The refinement procedure for the secondary or tertiary structure is identical: Each of the structures allowed by constraints derived from standard 2D NOE experiments is used to calculate the <u>NOE build up rates</u> for all local interactions in the case of secondary structure and for all long range interactions in the case of tertiary structure, <u>taking all alternative pathways into account</u>. The subset of structures (one or more) from which the NOE build up rates can be predicted correctly are then accepted as valid.

## A. Basic Information

- A determination of the solution structure of macromolecules from NMR and other physical measurements requires the following information:

    1. The primary structure.

    2. The average size and shape.

    3. The correlation times.

    4. The identity of surface exposed residues.

To be determined are:

    1. The location of the secondary structures in the primary sequence.

    2. The tertiary structure (the geometric arrangement of the secondary elements)

    3. The range of conformational space accessible to secondary elements and individual amino-acid residues.

1. <u>The primary structure</u> , as determined by standard methods is taken as a given.

2. <u>The size and shape</u> : The anhydrous volume of a macromolecule is given by the product of the molecular weight and the partial specific volume, which can either be measured [11], or estimated with good accuracy from the amino acid composition [12, 13], provided there is no carbohydrate or prosthetic group present. It is important to estimate the shape of the molecule, not only to determine whether or not it is compact, but also because it provides a constraint on the model building process. The shape can be roughly estimated from measurements of the diffusion constant or the sedimentation constant, which actually yield the translational friction coefficient, f , or Stokes' radius. Comparing f with that expected for a hydrated sphere allows one to determine the departure from spherical symmetry. It is usually found that small proteins can be adequately described by ellipsoids with axial ratios of 2:1 or less [14].

3. <u>The rotational correlation time and internal motions</u> : For the analysis of NMR relaxation data, it is important to estimate the apparent rotational diffusion constant, or equivalently, the rotational correlation time, and to estimate the extent of large scale internal motions. In principle, the anisotropy of the decay of the fluorescence of aromatic residues yields such information, though in practice, the data are difficult to interpret.

Measurements of the time-correlated anisotropy of scattered laser light gives an unambiguous estimate of the effective tumbling time, provided that sufficiently concentrated solutions can be obtained, without aggregation. Measurements of $^{13}C$ relaxation times allow one to determine the correlation times of individual carbon nuclei [15], though the requirement for high concentrations often results in aggregation, and overestimates of the overall tumbling time [15]. An alternative is to use 1H NMR. Measurements of the cross relaxation rate between protons that have a fixed internuclear separation (e.g. on aromatic rings or diastereotopic CH2's) as a function of temperature allow one to determine both the effective overall tumbling time ( an average over the principal axes of rotation for non-spherical molecules), and the presence of internal motions, with their amplitudes and frequencies [16]. The tumbling time should agree with that calculated from $f/f_0$ and the Perrin equations. The tumbling time is necessary for calculating NOEs used in the refinement of the structure (see below). As the analysis of NOE data is greatly complicated by the presence of internal motions, it is essential to determine the extent of such motions, so that it is possible to decide upon the effect they may have on the structures determined.

4. Identification of surface residues : The search for the tertiary structure will be greatly accelerated if residues are identified as being on the surface, or otherwise. There are many methods for identifying such residues, each relying on different properties. It is not surprising that the different methods can give different answers. This does not mean that the data are incorrect, merely that the question is not precisely formulated, or alternatively, the surface is not a simple, smooth entity. It is therefore necessary to use a wide variety of techniques, so that a consensus can be reached, before the data can be used for a structure determination.

The methods fall into two kinds; those based on accessibility to externally added reagents, and those based on the relaxation properties of the residues.

(i) accessibility to reagents:

One of the commonest experiments in protein NMR is to measure the titration curves of histidine, tyrosine and lysine residues (i.e. access to OH⁻ or H3O⁺). In unstructured peptides, these residues have characteristic chemical shifts, multiplicities, pK values, and titration steps. If a residue in a protein has such properties similar to those in small peptides then the residues can be unequivocally assigned to the surface, as it is clearly completely accessible to solvent, and has no interaction with other residues. The converse, however, is not true, as interactions with other residues may well change the chemical shift and the pK value, but the residues could nevertheless reside on the surface.

It is possible to nitrate, for example, tyrosine residues. The observation of nitration of some, but not others is generally taken to imply surface or buried locations. However, the same strictures apply here as to the titration data, and the effect of bulky substituents can sufficiently perturb the structure as to render the findings ambiguous.

PhotoCIDNP relies on the accessibility of aromatic residues to a dye, usually a flavin derivative. The size of this molecule is sufficient that it is unlikely to penetrate deeply into the protein. As there is no permanent chemical reaction, the interpretation of CIDNP experiments is perhaps more straightforward than chemical modification experiments. It is, of course, limited to tyrosine, tryptophan and histidine [15].

Tryptophan residues can be probed by accessibility to fluorescence quenching reagents. It is desirable to use at least two kinds of reagent, differing in charge, to eliminate the possibility of specific binding effects [16, 17].

Possibly more general is the use of paramagnetic ions such as manganese. The increase in line width depends on residence time of the ion [15], which is expected to be significant only for those residues exposed at the surface. A titration with $Mn^{2+}$ should produce differential line broadening. Those broadened the most are the most accessible, and by implication, closest to the surface, as charged species do not penetrate the interior of proteins [18]. The general rule for the interpretation of all such findings is that susceptibility to perturbation can be taken as evidence for a surface location, but failure to respond to a perturbation cannot be taken as evidence against a surface location.

(ii) Methods based on relaxation times:

It is well known that line widths and spin-lattice relaxation times depend on the correlation time and the number and distances to nearest neighbors. In the interior of proteins, one can expect on average a relatively large number of nearest neighbors, and a relatively small degree of internal motion, giving rise to broader lines, and short $T_1$ values. Surface residues tend to have fewer neighbors, and consequently may have additional degrees of motional freedom and therefore narrower lines and longer $T_1$ values.

For a rigid macromolecule, the line-width and reciprocal spin lattice relaxation time, $\rho$, should be directly proportional to the ratio of the bulk viscosity to the absolute temperature. Hence, a plot of the relaxation rate versus $\eta/T$ should be linear (Perrin plot) . Further, if the viscosity is varied by changing the temperature, an Eyring plot should also be linear, with an apparent activation energy of about 4.5 kcal/mole (for D2O). Therefore, lines that are substantially sharper than average that give non-linear Perrin plots, and activation energies substantially different from 4.5 kcal/mole are likely to be on the surface. The apparent activation energy can be larger than 4.5 kcal/mole, if there are changes in structure over the range of temperature studied. This information is also valuable, as it implies that a single conformation does not necessarily exist, so that the determined structure becomes an average over several states.

The temperature dependence of the cross relaxation rate for protons that are known to have a fixed internuclear separation (for example intraring NOEs, or diastereotopic $\beta$-protons [19]) are not sensitive to changes in structure in the same way, only to the correlation time. This therefore provides a means of estimating the correlation time for the motion, and the amplitude.

Finally, one can predict that the charged residues (especially arginine, lysine, glutamate and aspartate) will be exposed at the surface, because of the energetic cost of burying them in a region of low effective dielectric constant. When such residues are buried, anomalies of their chemical shifts are usually observed. If there are no anomalies in the spectrum, likely surface exposed and buried regions can then be identified by examining the local charge density in the primary structure. However, such information is not compelling and is best used only to corroborate conclusions that can be drawn directly from experimental data.

# B. Secondary Structures

Those proteins that have a high content of secondary structure (say >50%) are easier to treat than those that have only a small fraction of periodic structures. It is therefore important to determine how much, what kinds, and where they are in the primary sequence.

1. Content and nature of secondary elements: Despite the limitations of far UV CD, in the absence of disulphide bridges and carbohydrate an estimate of the probable total amount of periodic structures can be obtained by this method. If helix is the dominant type of periodic structure present, the helical fraction can be determined with moderate

accuracy. The same is not true for β-structures. However, sheet can often be identified from the chemical shifts of the αCH protons, as they tend to resonate downfield of the other α-protons [20]. IR measurements can now be made on solutions, and this may provide a more reliable estimate of the amounts of secondary structure than CD. Certainly, the measurements should be made under both native and denaturing conditions, which can also provide an estimate of the thermodynamic stability of the protein.

Another test of the amount of secondary structure is the rate of exchange of amide protons. To a reasonable first approximation, those protons that exchange with rate constants much smaller than the intrinsic rate constant can be considered to participate in hydrogen bonds, whether they are "buried" or not [26]. A convenient method of measuring these rates is NMR, which has the additional advantage that many of the protons can be assigned to particular residues (see below). The measurements should be made under a variety of conditions, such as pH, temperature, and pulse sequence. The pulse sequences include the effect of saturating the solvent in $H_2O$ solutions on the number of amide protons present and the number of amide protons present immediately after dissolution in $D_2O$. Solvent saturation will decrease the intensities of those protons that exchange with a rate constant of the order the reciprocal spin-lattice relaxation time. The total number of slowly exchanging protons is expected to agree with the estimates of secondary structure content from the other methods.

2. Location: A reasonably reliable method of determining the location of types of secondary structure elements in the primary sequence is that originally developed by Gibbons [21, 22], and subsequently refined by Wuthrich and colleagues [23, 24]. In this method, patterns of NOEs between amide, αCH and β protons are compared with three bond coupling constants ($^3J_{NH-\alpha H}$), and rates of exchange of the amide protons. The first step is to assign the resonances to particular protons. This is by no means a trivial task, but can be achieved for proteins of about 60 amino acid residues at present, and given the pace of technical development, can be expected to be extended to substantially longer polypeptides. The rate constants for exchange of amide protons are compared with the intrinsic amide exchange rate constants for unstructured peptides under the same conditions of temperature, pH and base concentration, with appropriate corrections for nearest neighbor effects [25]. Amide protons that exchange more than an order of magnitude more slowly than the intrinsic rate can be assumed to participate in hydrogen bonds, a feature of secondary structures.

Some additional information on the location of secondary structure can be obtained from coupling constants. Coupling constants generally follow a Karplus curve, and there have been several studies that have attempted to parametrize the Karplus equation for peptides having known geometries. Although the shapes of these curves are consistent with the Karplus equation, the particular model peptides chosen in the different studies yield substantially different values for the parameters. Hence, coupling constants can be used semi-quantitatively at best. Large values of J (i.e. >7 Hz) strongly indicate a relatively narrow range for the value of the peptide torsion angle $\phi$. On the other hand, small values of J ($\approx$ 4 Hz) could imply either that $\phi$ has a particular value, or that the structure is averaging over a wide range of angles. Wuthrich [23, 24] has suggested that the values of J be used as indicators, based on a statistical analysis of observed coupling constant and secondary structures in BPTI.

The pattern of NOE intensities is quite characteristic for different structures. The intensities are very sensitive to the internuclear separation. Accordingly, Wuthrich and coworkers have defined a set of distances d1, d2, d3 shown in figure 1, that can in principle be derived from NOE measurements. For example, in an α-helix, short distance (large intensities) are expected for d2, and somewhat larger distances for d1 and d1,i+3. On the other hand, in β-strands, one expects short distances for d1. In periodic structures of this type, short distances can generally be associated with large NOE intensities, subject to the refinement procedure described below. This method seems to work quite well, except that the ends of the periodic segments are not precisely defined ($\approx$ ± 2 residues, [24]).

A similar strategy exists for oligonucleotides [27, and see below].

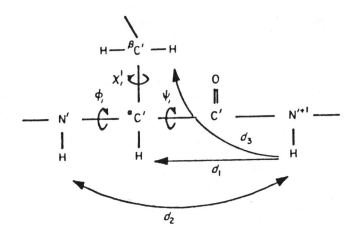

**Figure 1:** Polypeptide backbone segment. The through-space distances $d_1$, $d_2, d_3$ used in the determination of helical structure are indicated by arrows.

3. Refinement of secondary structures: It has been customary to assume that the elements of secondary structure are regular, that is, that they have essentially ideal geometries. While this may be reasonable for helices (but beware of bent $\alpha$-helices and $3_{10}$ or $\pi$-helices !), it is certainly not for $\beta$-strands. As a matter of fact, ideal $\beta$-strands are very rare, and usually they are twisted, forming curved sheets or barrel structures [28, 29]. Hence, even to define the secondary architecture of the protein, one must determine the regularity or irregularity of the secondary elements.

To do this, it is necessary to probe the structures of periodic elements in greater detail. In principle, the coupling constants could be useful, though in practice, there are too many ambiguities, such as the imprecision of standard curves of J versus $\phi$, and the problem of averaging. Motions need only to be of the order a few tens of Hz to average coupling constants; on this time scale relatively large amplitudes of motion are intrinsically probable. The alternative is to measure cross relaxation rates, which are proportional to $r^{-6}$. The simplest possible case is two spins, embedded in a rigid body. The transfer of magnetization between the spins , in this case, obeys simple first order kinetics, leading to a single exponential for the time course. The initial slope of the time course is the cross relaxation rate, which is related to the distance as:

$$\sigma = \alpha[6J(\omega_1+\omega_2)-J(\omega_1-\omega_2)]/r^6 \tag{1}$$

where $\alpha$ is a magnetic constant whose value for protons is 5.692 $10^{-38}$ cm$^6$ s$^{-2}$, and J are the spectral density functions. For protons, it is permissible to replace $J(\omega_1-\omega_2)$ and $J(\omega_1+\omega_2)$ by $J(0)$ and $J(2\omega)$, respectively. For a rigid macromolecule whose rotational correlation time is say 2 ns, $6J(2\omega)$ is 0.07 ns at 500 MHz, i.e is negligible with respect to $J(0)=\tau_R$. This forms the basis of estimating internuclear distances in macromolecules [15].

If this formulation were a reasonably accurate representation of macromolecules, then it would be a very simple matter to determine geometries from distances estimated from cross relaxation rates. Unfortunately, most macromolecules cannot be reasonably treated as rigid bodies consisting of nicely isolated pairs of protons. Even in a linear polypeptide chain, the C$\alpha$-proton generally has three or four near neighbours; the C$\beta$-protons, the C$\alpha$NH and the neighbouring C$\alpha$ proton. Hence, although in principle the torsion angle $\phi$ could be determined by estimating the distance between C$\alpha$H and NH, in practice one must take into account the relaxation of the NH and the possibility of alternative pathways of transfer of magnetization (see below). The true initial rate becomes difficult to measure because of relaxation, and the presence of alternative pathways means that the apparent cross relaxation rate is not simply related to a single internuclear distance. Taking the sixth root as Eq (1) suggests gives the result r = 3±1 Angstroms . Even if one could improve the precision of the measurements, there would always be a probable error of at least 0.5 Angstrom. We note that one should never confuse precision with accuracy. The former is defined by the quality of the experimental measurement, the latter by the validity of the assumptions used for interpretation. Now the extreme values of r(NH-CαH) are 2.2 Angstroms and 3.5 Angstroms. A probable error of 0.5 Angstrom would not fix the value of $\phi$ with sufficient accuracy for a structure determination. Hence, an alternative means of data analysis is required.

Provided that NOEs are measured in the high power limit [30], the changes in magnetization after saturating one spin still obey simple first order kinetics, and can be described using the Bloch equations. These equations can be integrated analytically, giving a sum of exponentials whose relaxation times are complicated functions of cross relaxation rates and spin-lattice relaxation times. These eigenvalues are not very useful. It is more meaningful to calculate the entire NOE build up curve for the minimum number of spins that describe the system, for an assumed structure. The structure is then varied, until the calculated and observed build-up curves agree. (This can be done iteratively, using a gradient search or other optimization algorithms). Note that this method automatically takes into account both spin-lattice relaxation and alternative pathways of magnetization transfer, so that it is not necessary to measure NOEs at vanishingly small irradiation times. As the relaxation times are also calculated, one can improve the performance by including measured intrinsic spin-lattice relaxation rate constants in the fitting routine. Fig. 2 shows the NOEs calculated a)using the 2 spin approximation and b)taking all alternative pathways into account. Obviously, there is no simple correlation between distance and the magnitude of the NOE, even in secondary structures.

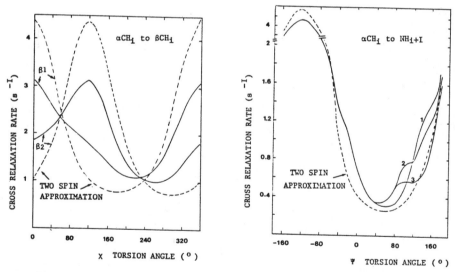

**Figure 2:** Cross relaxation rates in a dipeptide as a function of torsion angles. Rates were calculated according to the text, with $\tau_R$ = 10 ms.

For the periodic elements, one obviously has a good starting point; the algorithm will find the deviations from the ideal structure, which is precisely what one wants to find. For non-periodic elements, the structure may still be well defined, but merely irregular. Here, a more extensive search will be necessary, and places greater demands on the number of data and their precision.

Apart from the internuclear distances, the relaxation rates depend also on the correlation time(s). It is therefore essential to have a reliable estimate of the(ir) value(s). As the error on individual NOEs is likely to be at least ±10%, the correlation times do not have to be determined with greater precision. The overall tumbling time can often be calculated with this precision using simple hydrodynamic arguments. If the molecular weight, partial specific volume and $f/f_0$ are known (see above), the probable error on the apparent correlation time is less than ±20%. This is because globular proteins are densely packed, and do not depart greatly from spherical symmetry [14]. It is also possible to estimate the effective tumbling time from NMR [see above and 16].

It is also wise to make the measurements as a function of temperature, as this may allow certain internal motions to be detected. If extensive internal motions are present, a complete analysis is probably impossible: although the effect on the correlation time can be adequately accounted for, the effect of averaging internuclear distances in general cannot, with these data alone. This is because one cannot know a priori the number of states being averaged, and the relevant internuclear distances in each state.

If internal motions are detected, then one must seek physically reasonable models for the motions, and decide what the averaging includes. At the very least, an additional parameter is introduced in the fitting process. However, trends in data, even if not completely quantitative, can often be used to estimate the regularity or irregularity of segments of polypeptides. This is especially important for $\beta$-strands, because if they are significantly twisted or bent, using a linear chain will result in an incorrect structure (see below).

We will illustrate the refinement of a secondary structure using our data on the trp operator of *E.coli*. The sequence of the 20 base pair fragment is: CGTACTAGTT.AACTAGTACG. The point represents the position of palindromic symmetry. The assignments of the non-exchangeable protons were made by standard two-dimensional methods, and confirmed by one dimensional NOE measurements. CD spectra showed that the DNA belongs to the B family of conformations. The correlation time measured by cross relaxation rates for the cytosine and thymine residues indicated that it is double stranded, and that the bases do not undergo significant internal motions on the nanosecond time scale.

Measurements of the coupling constants H1' to H2' and H2" allows the basic pucker type to be determined (Fig. 3). NOE build up curves were obtained for irradiating the H1', H2' and H2" of each d-ribose. Fig. 4 shows the apparent cross relaxation rate as a function of the glycosidic torsion angle and pseudorotation phase angle for each irradiated proton. The dotted lines in Fig. 4 show the expected cross relaxation rate for two spins only; the full lines were computed using 6 spins. Clearly, the two spin approximation is wholly inadequate. Using such curves, it is possible to determine the glycosidic torsion angle, X, and the phase angle, P, for each d-ribose in the molecule. Initial values were then further refined using a simultaneous fit of the data to the calculated NOEs, with a gradient search method. The results are given in Table 1. The relative orientations of the nucleotide units were determined using internucleotide NOEs, again with the help of the gradient search algorithm. The parameters are also given in Table 1. As Table 1 shows, the basic pucker of the purines is largely in the south (C2'endo), whereas that of the pyrimidines is more toward the north (C3'endo). We also took into account averaging of the sugar puckers by pseudorotation. The cross relaxation rate for H1' to H2" depends on the correlation time, as the distance is independent of the value of P. The amplitude of this motion is about 23° projected on the long axis of the molecule, and compares well with a calculation, which gives 21°. The three NOE measurements and the coupling constants are sufficient to determine X and P, as well as the fraction C2' endo, assuming that only C2' endo and C3' endo are significantly populated.

There are quite large deviations from the standard B-DNA conformation. We note, however, that the mean pitch is 3.4 Angstroms, and the mean twist angle is 36°, typical of B DNA [31]. Further, the local deviations from the idealized structure are in accord with the findings of Dickerson and coworkers, and the predictions of Calladine [32, 33]. This is shown in Fig. 5. Hence, the refinement procedure works very well, and can be applied similarly to polypeptides.

**Table 1:** Structural Parameters of the trp Operator DNA

| R1° | X° | p° | B [θT°] | θp° [θr°] | B [hÅ] | p° | X° | R2° |
|---|---|---|---|---|---|---|---|---|
| 13 | -25 | S(162) | C1 [38] | – [-] | G20 [3.4] | S(162) | -48 | - |
| -10 | -38 | N(60) | G2 [34] | -5 [-11.5] | C19 [3.6] | N(54) | -33 | 5 |
| 10 | -33 | N(54) | T3 [30!] | 12 [9.5] | A18 [3.4] | S(126) | -46 | 2 |
| 1 | -46 | S(---) | A4 [36] | 13 [-6.5] | T17 [3.6] | N(54) | -40 | 12 |
| 2 | -33 | N(14) | C5 [43] | 2 [-2] | G16 [3.2] | N(70) | -48 | 0 |
| 11 | -39 | N(54) | T6 [26] | 16 [6] | A15 [3.4] | S(---) | -51 | 5 |
| 5 | -51 | S(---) | A7 [43] | 16 [-2] | T14 [3.2] | N(54) | -39 | 11 |
| 1 | -48 | N(70) | G8 [36] | 4 [6] | C13 [3.6] | N(45) | -25 | 3 |
| -13 | -35 | N(20) | T9 [44] | -12 [-6.5] | A12 [3.3] | S(126) | -41 | 1 |
| 3 | -35 | S(---) | T10 [30] | 7 [-1] | A11 [3.6] | S(126) | -46 | 4 |
| 4 | -46 | S(126) | A11 | 7 | T10 | S(---) | -35 | 3 |

a) parameters defining the conformation of each base pair : X is the glycosidic torsion angle (defined as the torsion angle of C8,6-N9-C1'-C2') and p the phase of the pseudorotation which determine the pucker of the deoxyribose. S and N correspond to south and north conformations. The value in bracket after S or N indicates the value of p given by the calculation (p=18 : C3'endo, p=90 : O4'endo, p=162 : C2'endo). (---) means that acceptable fits are obtained for all the south conformations. R1 and R2 are the individual base roll angles and θp the propeller twist angle. These angles are defined in the text.

b) respective orientations between base pairs : θT is the twist angle, h the local pitch and θr the inter base pair roll angle calculated for each step.

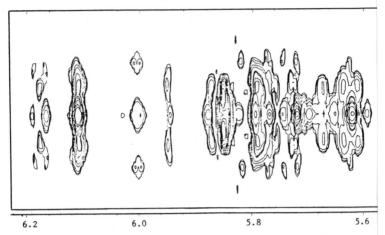

6.2          6.0              5.8              5.6

**Figure 3:** J-resolved spectrum of the trp operator. 2.8 mM trp ope
35°.C. H1' of purines are clustered at low field. Doublets cor
to C3'endo and triplet to C2'endo conformation.

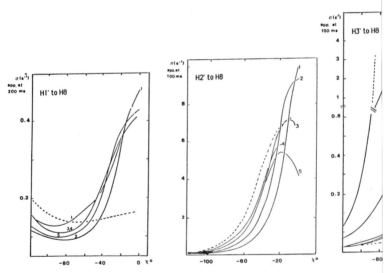

**Figure 4:** Intranucleotide cross relaxation rates as a function of t
glycosidic torsion angle and the pucker. The rates were calculate
to the text, using a correlation time of 6.4 ns. The numbers refe
of the pseudorotation angle, P, 1:P = 18, 2:P = 54, 3:P = 126, 4:
5:P = 190.

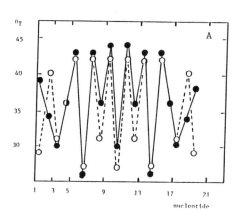
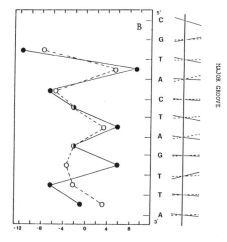

**Figure 5:** Predicted versus observed values of the roll and the helical twist.

A. Helical twist versus nucleotide number. [o] predicted,
[•] observed.

B. Roll angles versus nucleotide number. [o] predicted,
[•] observed. In
the ladder at the right, the solid line corresponds to the sequence shown and
the dotted line to its complement.

## C. Tertiary structure. Use of Artificial Intelligence in the Interpretation of NMR Findings

1. Determination of Topological Features: With the secondary structure defined, the task is to deduce the correct folding pattern from experimental data. The principal data are through-space distances between side chains of residues remote from each other in the sequence. They can be estimated either from Nuclear Overhauser effect measurements between side chain protons, or from relaxation parameters measured before and after substitution of a proton by a deuteron, or from relaxation measurements in spin labeling experiments. In principle distance estimates are possible from chemical shifts, but except for the case of aromatic ring current shifts, such estimates are difficult. This long-range distance information can be supplemented by experimental information on the shape of the molecule, its packing density and the identification of surface atoms.

To be rigorous, the method of deduction must take into account that distances obtained from spectroscopic measurements cannot be interpreted as static distances - i.e., unique distances characteristic of rigid structures. An NOE indicates proximity within, say 2.5 - 5 Angstroms, but proximity FOR A PERIOD OF TIME. Its magnitude does not distinguish between 50% of the time in Van-der-Waals contact and 100% of the time at 5 Angstroms, and therefore cannot be translated into a unique distance. The measurement reflects the dynamics of the structure as well as its geometry.

If the method of deduction is to remain true to the information content of the experimental measurement, it must aim to define the DYNAMIC STRUCTURE of the macromolecule - that is the relative orientation of the domains and their freedom of motion with respect to each other. Thus, the structure obtainable from spectroscopic data is in principle different from the average STATIC structure obtainable from X-ray crystallography. It is not likely to be as precise in defining the coordinates of each atom, but it can be accurate within the uncertainty limits of the spectroscopic method. An accurate deduction of the structure from solution data is not as straightforward as

59

the algorithmic calculation of a structure from the X-ray diffraction pattern. It requires the integration of multiple sources of information - such as molecular shape, long range distances, location of surface atoms. In addition, the method of deduction must take into account that the problem is likely to be underdetermined - i.e., that the number of constraints is likely to be too small to permit rapid convergence on a single structure in an algorithmic calculation which samples the entire configuration space at random. These aspects of the problem make it intractable from an algorithmic point of view and suggest the use of the more goal-directed and economical methods of Artificial Intelligence.

While it may be considered a weakness of NMR and other spectroscopic methods, that the data are not interpretable simply in terms of structure, but in terms of structure complicated by motion, it is also a major strength of the method that one can obtain from it a picture of the dynamic, rather than a static structure. Determinations of crystal structures have not produced as much insight into function, as had originally been expected, for lack of information on the internal dynamics of the macromolecules. Knowledge of the dynamic structure is essential to understand the interactive mechanisms between macromolecules - or macromolecules and ligands - which underlie biological function.

2. Fundamental Premises and Differences from Existing Approaches:    The difference between our approach and existing approaches based on distance geometry algorithms are fundamental:

- We do not assume, as do the distance geometry algorithms, that all constraints must be satisfied simultaneously. Spectroscopic data do not contain any information to justify this assumption, because of the problem of averaging.

- Our method of inference is independent of the notion that there necessarily must exist a single structure which corresponds to an energy minimum or an optimum of all constraints. The method allows the possibility that multiple structures may exist, which are not sub-states of a single minimum. Thus, the existence of a single structure (or of a very closely related family of structures) can be a conclusion, but is not an *a priori* assumption of the method.

- The common feature of all methods of inference is that a spectroscopic distance measurement (NOE, paramagnetic line broadening) signifies proximity whose approximate lower limit is a Van-der-Waals contact and the upper limit is ill-defined, but lies about 5-6 Angstroms for a relaxation effect and 15-20 Angstroms for a paramagnetic effect. In the distance geometry approach which minimizes an error function of all distances, this range has the significance that all distances must fall within it at all times, or the structure will not appear satisfactory. In the approach described here, the significance of the range is more limited: it is the range within which a given distance must fall during the time that a constraint is satisfied. The method aims to define an entire set of structures and all constraints must be satisfied by the set, but no individual structure is required to satisfy more than a subset of all distance constraints.

3. Method of Inference: Volume Refinement: Our basic strategy is to consider the long range distance constraints one by one and to define the entire range of mutual orientations of two - and subsequently more - domains defined by the secondary structure, which are compatible with a given constraint. The first step is to choose one domain (e.g., a helix or a $\beta$-sheet) and define its coordinate system. For a helix a convenient choice is to define the axis of the helix as the z-axis of a right handed Cartesian coordinate system and the x-axis as a perpendicular axis passing through the nucleus of the first (N-terminal) $\alpha$-carbon in the helix. The second step is to "anchor" a second structured domain to it by sweeping out the entire volume in which the second domain can be located and still satisfy the given constraint. This volume represents the limits of our knowledge about the structure defined by the one given

experimental constraint. The folding is deduced by a successive application of all available constraints in a similar manner and the method of inference can therefore be called the VOLUME REFINEMENT method.

The third step is to apply the next constraint and define the free volume compatible with it. The next step is to define the intersection of the two free volumes. If the volumes do NOT intersect, we can CONCLUDE that the two constraints cannot be satisfied simultaneously, and therefore that no single structure exists. If the two free volumes do intersect, we know that the constraints can be satisfied simultaneously and that a single structure MAY exist. We then have a choice: (1) to ASSUME that the constraints ARE satisfied simultaneously and proceed to work with the reduced intersected volume when exploring other constraints, or (2) to retain the entire free volume of the two constraints and proceed to define the free volume of the next constraint and its intersections with each of the preceding constraints individually. This procedure is considerably more time consuming, but can have an advantage in certain situations, where an intersection of the free volume of the third constraint has no intersection with the intersected volume of the first two, but does separately intersect each of them. This can be the case, for example in a protein structure fluctuating between two conformations, so that either constraints 1,3 or 2,3 are satisfied, but the combination 1,2 is not. It is worth noting that long range constraints contain information on the possible geometry of macromolecular conformations, but not on their energetics. Thus, the fact that the combination of constraints 1 and 2 is geometrically possible provides no information as to whether it is energetically feasible. This is an important limitation of the information content of a spectroscopic measurement and requires great caution in the use of the very tempting assumption that any two constraints which CAN be satisfied simultaneously ARE indeed satisfied simultaneously. The information contained in a spectroscopic measurement is LOCAL information and provides no basis for inferences about the remainder of the structure. The outlined method retains the option of reexamining this assumption for any pair of constraints, even if it has been introduced at some stage of the model building process.

The remaining constraints are then introduced sequentially and the free volumes and their intersections with the preexisting free volumes and intersections are defined, until the entire list of available experimental constraints between the two domains is exhausted. The two domains are then considered anchored to each other.

The next step is to choose a third domain and to anchor it to first one and then the other of the two preceding, defining the free volumes and allowed intersections until the list of structured domains is exhausted. This is followed by one or more steps of satisfying the constraints (if any are available experimentally) between any unstructured ("random coil") segments and the domains defined by secondary structure.

Two additional sources of information can be invoked to check the validity of the inferences based on long range distance constraints: (1) The shape of the macromolecule, as determined by small angle X-ray, or neutron scattering, hydrodynamic measurements or light scattering experiments, and (2) The identification of surface atoms by, for example, relaxation measurements in the presence of paramagnetic perturbations.

Any structure derived from long range distance constraints must be compatible with the overall dimensions of the macromolecule, as determined experimentally. The latter are only approximately known as ellipsoids of revolution, but significant asymmetries are usually apparent. To check for compatibility, the center of mass of the proposed structure can be computed and made to coincide with the geometric center of the corresponding, experimentally derived, ellipsoid of revolution. The ellipsoid can then be rotated around its three axes to circumscribe the proposed structure. Any major incompatibilities would cast doubts on the correctness of the structure. If the free volume of a domain (with all constraints considered) only partially overlaps the volume of the ellipsoid of revolution, one would have to examine the possibility of a breathing mode which for periods of time distorts the molecular shape from its experimentally apparent average. It should be possible to develop criteria, based on the number and nature of constraints, for determining the fraction of time each domain spends in each part of its free volume, but this has not as yet been attempted. If, on the other hand, the entire free volume (or a very large fraction) lies outside the ellipsoid of revolution defining the average molecular shape, the structure clearly cannot be correct.

The use of surface information may be regarded as the first step of refinement. The coordinate system in which the structure has been built can be subdivided into a grid of atomic size (~1 A³). All grid cells on or near the surface of the structure are labelled as "surface" and all atoms in the structure which are known to lie on the surface are labelled similarly. The domains within the structure are then rotated and/or translated until the two sets of labels match. While the precision of such matching may not be very great, it must be borne in mind that neither can the position of surface residues, which are known to move freely in solution, be specified very precisely. However, major incompatibilities can serve as indicators that the proposed structure can not be correct.

The free volumes for each of the structured and unstructured domains are, strictly speaking, measures of the uncertainty of spectroscopic data. This uncertainty has two principal sources: insufficient data and degrees of internal motional freedom. The existence of mutually exclusive structural constraints can be taken as definite evidence that internal motion is occurring, provided that a proper distinction between real and apparent constraints has been made, as discussed in the section on structure refinement. Apparent constraints can arise, for example, from the mistaken use of indirect NOEs as direct. However, detailed consideration of all alternative pathways, as described below, can eliminate such ambiguities. In the absence of truly incompatible constraints the distinction between insufficiency of the data and internal mobility is difficult and can only be made on additional experimental grounds. For example, if the relaxation of nuclei on domain A by nuclei on domain B does not follow the pattern that can be predicted from any single structure that can be instantiated within the free volume, it is possible to infer that internal motion must be occurring. Obviously, extensive additional experimental evidence is required to substantiate such conclusions.

4. The Order of Inference: The method of inference described above has several features that make it unsuitable for an algorithmic implementation:

- To remain true to the information content of each experimental measurement it does not invoke constraints that cannot be deduced from the data. Since the data do not indicate whether all observed constraints are or are not satisfied simultaneously, the use of global error functions which can be minimized is precluded. Thus, a hierarchical order for the sequential application and testing of the constraints becomes necessary. There is no reason to assume *a priori* that a unique hierarchical order will be universally applicable to all situations.

- The data on which the inferences have to be based are incomplete and imprecise by their very nature.

- The sequential construction of a macromolecular model from the available spectroscopic constraints requires that several choices be made to determine the sequence of operations. For example, it is necessary to choose 1) the order in which domains are anchored to each other 2) the order in which constraints are applied 3) whether to accept the intersection of the free volumes defined by two or more constraints as the only residual allowed free volume for the remainder of the model building process or not. There are also optional choices which may improve the efficiency of model building, but which may be allowed only in certain situations - for example whether to apply constraints individually or in groups, whether to anchor the third structured domain to the first two or to the second or fourth, thus creating substructures to be merged later, etc.

- While rigorously adhering to the information content of each set of experimental data, the method permits the use of data of different kinds, which are not easily combined in a single type of calculation - e.g., long range distance constraints obtained from NOE measurements, identity of surface atoms which cannot be translated into a distance without prior knowledge of the structure, in some cases - dihedral angles estimated from coupling constant measurements, mutual orientations of aromatic rings from chemical shift measurements, etc. The integration of multiple sources of knowledge is an essential feature of the method.

5. The PROTEAN Program: The foregoing features of the problem - the fact that a one-to-one correspondence between experimentally measured and molecular structural parameters does not hold for solution methods as it does in crystallography, the need to use symbolic, as well as numerical constraints, and multiple sources of knowledge, the incompleteness and irreducible uncertainty of the data and the resulting desirability of following more than one option in the analysis of the data - all suggest that the solution is best approached through Artificial Intelligence (AI). An AI program can be defined as a set - or system - of computer programs capable of symbolic inference and heuristic reasoning as well as of numerical calculation. Rather than following a rigid sequence of tasks, an AI program develops a line of reasoning using considerable knowledge of a task domain and applying it intelligently to the problem at hand. The system we have constructed for the determination of macromolecular structures in solution has been called PROTEAN. The system is still under development and at present contains programs for the determination of protein structures. However, incorporation of programs for the determination of nucleic acid (or other macromolecular) structures is possible within the framework of the same basic design.

PROTEAN is based on the Blackboard Model of an Expert System, and specifically on the model referred to as BB1. In this model the solution of the problem is broken up into a series of tasks, each of which is performed by a specific program or a sequence of linked programs. The choice of the order in which the tasks are performed is vested in a control program which incorporates heuristic rules of arbitrary complexity by which specific choices are made. the output of each task-specific program is recorded as an entry in the accessible part of the computer memory used to monitor the choices and the execution of specific tasks, and the progress of the solution. This block of memory remains accessible throughout the problem solving process and is called the Blackboard. The essential elements of the Blackboard model are therefore: the Blackboard itself (somewhat akin to the Strategy Room of an Army); the task-oriented programs, called the Knowledge Sources; their outputs -- the Blackboard Entries (representing partial solutions of the problem); and a Control Mechanism or Scheduler. The high-level programming language commonly used for the Blackboard model, and used for PROTEAN is LISP. Low level tasks can be programmed in FORTRAN or other languages.

The Blackboard is to begin with a two-dimensional construct, with a vertical dimension representing different levels of complexity (or abstraction) used in the solution of the problem and a horizontal dimension recording the degree of advancement of the problem solving process. It is possible to design blackboards incorporating additional dimensions, but thus far we have not found it necessary for our purposes.

A Knowledge Source is a high-level program which may contain commands to execute a sequence of low-level programs. Knowledge Sources are constructed to consist of two parts: a part designed to execute a specific tasks or series of tasks and a part designed to evaluate whether the conditions for their execution exists. They may therefore be regarded as CONDITIONAL programs, to be executed only if specific conditions for their execution are satisfied by an entry on the blackboard. When a Knowledge Source is activated and executed, its output is recorded as an entry on the Blackboard.

The appearance of an entry (or a new event) on the Blackboard triggers the Control Mechanism, which contains the Knowledge Source Activating Records (KSAR) specifying the conditions for the activation of each Knowledge Source and a program for evaluating the new blackboard entry as a trigger for the complete or partial set of Knowledge Sources, in accordance with specified heuristic rules. The result of this evaluation is then posted as an entry on the Blackboard and triggers the execution of one or more additional Knowledge Sources. It is worth noting that the Blackboard can be designed to execute tasks in sequence or in parallel, depending on the available computer capacity.

The Blackboard Model thus requires two levels of Knowledge Sources: DOMAIN or TASK-SPECIFIC Knowledge Sources which contain all the programs for performing all the tasks needed to solve a specific type of problem -- such as correctly deducing a protein structure from experimental data -- and CONTROL Knowledge Sources which contain programs for deciding on the order of procedure and evaluating a partial result on the basis of heuristic rules representing different types of information relevant to the solution of the problem. (In the context of PROTEAN the term task-specific is to be preferred to domain knowledge source to avoid confusion with the structured domains of a protein). The execution of a task and control decisions on the next step(s) can be carried out either in sequence or in parallel, depending on available computer capacity.

A very significant advantage of the Blackboard Model is that it provides a common framework for the use and correlation of the results of widely different Knowledge Sources. Some Knowledge Sources may represent sets of programs performing numerical computations using numerical constraints, such as long range distances. Others may perform symbolic reasoning, using constraints that can only be represented symbolically, such as the identity of surface atoms. Yet the inferences drawn by the two operationally unrelated methods can be correlated on the Blackboard and incorporated into the final solution of the problem. This feature is especially important in the determination of the solution structure of macromolecules: no single method, no single type of measurement, and therefore no single type of calculation contains adequate information to unambiguously deduce the structure, along with its degrees of internal motional freedom. However, concurrent use of information obtained from different types of measurements does make it possible.

6. The Principal Features of PROTEAN: A complete technical description of PROTEAN is beyond the scope of this presentation. However, its principal features and the underlying strategic concepts can be briefly illustrated by its application to the determination of the solution structure of the N-terminal, DNA binding domain of the lac-repressor (The lac-repressor headpiece). No crystal structure for this structured peptide (MW 6000) is available, but the principal topological features have been inferred from NMR data, using model building by hand and the essential features of the strategy subsequently incorporated into PROTEAN. Thus a basis for comparison of the results obtained by computer calculation and conventional model building is available.

The PROTEAN Blackboard at present consists of three levels of abstraction in the vertical dimension: (1) The solid level at which only the overall shape of the structured domains is considered, i.e., random coils are represented as lines, $\alpha$-helices as cylinders, and $\beta$-sheets as parallelepipeds (or one, two or three vectors respectively); (2) The hinge or "Blob" level, at which all covalent bonds around which rotation is possible are explicitly specified, the rotationally invariant parts of the structure being represented by superatoms -- e.g., alanine being represented as a string of three superatoms -- the peptide group, an $\alpha$-CH superatom and a CH3 superatom; and (3) The atomic level at which all atoms are represented individually. Partial solutions at varying degrees of advancement form the horizontal dimension. To construct the model of the lac-repressor headpiece, a knowledge source called POST-THE-PROBLEM must be activated first. This makes available to the Expert System all the pertinent information permanently stored in libraries: the primary sequence, the elements of amino acid and peptide bond geometry, the Van-der-Walls radii of all atoms in the sequence, and the information on the secondary structure, which in this case means the specification of the three $\alpha$-helices as comprising segments 6-14, 17-25, and 35-45 in the primary sequence. A choice of the helix to be used as an anchor has to be made and a knowledge source POST-THE-HELIX specifies the anchor and defines the initial coordinate system. A choice of the first helix to be anchored is required and a series of knowledge sources collectively called ANCHOR-HELIX is then activated to define the free volume of the anchoree helix that is compatible with each of the constraints. The relevant NOE constraints are taken from the data set represented in Fig. 6. In this case the intersection of the free volumes is taken to define the net allowed free volume of the anchoree with respect to the anchor. This free volume defines the allowed topological features of the partial structure consisting of the two helices. The same set of ANCHOR-HELIX knowledge sources is used to anchor the third helix with respect to the first and the intersection of the free volumes of the second and third helices is found by a set of knowledge sources called YOKE-HELIX. The result defines the main topological features of the entire molecule, as shown in Fig. 7, and the free volume within which the structure remains uncertain. The four random coil segments (Fig. 6) can then be sequentially anchored to this structure using the set of knowledge sources called ANCHOR-COIL. The residual free volumes indicate the extent to which the structure can be specified from the existing set of solution data (Fig. 8). The entire definition of the main topological features is initially carried out at the solid level of abstraction. It is seen from the figures that the residual free volumes are in this case sufficiently large to preclude a unique definition of a single structure, but also sufficiently small to define its main features so that they can be clearly recognized. A further refinement of this structure by a more detailed examination of the power of the existing experimental constraints at lower levels of abstraction is still in progress.

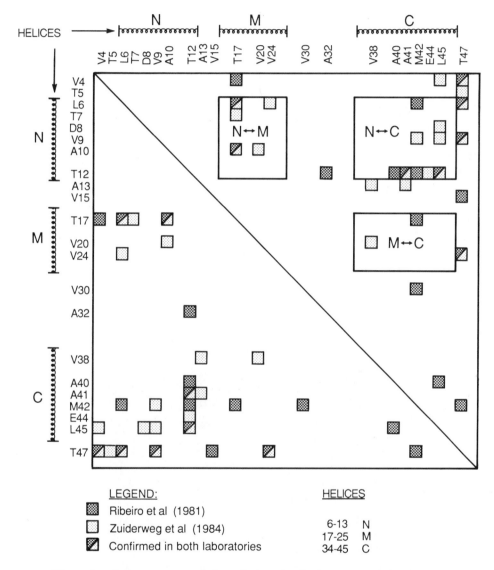

**Figure 6:** Long range proximity relations in the lac repressor headpiece.

The control mechanism of PROTEAN is at present still its least definitively defined feature and we are experimenting with alternative strategies of control. A central notion for choosing the order in which the anchoring of helices is done is the development of criteria for balancing the EASE and GAIN in performing each task. It is intuitively appealing that both the ease of model building and the relative gain will be maximal if the longest helix is chosen as an anchor and the helix with the maximal number of constraints to it is chosen as the first anchoree. However, if the second helix is short, and there exists a third helix that is longer (thus incorporating a larger number of secondary structure constraints), but has one or two fewer constraints, the long term gain (in terms of the efficiency of reaching the final solution) may be greater, if it is chosen as the first anchoree. Thus the efficiency with which one will ultimately be able to arrive at the final solution critically depends on the development and testing of a variety of EASE/GAIN functions.

Similarly, criteria for choosing whether to proceed with a given free volume intersection or to examine the intersection of each new free volume with each preceding or some of the preceding free volumes individually, are still under development. The principle of parsimony dictates the assumption that if two constraints can be satisfied simultaneously, they probably are. However the need to reexamine this assumption arises whenever incompatible constraints are found. Here the criteria to be used by the control mechanism have to depend on the number of constraints with which a given constraint is compatible and on the extent of overlap between the sets of compatible constraints.

For simple structures such as the lac-repressor headpiece, the issues of control are largely issues of efficiency. For more complex structures however they can become the difference between success in a finite time and failure. The issues of the level of abstraction at which the constraint satisfaction is carried out are issues of accuracy and precision. The volume refinement method is designed to overestimate but not to underestimate the free volume associated with each constraint. Therefore the residual free volume defined at the solid level defines the limits of accuracy within which the structure can be determined at that level. It will not generate a wrong structure, i.e. a structure incompatible with the constraints used. Redefinition at a lower level of abstraction can therefore be regarded as a refinement step. The final result is in any

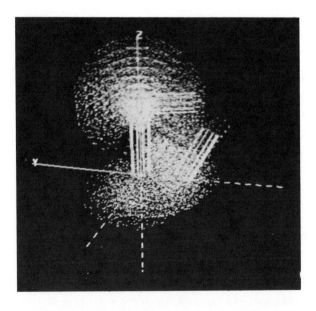

**Figure 7:** Free volumes of the M and C helices in the anchor space of the N helix of the lac repressor headpiece.

case the set of structures which can be rigorously deduced from the available experimental data, defined within the limits of a residual free volume that is irreducible within the limits of the available date set.

This set of structures can be subject to further refinement using additional experimental data obtained and analyzed as described in the following section.

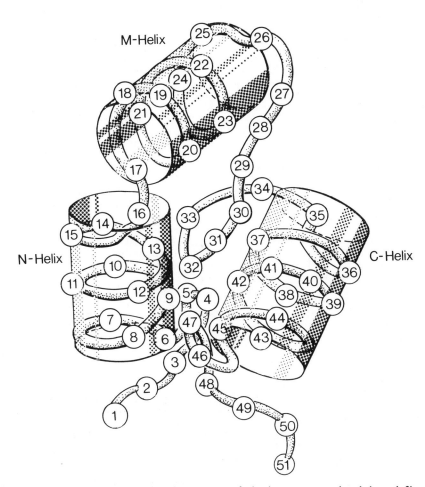

**Figure 8:**    Three dimensional structure of the lac repressor headpiece defined by NMR.

## D.Refinement of the Tertiary Structure

The tertiary structure(s) can be refined by the same procedure that is used to refine the secondary structure. The starting point of the refinement is the set of structures found by folding the domains of secondary structures using the method delineated above. From the proposed set of tertiary structures, one can design experiments to investigate contact points between domains and the equilibrium between the different extreme conformations. From each structure, one can predict NOEs between specific pairs of protons.   Measurement of NOE build up between these protons as well as of their intrinsic spin-lattice relaxation rate will constitute the data base for the refinement program. Some of the NOEs have already been observed and used as indicator of proximity between domains in PROTEAN, but it is more accurate for the refinement procedure to measure the time course of these NOEs (see below). Once the data on the time course are collected, it is a matter of modifying the structure of the contact residues (if necessary) and the orientation of the domains, until the observed and calculated NOEs (and not distances) agree. Structures of residues are defined by torsion angles. The position of a domain with respect to another one, fixed in a Cartesian coordinate system, can be given by translations along the three coordinate axes which bring the domain from a starting position to its final (best) position. Its orientation in space depends on rotations about two axes of the Cartesian coordinate system attached to its center. A gradient search routine varies the torsion angles of the residues, the translation increments and the rotation angles until the calculated set of NOEs gives the best agreement with the observed, minimizing $\chi^2$. If the differences between calculated and observed NOE values fall within experimental error, then the found structure represents the solution structure, or one of the solution structures of the protein. The refinement can be performed again from another starting conformation, to investigate whether the set of NOEs can also be satisfied by another tertiary structure, until the free volume defined by PROTEAN has been adequately sampled.

For purpose of the first refinement, we have assumed that the structure of the residues in contact and the respective orientation of the domains are fixed. However, structural variations at the level of each residue, as well as of the entire tertiary structure are expected. The rates of interconversion are likely to affect the relaxation processes in two ways already discussed above: decrease of the correlation time and averaging of the internuclear distances. The value of the correlation time for the specific region, taking internal motion into account, is necessary to completely interpret the NOE data. The dependence of NOEs on the conformation can be simulated by sweeping through extreme structures allowed by the PROTEAN folding procedure. If the NOEs calculated for the refined tertiary structure are too far from the experimental values, then those NOEs which are the most sensitive to the structure should be discarded from the data base of the refinement program. They can give an insight into the conformational equilibrium of the protein, as they are the most likely to be weighted averages of the NOEs occurring in the different structures. The problem of multiple conformational states is addressed in more detail in the next section. The refinement procedure can be applied iteratively, taking into account at each cycle, a new estimate of the fractional population in different conformations, as deduced from highly conformation dependent NOEs.

The number of required NOE data is theoretically determined by the number of structural parameters to be estimated. This number is often limited by the difficulty of obtaining well resolved NOEs, especially when severe overlap and/or line broadening are present. However, structural constraints discussed below and use of all the structural information included in an NOE tends to make the problem less undetermined than it could appear at first sight.

The search for refined structures is already confined within the limits defined by the tertiary structures given by the PROTEAN program. The structure and orientation of residues involved in contact points are also obviously restricted by van der Waals contact violations and by their attachment to the backbone.

In PROTEAN, observation of an NOE is only interpreted as an indication of proximity (within wide limits, e.g. 2.2-6 Angstroms). As stated above, the structural information contained in an NOE exceeds the simple distance estimate. A relayed NOE includes more structural parameters than a direct NOE, as it involves more protons. Relay of magnetization affects the NOE values even at short irradiation times. At moderately long irradiation times, the relaxation of the observed proton by its neighbors tends to decrease the NOE value. The dependence of the spin-lattice relaxation on the structure is too ambiguous to be used alone for structural determination, it will however confine the search to certain limits. Therefore, it is desirable to measure thoroughly the time course of the NOEs as well as the spin lattice relaxation rates of the observed protons and their neighbors. If adequately analyzed, these relaxation parameters provide a wealth of structural information which is only partially and often erroneously used in distance geometry algorithms. Lastly, it should be realized that PROTEAN is a necessary step before the refinement of the structure.

When starting from an arbitrary tertiary structure, the refinement procedure by itself cannot find the correct folding pattern, as NOEs are detectable only in a small distance range. Until the contact points are established, the gradient search which uses the NOE values is totally inefficient. Besides the starting structure, PROTEAN provides also the limits of the search, and a first idea of the dynamics of the protein.

## E. An Approach to the Problem of Multiple Conformational States.

The existence of more than one well defined conformational state is quite likely for many macromolecules. This may become immediately apparent if incompatible constraints -e.g. NOEs that cannot be satisfied simultaneously- are found in the set of constraints used for the structure determination. However, even if all constraints can be satisfied simultaneously (i.e. there is a free volume overlapping all constraints), the existence of different conformations within these free volume can not be ruled out. In this case, information from chemical shifts and line widths, which is not quantitative enough for calculating structures, may be used to define the individual states.

Consider a simple case, in which n conformational states exist, but which are in rapid exchange. If S is the observed signal, $X_i$ are the mole fractions of each state, and $s_i$ are the intrinsic signals of each state, then

$$S = \Sigma s_i X_i \tag{2}$$

The mole fractions are related to the equilibrium constants Ki as

$$X_i = 1/(1 + K_i) \tag{3}$$

and

$$K_i(T) = K_i^* \exp\{-\Delta H(1/T - 1/T^*)/R\} \tag{4}$$

where $\Delta H$ is the enthalpy difference, and the asterisk denotes a reference state. Because the $K_i$ are temperature dependent, so are the mole fractions, so that varying the temperature will lead to changes in the observed signal, S. Hence, measurements of the chemical shift, spin-lattice relaxation time, line widths and cross relaxation rate constants as a function of temperature may permit the determination of the minimum number of states accessible to the molecule in the range of temperature studied. It is obviously necessary to work at temperatures substantially below the melting temperature for global unfolding.

In some instances, the variation of the chemical shift alone can be sufficient to indicate the minimum number of conformational states. It is then possible to determine purely phenomenologically the enthalpy differences, and the populations at any given temperature. If the populations can be derived from chemical shift measurements, then relaxation measurements at well chosen temperatures can be used to define some of the conformational features; the intrinsic values of $s_i$ can be obtained if the $X_i$ are known. Obviously, the cross relaxation rate constants are the most useful for structural purposes, but as we have already pointed out, the spin-lattice relaxation times are also useful. The relaxation rates are themselves temperature dependent, owing to the changes in viscosity. However, this dependence is predictable for macromolecules, and can be allowed for in the calculations.

The line widths in the absence of exchange contain the same information as the spin-lattice relaxation time. However, in the presence of exchange, depending on the rate constants and the chemical shift differences, the line widths also contain a contribution from the exchange rate constants. The spin-lattice relaxation rate constant is then a useful reference for subtracting out the purely conformational effects, so that the excess line width can be calculated. The excess line width can be analyzed to give approximate values of the exchange rate constants. This is obviously important for analyzing the cross relaxation data.

It remains possible that each state is conformationally mobile, i.e. there is averaging about the potential minimum of each state. The structures derived for each state are then apparent (see above). The extent of averaging about each state should also be investigated. One possibility is $^{13}C$ relaxation times at appropriate temperatures (but see above for complications). Another is to vary the overall tumbling time at constant temperature, by adding ,for example, glycerol. Internal motions should be relatively less damped, so that the observed correlation times for different residues will not give a linear Perrin plot (see above and 16). Such plots would have to be constructed at different temperatures to account for the different populations.

In general, the problem is intractable. Suppose that there are n conformational states, with averaging about the potential minimum of each state, and there are alternative pathways for magnetization transfer. Then the observed cross relaxation rate constant will be:

$$\sigma_{obs} = \alpha\{\Sigma X_k\langle\tau_i/r_i^6\rangle + \Sigma\Sigma X_k\langle\tau_j/r_j^6\rangle\} \tag{5}$$

The first term is the direct pathway averaged over all conformation states, with $\tau_i$ the effective correlation time, and $r^6$ is averaged over the distances sampled during the motion. The second term is a similar average over the alternative pathways. In this case, the uncertainty on the structure determination will define the range of variation, but the definition of individual states will not be possible.

Despite the potential complexity, a fairly complete analysis may be possible in practice. We have analyzed the temperature dependence of the chemical shifts and relaxation rate constants of the trp operator. Of the 20 bases, only two show anomalous behavior, they are A11 and A12 in the Pribnow box. The dependence of the chemical shifts of the H8 and H2's of these bases indicated a minimum of three conformational states being accessible in the range $0 < T < 40°C$. The transition temperatures were 9 and 30 °C, so that at 0°C and 40°C, essentially pure states exist. The enthalpy differences were surprisingly large, 40 and 60 kcal/mole, respectively. At 25°C, the intermediate state accounted for 80% of the molecules. It was therefore a simple task to determine the relaxation times (T1 and T2) of each state. Further, we could estimate the cross relaxation rate constants between these and other protons in each state, so that the principle conformational features could be determined. The changes involved a simultaneous change in the pitch and helical twist angle for one transition, and an increase in the propellor twist of A11 for the other transition.

The excess line width of A11H2 first increased and then decreased ($\Delta_{max} \approx 12$ Hz), i.e. intermediate exchange. Analysis showed that the rate constants for the transitions at the mid-point temperatures must be about 1000 $s^{-1}$. Internal motions were shown to be insignificant for these bases by measuring the cross relaxation rate constant AH2 to NH (r=2.85 Angstroms) at different temperatures.

Hence, we were able to identify different conformational states, and analyze their structures. The structural change may well be of physiological significance. It is limited to the Pribnow box of the trp promoter which is intimately involved in the binding of the RNA polymerase and the repressor to the operator. The correlation of the binding and transcription properties with the occurrence of the TAA sequence on this position strongly suggests that the conformational instability in the sequence is a requirement for good promoters [34].

# Conclusion

It is desirable to achieve the highest possible level of detail in the structural description of biologically active macromolecules. Deviations from canonical structures (such as alpha helix, beta sheet in proteins, and A, B, C or Z forms in nucleic acids) are expected to occur, due to sequence dependent constraints. The biological activity of the molecule depends on the location of groups involved in the binding or active site. A displacement of 0.5 to 1 Angstrom is sufficient to break hydrogen bonds or to decrease by 15 to 30% the electrostatic energy between two charged groups at 3 Angstoms distance (in H2O). On the other hand, such variations in the position of atoms can be produced by variations in torsion angles already observed in known structures. For example, depending on the sequence, twist angles in DNA can vary up to $13°$ from one step to the next [29 and see results on the trp operator DNA above]. This will change the positions of groups in the major or the minor groove by about 0.8 Angstrom, compared with a standard B structure. A change of $10°$ in the $\Phi$ or $\Psi$ angle in a peptide unit will move atoms of the next nearest peptide unit 0.5 to 0.8 Angstrom away from their previous positions. Antiparallel or parallel $\beta$-pleated sheets can be twisted by changing the $\Phi$ or $\Psi$ angles respectively, by about $20°$. It is therefore necessary to define macromolecular structures to this level of accuracy.

The major points of the new methods developed here are 1) the search of folding patterns and 2) the refinement of the structures (secondary and tertiary), neither of which rely on any classical distance geometry algorithm.

A goal-directed Artificial Intelligence program (named PROTEAN) is developed to obtain folding patterns of the domains of secondary structure. The method uses different constraints which progressively restrict the respective positions of the domains to a limited set of structures. This set represents the residual uncertainty in the structure of the molecule, after all constraints have been applied.

In the refinement procedures, the NOEs are simulated from the calculated coordinates of the protons for an instantiated structure, taking into account alternative pathways and intrinsic spin-lattice relaxation. The structure of the molecule is changed until an agreement is found between calculated and observed NOE. Refinement of secondary structure is performed beginning with canonical structures (for example $\alpha$-helix, $\beta$-sheet in protein). Refinement of tertiary structures starts from the set of conformation defined by PROTEAN. For nucleic acid we have already shown that, using this refinement procedure, new insight can be obtained on significant deviations from the standard structure, and on the existence of minor conformations.


## ACKNOWLEDGMENTS

We acknowledge NIH grants RR00711 and GM 18098, and NSF grants GP 23633 and DMB 84-02348.

## REFERENCES

1. Jardetzky, O. (1965) Proc. Int. Conf. Mag. Res., Tokyo, Japan N-3-14: 1-4.
2. Campbell, I.D., Dobson, C.M., Williams, R.J.P. and Xavier, A.V. (1973) Ann. Rev. NY Acad. Sci. 222, 1963.
3. Wagner, G. and Wuthrich, K. (1982) J. Mol. Biol. 155, 427-466.
4. Braun, W., Bosch, C., Brown, L.R., Go, N. and Wuthrich, K. (1981) Biochim. Biophys. Acta 667, 377.
5. Braun, W., Wider, G., Lee, K.H. and Wuthrich, K. (1983) J. Mol. Biol. 109, 921-948.
6. Zuiderweg, E.R.P., Billeter, M., Boelens, R., Scheek, R.M., Wuthrich, K. and Kaptein, R. (1984) FEBS Lett. 179, 243-247.
7. Kaptein, R., Zuiderweg, E.R.P., Scheek, R.M. and Boelens, R. (1985) J. Mol. Biol. 182, 179-182.
8. Jardetzky, O. (1980) Biochim. Biophys. Acta 621, 227-232.
9. Jardetzky, O. and Roberts, G.C.K. (1981) "NMR in Molecular Biology", Academic Press, New York, Ch. 4.
10. Jardetzky, O. (1984) in "Progress in Bioorganic Chemistry and Molecular Biology", Yu. A. Ovchinnikov, ed., Elsevier Science Publishers B.V., Amsterdam, pp. 55-63.
11. Kratky, O., Leopold, H. and Staubinger, H. (1973) Meths. Enzymol. 270, 98-110.
12. McMeekin, T.L. and Marshall, K. (1952) Science 116, 142-144.
13. Lane, A.N. and Kirschner, K. (1983) Eur. J. Biochem. 129, 675-684.
14. Lane, A.N. (1982) J. Theor. Biol. 97, 511-527.
15. Jardetzky, O. (1981) Accts. Chem. Res. 14, 291-298

16. Lane, A.N. (1983) Eur. J. Biochem. $\underline{133}$, 531-538.

17. Calhoun, P.B., Vanderkooi, J.M., Woodrow, G.V. and Englander, S.W. (1983) Biochem. $\underline{22}$, 1526-1532.

18. Paul, C.H. (1982) J. Mol. Biol. $\underline{155}$, 53-62.

19. Lane, A.N., Lefevre, J-F. and Jardetzky, O. (1985) submitted to J. Mag. Res.

20. van de Ven, F.J.M., de Bruin, S.N. and Hilbers, C.W. (1984) FEBS Lett. $\underline{169}$, 107-111.

21. Jones, C.R., Sikakana, C.T., Henir, S.P., Kuo, M.C. and Gibbons, W.A. (1978) Biophys. J. $\underline{24}$, 815-824.

22. Jones, C.R., Sikakana, C.T., Henir, S.P., Kuo, M.C. and Gibbons, W.A. (1978) J. Am. Chem. Soc. $\underline{100}$, 5960-5967.

23. Billeter, M., Braun, W. and Wuthrich, K. (1982) J. Mol. Biol. $\underline{155}$, 321-346.

24. Zuiderweg, E.R.P., Kaptein, R. and Wuthrich, K. (1983) Proc. Natl. Acad. Sci. $\underline{80}$, 5837-5841.

25. Molday, R.S., Englander, S.W. and Kallen, R.G. (1972) Biochem. $\underline{11}$, 150-161.

26. Wagner, G. (1983) Q. Rev. Biophys. $\underline{16}$, 1-57.

27. Hare, D.R., Wemmer, D.E., Chou, S-H., Drobny, G. and Reid, B.R. (1983) J. Mol. Biol. $\underline{171}$, 319-336.

28. Richardson, J. (1980) in "Protein Folding", Jaenicke, R., ed., Elsevier Science Publishers B.V., Amsterdam, pp. 41-52.

29. Finney, D. (1979) in "Water", vol. 6, Franks, F., ed., Plenum Press, New York, Ch. 2.

30. Bothner-By, A.A. and Noggle, J.H. (1979) J. Am. Chem. Soc. $\underline{101}$, 5162-5170.

31. Saenger, W. (1984) "Principles of Nucleic Acid Structure", Springer Verlag, New York.

32. Fratini, A.V., Kopka, M.L., Drew, H.R. and Dickerson, R.E. (1982) J. Biol. Chem. $\underline{257}$, 14686-14707.

33. Calladine, C.R. (1982) J. Mol. Biol. $\underline{161}$, 343-352.

34. Lefevre, J-F., Lane, A.N. and Jardetzky, O. (1985) in press FEBS Lett.

# NMR STUDIES OF PROTEIN-LIGAND INTERACTIONS: DIHYDROFOLATE REDUCTASE

G.C.K. Roberts

Division of Physical Biochemistry
National Institute for Medical Research
Mill Hill, London NW7 1AA, U.K.

## INTRODUCTION

The study of protein-ligand interactions has proved to be one of the more fruitful applications of high-resolution nmr to biological problems. The specific recognition of small molecules by proteins is fundamental to a wide range of biological phenomena, from enzyme action and its regulation, through the control of gene expression to the action of hormones and neurotransmitters. Nmr can provide a variety of information on both structural and dynamic aspects of the recognition process in the solution state. In this article I shall describe some of the different kinds of information which can be obtained, drawing illustrations from work on the enzyme dihydrofolate reductase, which we have been studying for a number of years. A broader view of the wide range of experiments which have been done on other systems can be found in ref. 1, while fuller references to the work on dihydrofolate reductase are given in ref. 2. Operationally, two kinds of experiments can be distinguished, depending on whether one studies resonances of the small molecule or of the protein, and examples of both will be discussed. First, however, we must consider, briefly, the effects of chemical exchange processes on nmr spectra and their interpretation. Whenever we study a small molecule binding to a protein, we are studying a system in which chemical exchange plays an important part, and the first step in understanding the nmr spectra obtained from such a system must be to understand the effects of this exchange upon them. For simplicity, these effects will be discussed in the context of studies of ligand resonances; analogous effects are obviously seen on protein signals.

## CHEMICAL EXCHANGE

As is well known (see e.g. 1) the appearance of the spectrum of a molecule which is exchanging between two states depends upon the lifetime of the molecule in each of the two states. If the exchange is slow, separate signals are seen for the molecule in each state, while if the exchange is fast, a single (averaged) signal is observed. 'Fast' and 'slow' here refer not to any absolute time scale but to the 'nmr time scale' - that is, fast or slow relative to the <u>difference</u> in the observed nmr parameter (chemical shift, coupling constant or relaxation rate) between the two states. Thus if one is looking at more than one resonance from the same molecule, one can find that exchange is perhaps fast for one resonance and slow for another in the same molecule. The condition for slow exchange with respect to chemical shift, for example, is

$$1/\tau \ll |\,\delta_A - \delta_B\,|$$ (1)

where $\tau$ is the exchange lifetime, and $\delta_A$ and $\delta_B$ are the chemical shifts of a given nucleus in the two states, A and B. In considering the meaning of the 'exchange lifetime', $\tau$, it is important to distinguish between first-order and second-order exchange processes.

First order $\quad 1/\tau = k_{AB} + k_{BA}$ (2)

Second order $\quad 1/\tau = k_{off}\,(1 + p_A/p_B)$ (3)

Thus for a ligand binding to a protein, a second-order process, the apparent exchange rate depends upon the the dissociation rate constant and concentration of the species present (where $p_A$ and $p_B$ represent the fraction of the ligand molecules in the complex and the free state, respectively, with $p_A + p_B = 1$).

To illustrate the kinds of behaviour observed for different exchange rates, I shall use some $^{31}$P studies of the binding of analogues of the coenzyme, NADP$^+$, to dihydrofolate reductase (3,4). The coenzyme 'fragment', adenosine 2'-monophosphate, binds to the enzyme in 'very fast' exchange, i.e.

$$1/\tau \gg |\delta_A - \delta_B|,\ \ |1/T_{2A} - 1/T_{2B}|$$ (4)

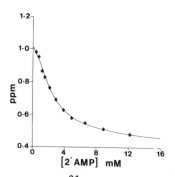

Figure 1  The dependence of the $^{31}$P chemical shift of adenosine 2'-monophosphate (2'AMP) on the concentration of 2'AMP in the presence of 1.25 mM dihydrofolate reductase at pH 7.0.  The line is the best-fit theoretical curve, calculated with $\delta_{bound}$ = 1.21 ppm and K = 3.6 $10^3$ M$^{-1}$.  From (3).

74

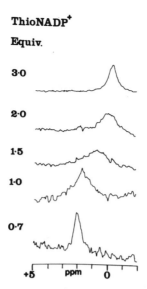

ThioNADP⁺

Equiv.

3·0

2·0

1·5

1·0

0·7

+5    ppm    0

<u>Figure 2</u>  The 2'-phosphate $^{31}$P resonance of thioNADP$^+$ in the presence of dihydrofolate reductase as a function of thioNADP$^+$ concentration, expressed as moles thioNADP$^+$/mole enzyme.  From (4).

The chemical shift of the $^{31}$P signal is a simple weighted average of the chemical shifts of the bound and free states.

$$\delta_{obs} = P_A \delta_A = P_B \delta_B \qquad (5)$$

Thus a plot of the chemical shift as a function of ligand concentration at constant enzyme concentration (Figure 1) is a rectangular hyperbola from which the binding constant can be determined.  Extrapolation to infinite ligand concentration ($P_A \rightarrow 1$) gives the chemical shift in the free state, while extrapolation to zero ligand concentration ($P_B \rightarrow 1$) gives the shift in the bound state.  (Note that it is essential to obtain data at the lowest possible ligand concentrations so as to minimise the length of the extrapolation needed to obtain the bound chemical shift.)  The bound shift thus obtained can then be interpreted in terms of the environment of the bound ligand.  For example, a series of binding curves for adenosine 2'-phosphate such as that in Figure 1 was obtained at different pH values, and the pH-dependence of the bound $^{31}$P chemical shift, and hence the pK of the bound 2'-phosphate, was derived (3).

If the exchange rate is somewhat slower, we reach the region of 'moderately fast' exchange, illustrated in Figure 2 by the behaviour of the 2'-phosphate resonance of thioNADP$^+$.  Once again, the chemical shift changes progressively from that of the bound state to that of the free state as the ligand concentration is increased.  The linewidth, however, does not change monotonically as a function of ligand concentration, but rather passes through a maximum; this reflects an exchange contribution to the linewidth, as indicated in the expression for $1/T_2$:

$$\frac{1}{T_{2,obs}} = \frac{p_A}{T_{2A}} + \frac{p_B}{T_{2B}} + \frac{p_A(1-p_A)^2 \, 4\pi^2(\delta_A - \delta_B)^2}{k_{off}} \qquad (6)$$

The first two terms on the right-hand side represent the weighted average of the relaxation rates in the two states (as would be observed in 'very fast' exchange), while the third term is the exchange contribution. Since this third term includes $k_{off}$, the dissociation rate constant, analysis of the concentration dependence of the linewidth allows one to determine the value of this rate constant. At the same time, determination of the bound chemical shift gives structural information. The concentration-dependence of the chemical shift in 'moderately fast' exchange again looks like a simple rectangular hyperbola. However, analysis using eq. 5, appropriate for 'very fast' exchange, can give incorrect values for the binding constant if applied to a system in 'moderately fast' exchange (5). The full lineshape equation must be used. This is even more important in intermediate exchange, $1/\tau \sim |\delta_A - \delta_B|$, where a complex series of line shape changes are observed.

Finally, in slow exchange, separate resonances are observed for the bound and free states, as illustrated for the 2'-phosphate signal of $NADP^+$ in Figure 3. The signal from the bound state does not change as the ligand concentration increases, while that from the free state increases in intensity but does not change in position. In this exchange region, too, the dissociation rate constant can be determined by analysis of the linewidths:

$$1/T_{2A,obs} = 1/T_{2A} + k_{off}$$

$$1/T_{2B,obs} = 1/T_{2B} + \frac{p_B \cdot k_{off}}{p_A}$$

(note that the linewidth of the signal from the free ligand is concentration-dependent, while that of the bound ligand is not). Studies in the slow-exchange region have the real advantage that the resonance parameters of the bound stage can be measured directly, without the need for the extrapolations required in the fast-exchange region.

In discussing these exchange processes, I have made the implicit assumption that we are dealing with a simple two-site exchange process — that is the ligand molecule exists either in the free state or in the bound state. Obviously this may not always be true. In particular, there may be more than one conformational form of the complex, giving rise to a more complicated exchange process. For slow exchange, in favourable cases it may be possible to see separate resonances from the different conformational forms (6-9). In fast exchange, however, the observed resonance is an average over all the states of the system, and the values obtained for the binding constant and the chemical shifts are only meaningful to the extent that the data are analysed in terms of the correct model. Thus if a two-site analysis is used for a process which actually involves exchange between three or four sites, the bound shifts obtained will not be characteristic of any real species.

MAGNETISATION TRANSFER

The advantages of working in the slow exchange regime have been mentioned above. Its major disadvantage is seen in $^1$H nmr, where the resonances from the bound ligand are likely to be obscured by the multitude of $^1$H resonances from the protein. This can be overcome by an important

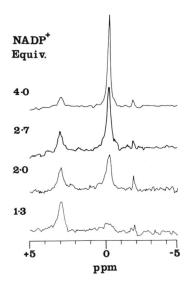

Figure 3  The 2'-phosphate $^{31}$P resonance of NADP$^+$ in the presence of dihydrofolate reductase as a function of NADP$^+$ concentration, expressed as moles NADP$^+$/mole enzyme. From (4).

class of experiments known as magnetisation transfer experiments (e.g., 10), in which information about the bound ligand can be obtained indirectly, by observation of resonances of the free ligand.

Consider a sample containing a ligand molecule in excess over the protein, so that both bound and free ligand will be present. Ligand molecules will be exchanging between these two states, but if this exchange is reasonably slow, separate signals will be observed for the two states. Now if a perturbation, such as saturation by a selective r.f. field, or inversion by a selective 180° pulse, is applied to a resonance of the bound ligand, this has the effect of labelling the nuclei in this state, by perturbing their energy level populations. If a bound molecule exchanges to the free state this 'label' will be observed in the free state (as a perturbation of the intensity of the corresponding resonance of the free molecule) provided only that the rate of exchange is at least comparable to the rate of 'decay' of the 'label' (the spin-lattice relaxation rate in the free state). These experiments can be used to measure the dissociation rate constant of the small molecule from the protein (e.g. 11), though once again

care is required in systems involving exchange between more than two sites
(7,12,13). A practical benefit of this experiment lies in the fact that it
allows one to locate the resonances of a bound ligand without having to
observe them directly. In the case of the saturation transfer experiment,
systematic irradiation through the relevant region of the spectrum allows
one to locate resonances of the bound ligand by observing selective
decreases in intensity of the corresponding resonance of the free ligand
(see Fig. 5 below). This experiment has a wide range of application – to
proteins of $M_r > 100,000$, and at protein concentrations as low as $50 \mu M$. The
chemical shifts obtained can be used to compare the binding of related
ligands (e.g., 11), to determine the ionisation state of the bound ligand,
and, in favourable cases, to determine its conformation (e.g., 14).

A systematic search through even a limited region of the spectrum can
obviously be time-consuming, and the information can be obtained more
efficiently by using a two-dimensional magnetisation transfer experiment.

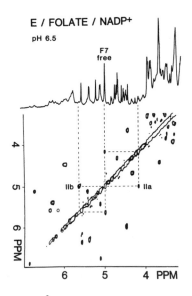

Figure 4  Part of the 500 MHz [1]H 2D exchange spectrum obtained from a sample
containing the dihydrofolate reductase-folate-NADP[+] complex and excess
(free) NADP[+] and folate. The spectrum was recorded with a mixing time of 25
ms, and contoured so that only exchange cross-peaks appear; those indicated
are for the pteridine 7-proton of folate. (B. Birdsall et al., unpublished
work).

(Though it should be noted that the one-dimensional experiment has greater sensitivity when very low protein concentrations and a large excess of ligand are being used.) The 2D exchange epxeriment employs just the same pulse sequence as the NOESY experiment. Exchange cross-peaks are often more intense than NOE cross-peaks, especially if exchange is reasonably fast, allowing a short mixing time to be used. They can always be identified, since they are present only when both states are substantially populated – not, for example, when only the complex and no free ligand is present. Part of a 2D exchange spectrum is shown in Figure 4, illustrating the determination of the pteridine 7-proton chemical shift of bound folate in the dihydrofolate reductase-folate-NADP$^+$ complex (note that two bound shifts are found, since this complex exists as a mixture of two conformations under these conditions; 7,9). Although signals from only one proton are indicated in Fig. 4, the important feature of the 2D experiment is that all the resonances of the bound ligand can be located in a single experiment.

As well as, effectively, transferring chemical shift information from the bound state to the free state, we can also transfer cross-relaxation (NOE) information in the same way. This 'transferred NOE' experiment (15) is illustrated, again by coenzyme binding to dihydrofolate reductase, in Figure 5. The difference spectrum (c) shows that irradiation at 2.04 ppm leads to a substantial decrease in intensity of the resonance, at 2.34 ppm, from the nicotinamide ribose 1'-proton of free NADP$^+$, thus identifying the resonance position of this proton in the bound state. There is also a clear decrease in the intensity of the nicotinamide 2-proton signal of free NADP$^+$ at 5.55 ppm. This arises from cross-relaxation between the ribose 1'- and nicotinamide 2-protons; since a negative NOE is observed, this cross-relaxation must be taking place in the bound coenzyme. Saturation of the H1' resonance of free NADP$^+$ leads to a transfer of magnetisation to the H1' resonance of the bound coenzyme by chemical exchange; cross-relaxation in the bound state effectively transfers part of this magnetisation to the H2 signal of bound NADP$^+$ and thence, by exchange, to the H2 signal of free NADP$^+$, where it is observed. Efficient cross-relaxation between the ribose H1' and the nicotinamide H2 implies that these two protons are close together in space in the bound coenzyme, and hence that the conformation about the nicotinamide glycosidic bond is anti. These transferred NOE effects (which are also observed in the 2D exchange experiment) can be quantitated (16,17) and have proved to be a powerful approach to the determination of the conformations of small molecules bound to proteins.

IONISATION STATE AND DYNAMICS OF BOUND LIGANDS

Two valuable kinds of information about small molecules bound to proteins which are not available from X-ray crystallography but are readily obtained by nmr are the charge state (the presence or absence of a proton at a specific site) and the dynamics – both the dissociation rate of the complex discussed above, and the 'intra-complex' conformational dynamics.

The ionisation state of a molecule is often indicated quite clearly simply by the chemical shifts of appropriate nuclei. Consider the case of trimethoprim (2,4-diamino-5-(3,4,5-trimethoxy-benzyl) pyrimidine) (I) binding to dihydrofolate reductase.

X-ray crystallography shows that this molecule binds to the E. coli enzyme with its N1 and 2-NH$_2$ groups close to the carboxyl group of Asp 27 (18; the homologous residue in the L. casei enzyme is Asp 26). This suggests the

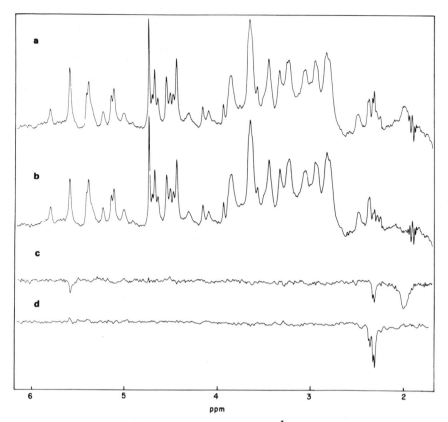

**Figure 5** The aromatic region of the 270 MHz [1]H nmr spectrum of dihydrofolate reductase in the presence of 5 molar equivalents of NADP[+] and 1 molar equivalent of methotrexate; sample temperature 40°C. (a) Control; (b) irradiation at 2.04 ppm; (c) spectrum (b) minus spectrum (a). (d) After addition of 1 molar equivalent of NADPH to displace the NADP[+] from the enzyme; difference between a spectrum obtained with irradiation at 2.34 ppm (N1' proton of free NADP[+]) and the control spectrum. All spectra have the same vertical scale. From (15).

possibility that bound trimethoprim is protonated on N1, and that hydrogen-bonds are formed between N1-H, the 2-$NH_2$ and the carboxylate oxygens. Evidence for this is obtained from studies of 2-[13]C-trimethoprim (19). In free trimethoprim, the 2-[13]C chemical shift changes from 95.06 ppm to 87.97 ppm as the molecule is protonated on N1 (pK 7.7), establishing that this shift is very sensitive to the charge state of the molecule. When the

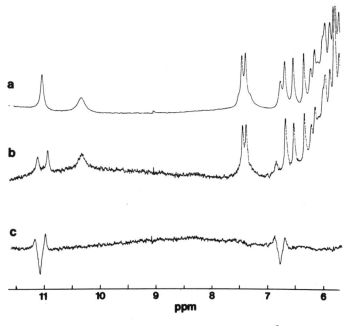

Figure 6 Comparison of the low-field region of the [1]H NMR spectra, in 90% H₂O/10% [2]H₂O, of the complexes of dihydrofolate reductase with (a) trimethoprim and (b) [[15]N₃]trimethoprim. The difference (b)-(a) is shown in (c), and reveals the resonances of the N1-H (at 11.07 ppm) and one 2-NH₂ (at 10.31 ppm). Chemical shifts from dioxan. From (22).

ligand is bound to the enzyme, the 2-[13]C signal appears at 89.26 ppm, and is independent of pH over the range 5-8. Since the bound chemical shift is 1.29 ppm from that of the protonated trimethoprim but 5.80 ppm from that of the unprotonated molecule, it is reasonable to conclude that bound trimethoprim is protonated (with a pK ⩾ 10.5). The 1.29 ppm difference in shift from free protonated trimethoprim would then be ascribed to the changes in environment on binding (e.g., the proximity of Asp 26). This is a very reasonable (and, it turns out, correct) interpretation; however, it is impossible to rule out the alternative that trimethoprim is unprotonated when bound, and the 2-[13]C experiences a much larger, 5.8 ppm, 'environmental' shift.

Unambiguous evidence for the charge state of bound trimethoprim can, however, be obtained by showing that there is a proton attached to N1. In the [15]N spectrum of bound [1,3,2-NH₂-[15]N₃]-trimethoprim, obtained by the INEPT polarisation transfer method (20,21), the [15]N1 resonance appeared as a 90Hz doublet, showing clearly that a proton is directly bonded to this nitrogen (22). The resonances of this proton and of one of the 2-NH₂ protons can be observed directly in [1]H spectra obtained in H₂O solution, as shown in Fig. 6; their chemical shifts are entirely consistent with the proposal of hydrogen-bonds between N1, the 2-NH₂ and Asp 26.

The observation of a separate signal for the N1-proton obviously indicates that exchange of this proton with the solvent is slow on the nmr timescale. The temperature dependence of the linewidth of this resonance allows us to measure this exchange rate (22); it is found to be $160s^{-1}$ at 313 K. This is much faster than the rate of dissociaton of trimethoprim from the complex (3 $s^{-1}$ at 318 K; 23), and is thus a measure of the rate at which the structure around the N1-H-Asp 26 hydrogen bond fluctuates in the complex.

A further kind of fluctuation in the structure of protein-ligand complexes is that which permits 180° 'flips' of symmetrically substituted aromatic rings. This kind of motion is almost universally observed for tyrosine and phenylalanine rings in proteins (see, e.g., 24-26), and has also been observed for the aromatic rings of a number of bound ligands (23,27-29). In those cases where high-resolution crystallographic information is available, it is clear that this ring flipping can only occur if there are appropriate fluctuations in the position of neighbouring amino-acid residues of the protein. Studies of ring flipping can thus provide useful information on local dynamic behaviour. For example, $^{19}$F nmr studies of 3',5'-difluoromethotrexate bound to dihydrofolate reductase showed that its symmetrically substituted benzoyl ring flips at a rate of 7.3 $10^3$ $s^{-1}$ (at 298 K). Addition of coenzyme to form the ternary complex, in which methotrexate binds more tightly to the enzyme, leads to an increase in this rate of flipping to 20 $10^3$ $s^{-1}$ (28). This clearly indicates that coenzyme binding has produced conformational changes in the vicinity of the benzoyl ring binding site which permit larger and/or more frequent fluctuations of the local structure.

Although these experiments demonstrate the existence of coenzyme-induced conformational changes, to define these we must turn away from studies of ligand resonances and examine the spectrum of the protein itself.

PROTEIN RESONANCES - ASSIGNMENTS

An essential preliminary to obtaining detailed structural information from the $^1$H nmr spectrum of a protein is, of course, the resolution and assignment of resonances to individual residues in the sequence. For all but the smallest proteins, resonance assignment remains the single most difficult stage in the study of a protein by nmr, although 2D nmr methods have considerably improved the situation. Space does not permit a detailed discussion of the various methods here, but a brief outline of the principal approaches will be presented, to give an indication of the present 'state of the art'.

For small proteins, $M_r < 12000$, the elegant sequential assignment procedure developed by Wuthrich and his colleagues (30-33) provides a general solution. In this approach, NOEs are used to connect the spin-systems of residues adjacent in the sequence. After identification of the residue type from the nature of the spin-system, the sequentially connected residues can then be assigned by reference to the amino acid sequence.

This approach requires that essentially all the resonances in the spectrum be resolved, and at presently available field strengths it does not seem to be feasible for proteins of $M_r > 15000$. A number of general approaches to the assignment problem for larger proteins can be envisaged, involving large-scale isotopic substitution and/or site-directed mutagenesis, but these have yet to be put into practice on more than a trial basis.

The strategy we have used for making assignments in dihydrofolate reductase, $M_r$ 18,500, (which is generally similar to that used by Dobson and his colleagues for lysozyme; e.g. 34,35) is as follows. First, resonances are assigned to amino-acid type either by identifying the spin-systems in 2D COSY and RELAY spectra (36,37) or by selective deuteration (38-40). Second, groups of residues which are close together in space are identified in phase-sensitive 2D NOESY spectra (41). Reference to the crystal structure then allows the residues in these groups to be identified; it is important to note that the crystal structure is used only semi-quantitatively, so that a precise identity of crystal and solution structures need not be assumed. Finally, assignments are transferred between spectra of different complexes by 1D or 2D magnetisation transfer experiments (see above). A detailed description of the use of these procedures for the assignment of resonances from about 20% of the residues of dihydrofolate reductase is given elsewhere (42).


INDIVIDUAL PROTEIN-LIGAND INTERACTIONS

Once resonances from residues in the binding site have been assigned, they can be used to monitor individual protein-ligand interactions, just as the trimethoprim signals were used to monitor the N1-H-Asp 26 ion pair (see above). For example, the $\gamma$-carboxylate of methotrexate forms an ion-pair with His 28, and the accompanying 1 unit increase in the imidazole pK can readily be measured by using the assigned $C_{\varepsilon 1}H$ signal of this histidine. The hydrophobic interactions between the protein and the pteridine and benzoyl rings of methotrexate can be monitored by protein-ligand NOEs. For example, Figure 7 shows part of the 2D NOESY and COSY spectra of the enzyme-methotrexate complex indicating the NOE cross-peaks between the pteridine H7 and three methyl resonances, a-c, which have been assigned to the two $C_\delta H_3$ of Leu 19, and one $C_\delta H_3$ of Leu 27 (42).

In order to determine the energetic contribution of each of these interactions to the overall binding it is necessary to make modifications either to the ligand or, using site-directed mutagenesis, to the protein designed to 'block' one specific interaction. A crucial step in this process is to compare the native and modified complexes so as to establish that only the one desired interaction has been disrupted, and nmr can be very useful in making this comparison. This can be illustrated by considering the two ion-pairs formed by the glutamate moiety of methotrexate: the $\alpha$-carboxyl with Arg 57, and the $\gamma$-carboxyl with His 28. To estimate the energetic contributions of these two ion pairs, we examined the binding of the $\alpha$- and $\gamma$-amides (43). The $\gamma$-amide binds about 10-fold more weakly than methotrexate, and, as expected, produces no increase in the pK of His 28. Apart from this, and a small shift in the resonances of the neighbouring Leu 27, assigned resonances in the $\gamma$-amide complex are the same as in the complex of methotrexate itself, indicating that only this one interaction has been broken. It's energetic contribution can thus be estimated as about 5.5 kJ mole$^{-1}$. The $\alpha$-amide, by contrast, binds 100-fold less tightly, apparently indicating a stronger ion-pair with Arg 57. However, examination of the nmr spectrum indicates, first that the pK of His 28 is not increased, indicating that the $\gamma$-carboxylate-His 28 ion-pair has been disrupted (43) and, second, that a number of other residues around the benzoyl ring binding site, including Leu 19 and Leu 27, are also affected (Birdsall et al., unpublished work). Thus the modification of the $\alpha$-carboxylate has substantially affected the mode of binding, and the decrease

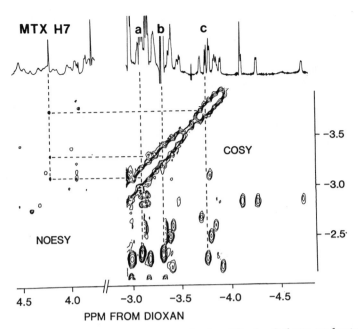

<u>Figure 7</u>  Part of the NOESY spectrum of the dihydrofolate reductase-
methotrexate complex showing the nOes from the H7 of methotrexate to three
methyl groups at high-field (a, b and c).  The region of the COSY spectrum
pertinent to these methyl groups is shown below the diagonal.  Resonances a
and b have been assigned to the two C $H_3$ of Leu 19, and resonance c to a C
$H_3$ of Leu 27.  From (42).

in binding constant is clearly not attributable solely to the blocking of
the $\alpha$-carboxyl-Arg 57 ion pair.

This ability to monitor individual interactions is also valuable in the
design of improved inhibitors (44).

LIGAND INDUCED CONFORMATIONAL CHANGES

When ligand binding produces changes in chemical shift of resonances
assigned to residues remote from the binding site, these can be ascribed to
changes, possibly only slight, in protein conformation.  In dihydrofolate
reductase, we are particularly interested in the way in which coenzyme
binding affects the binding constants for substrates and inhibitors, an
effect which is, at least in part, due to coenzyme-induced conformational
changes.

As described above, the experiments with 3',5'-difluoromethotrexate
show that one of the changes produced by coenzyme binding is in the binding
site for the benzoyl ring of methotrexate.  One of the residues in contact
with the benzoyl ring is Phe 49, whose resonances are significantly shifted

on coenzyme binding. This residue is at the C-terminal end of the short helix C, residues 42-49, which seems to be a good candidate for transmission of effects from the coenzyme site to the methotrexate site, since Arg 43, Arg 44 and Thr 45 are all involved in binding the coenzyme. A small (axial) shift of this helix on coenzyme binding could move Phe 49 and allow the benzoyl ring to flip more readily. In support of this hypothesis, we have found that the signals of Tyr 46 (on helix C) and of Val 61 and Tyr 68 (whose side-chains are in contact with side-chains of residues in helix C) are all affected by coenzyme binding (42). Confirmation of this hypothesis, and a precise description of the changes, will have to await the results of quantitative NOE experiments now in progress, but it is clear that nmr methods are capable of describing such conformational changes in atomic detail.


ACKNOWLEDGEMENTS

I am most grateful to a number of past and present colleagues at Mill Hill and elsewhere for their collaboration in the experiments described here, most particularly to Jim Feeney, Berry Birdsall and Gill Ostler.

REFERENCES

1.  Jardetzky, O. and Roberts, G.C.K. (1981). Nmr in Molecular Biology. Academic Press, New York.
2.  Feeney, J. (1985) in "Nmr in Living Systems" (Proc. NATO ASI) D. Reidel, Dordrecht, in press.
3.  Birdsall, B., Roberts, G.C.K., Feeney, J. and Burgen, A.S.V. (1977) FEBS Lett., 80:313.
4.  Hyde, E.I., Birdsall, B., Roberts, G.C.K., Feeney, J. and Burgen, A.S.V. (1980) Biochemistry, 19:3746.
5.  Feeney, J., Batchelor, J.G., Albrand, J.P. and Roberts, G.C.K. (1979) J. Mag. Reson., 33:519.
6.  Gronenborn, A.M., Birdsall, B., Hyde, E.I., Roberts, G.C.K., Feeney, J. and Burgen, A.S.V. (1981) Molec. Pharmacol., 20:145.
7.  Birdsall, B., Gronenborn, A., Hyde, E.I., Clore, G.M., Roberts, G.C.K., Feeney, J. and Burgen, A.S.V. (1982) Biochemistry, 21:5831.
8.  Birdsall, B., Bevan, A.W., Pascual, C., Roberts, G.C.K., Feeney, J., Gronenborn, A. and Clore, G.M. (1984) Biochemistry, 23:4733.
9.  Birdsall, B., Hammond, S., De Graw, J.I., Roberts, G.C.K. and Feeney, J. (1986) Submitted for publication.
10. Forsen, S. and Hoffman, R.A. (1963) J. Chem. Phys., 39:2892.
11. Hyde, E.I., Birdsall, B., Roberts, G.C.K., Feeney, J. and Burgen, A.S.V. (1980) Biochemistry, 19:3738.
12. Clore, G.M., Roberts, G.C.K., Gronenborn, A., Birdsall, B. and Feeney, J. (1981) J. Mag. Reson., 45:141.
13. Birdsall, B., Hyde, E.I., Burgen, A.S.V., Roberts, G.C.K. and Feeney, J. (1981) Biochemistry, 19:3732.
14. Birdsall, B., Roberts, G.C.K., Feeney, J., Dann, J.G. and Burgen, A.S.V. (1983) Biochemistry, 22:5597.
15. Albrand, J.P., Birdsall, B., Feeney, J., Roberts, G.C.K. and Burgen, A.S.V. (1979) Int. J. Biol. Macromol., 1:37.
16. Clore, G.M. and Gronenborn, A.M. (1982) J. Mag. Reson., 48:402.
17. Feeney, J., Birdsall, B., Roberts, G.C.K. and Burgen, A.S.V. (1983) Biochemistry, 22:628.
18. Baker, D.J., Beddell, C.R., Champness, J.N., Goodford, P.J., Norrington, F.E.A., Smith, D.R. and Stammers, D.K. (1981) FEBS Lett., 126:49.

19. Roberts, G.C.K., Feeney, J., Burgen, A.S.V. and Daluge, S. (1981) FEBS Lett., 131:65.
20. Morris, G.A. and Freeman, R. (1979) J. Am. Chem. Soc., 101:760.
21. Morris, G.A. (1980) J. Am. Chem. Soc., 102:428.
22. Bevan, A.W., Roberts, G.C.K., Feeney, J. and Kuyper, L. (1985) Eur. Biophys. J., 11:21.
23. Cayley, P.J., Albrand, J.P., Feeney, J., Roberts, G.C.K., Piper, E.A. and Burgen, A.S.V. (1979) Biochemistry, 18:3886.
24. Campbell, I.D., Dobson, C.M. and Williams, R.J.P. (1975), Proc. Roy. Soc. B., 189:503.
25. Wuthrich, K. and Wagner, G. (1975) FEBS Lett., 50:265.
26. Karplus, M. and McCammon, J.A. (1981) CRC Crit. Rev. Biochem., 9:293.
27. Feeney, J., Birdsall, B., Albrand, J.P., Roberts, G.C.K., Burgen, A.S.V., Charlton, P.A. and Young, D.W. (1981) Biochemistry, 20:1837.
28. Clore, G.M., Gronenborn, A.M., Birdsall, B., Feeney, J. and Roberts, G.C.K. (1984), Biochem. J., 217:659.
29. Cheung, H.T.A., Searle, M.S., Feeney, J., Birdsall, B., Roberts, G.C.K., Kompis, I. and Hammond, S. (1986), Biochemistry, in press.
30. Wuthrich, K., Wider, G., Wagner, G. and Braun, W. (1982), J. Mol. Biol., 155:311.
31. Billeter, M., Braun, W. and Wuthrich, K. (1982), J. Mol. Biol., 155:321.
32. Wagner, G. and Wuthrich, K. (1982) J. Mol. Biol., 155:347.
33. Strop, P., Wider, G. and Wuthrich, K. (1983), J. Mol. Biol., 166:641.
34. Dobson, C.M., Howarth, M.A. and Redfield, C. (1984), FEBS Lett., 176:307.
35. Delepierre, M., Dobson, C.M., Howarth, M.A. and Poulsen, F.M. (1984) Eur. J. Biochem., 145:389.
36. Aue, W.P., Bartholdi, E. and Ernst, R.R. (1976), J. Chem. Phys., 64:2229.
37. Eich, G., Bodenhausen, G. and Ernst, R.R. (1982) J. Am. Chem. Soc., 104:3732.
38. Feeney, J., Roberts, G.C.K., Birdsall, B., Griffiths, D.V., King, R.W., Scudder, P. and Burgen, A.S.V. (1971), Proc. Roy. Soc. B., 196:267.
39. Feeney, J., Roberts, G.C.K., Thomson, J., King, R.W., Griffiths, D.V. and Burgen, A.S.V. (1980), Biochemistry, 19:2316.
40. Birdsall, B., Feeney, J., Griffiths, D.V., Hammond, S., Kimber, B., King, R.W., Roberts, G.C.K. and Searle, M.S. (1984), FEBS Lett., 175:364.
41. Williamson, M.P., Marion, D. and Wuthrich, K. (1984), J. Mol. Biol., 173:341.
42. Hammond, S.J., Birdsall, B., Searle, M.S., Roberts, G.C.K. and Feeney, J. (1986), J. Mol. Biol., in press.
43. Antonjuk, D.J., Birdsall, B., Burgen, A.S.V., Cheung, H.T.A., Clore, G.M., Feeney, J., Gronenborn, A., Roberts, G.C.K. and Tran, T.Q. (1984), Brit. J. Pharmacol., 81:309.
44. Birdsall, B., Feeney, J., Pascual, C., Roberts, G.C.K., Kompis, I., Then, R.L., Muller, K. and Kroehn, A. (1984), J. Med. Chem., 27:1672.

# DIVERSITY OF MOLECULAR RECOGNITION: THE COMBINING

## SITES OF MONOCLONAL ANTI SPIN LABEL ANTIBODIES

Harden M. McConnell, Tom Frey, Jacob Anglister, Mei Whittaker

Stauffer Laboratory for Physical Chemistry
Stanford University
Stanford, CA 94305

## INTRODUCTION

Physical chemistry includes the study of how atoms come together to form molecules, and how combinations of molecules can interact with one another to form aggregates, crystals, and macromolecules. One of the most challenging problems in the area of macromolecules is the problem of protein structure, the problem of finding the "code" that specifies how a given amino acid sequence gives rise to a three-dimensional protein structure, such as an enzyme, with a highly specific biochemical function. This problem has been already attacked with considerable success using NMR methods, through studies of the folding-unfolding of polypeptides and proteins.[1] Another important facet of the problem of protein structure, and the evolution of protein structures, concerns the manner in which amino acid sequences corresponding to exons, are assembled as structural units ("modules") to form three-dimensional structures with specific functions.[2]

The purpose of the present article is to indicate that one can use NMR to study the structure of the combining sites of monoclonal antibodies. These combining site structures involve both the protein folding problem, the "module assembly problem," and the molecular complementarity problem-- the "fit" of hapten/antigen to the combining site. Antibodies constitute a unique class of proteins for studying these problems.

Our NMR technique for studying the structure of antibody combining sites employs an intrinsic probe. We use a paramagnetic spin label hapten to facilitate the identification of the amino acids in combining sites, and to obtain structural information based on hapten-amino acid distances. As discussed later, our method in essence provides a "fingerprint" of the antibody combining site region, this fingerprint depending in a sensitive way on both the amino acid composition and structure of the combining site. Our paramagnetic spin label hapten is the natural target for the antibody combining site, since the antibody is derived from the cells of mice immunized with the hapten. Thus, there is no issue as to whether our paramagnetic nitroxide group "perturbs" the native structure of the protein. A second unique feature of antibodies is their diversity--not only can antibodies be formed against almost any substance, but typically, many different antibodies can be formed that bind to one single substance--in our case, the paramagnetic hapten. A particularly relevant study of antibody diversity against a specific hapten has been carried out in connection with the maturation of immune responses.[3] It is known that the diversity of the antibody response against a hapten or antigen originates in a number of ways: (1) There is a multiplicity of heavy chain germ line genes ($V_H$, D, J) and light chain germ line genes ($V_L$, $J_L$). One source of diversity is that different antibodies employ different genes to bind a given specific hapten. (2) There is a combinatorial diversity brought about by different combinations of these genes within each chain, and different combinations of the heavy and light chains. (3) A further diversity is generated by joining these various genes at different sites. (4) Finally, diversity is created by somatic mutations of the individual genes.

Thus, from these considerations we anticipate that using the hybridoma technique of Milstein and Kohler[4] to generate monoclonal antibodies of defined specificity, we will have available to us a repetoire of antibodies that bind to our paramagnetic hapten, some of which differ one from another by small changes in amino acid sequence (e.g., "variants" arising from somatic mutations) as well as other antibodies that differ one from another by many changes in amino acid sequence (e.g., different germ line gene products). We anticipate that this may be an effective means of investigating the structure-function aspects of protein structure, and may perhaps provide insight into the relation between protein structure and the genetic events involved in generating diversity.

ANTIBODY STRUCTURE

At the present time, much is known, and much is not known about the structures of antibody molecules. We focus on the IgG class of antibody molecules that have two heavy chains and two light chains, and that have two equivalent combining sites. For a review on antibody structure see especially Davies and Metzger[5], and Amzel and Poljak.[6] For purposes of both X-ray diffraction and NMR experiments, Fab fragments, containing single combining sites, are frequently employed. Fab fragments can be obtained from the IgG molecule by proteolytic digestion. The structures of three Fabs determined by X-ray crystallography have been published.[6] These structures, together with other information on protein structures, now make it possible to make approximate models of antibody structures, since certain structural features of these molecules appear to be highly conserved. Thus, with computer modeling, one can obtain approximate "theoretical" models of an antibody molecule (M. Levitt, private communication). However, a knowledge of the amino acid sequence, plus computer modeling, has not reached the point where one can say with any assurance where the combining site is, or what the appropriate hapten or antigen might be. Of course, given a Fab fragment that makes good crystals together with the appropriate hapten, this information could be obtained from X-ray diffraction data.

Early studies of antibody combining site structures using magnetic resonance methods were made by Dwek and collaborators[7], and by Goetze and Richards.[8] The applicability of magnetic resonance methods to the combining site structure problem is now even more attractive, due in large part to the development of the hybridoma method of Kohler and Milstein[4], to the increase in understanding of the genetic basis of antibody diversity[9], and to the development of improvements in magnetic resonance instrumentation.

NMR Approach to Antibody Combining Site Composition and Structure

The hybridoma technique of Milstein and Kohler[4] makes possible the production of monoclonal antibodies of defined specificity in sufficient quantities to be practical for NMR experiments. Some time ago, a hybridoma

ANO2 was produced in this laboratory that binds the paramagnetic spin label hapten **I**.[10]

NO$_2$

NO$_2$ — NH — (piperidine ring) N — O    I

NH$_2$CH$_2$CH$_2$NH

SPIN-LABEL HAPTEN

The spin label I was used as an adventitious hapten in some of the studies of the myeloma protein MOPC315 by Dwek and collaborators.[7]

We have pursued the following strategy for studying the structure of the combining site for ANO2.

1. _Difference spectra._ By recording the spectrum of the Fab fragment of ANO2, and subtracting the spectrum of the Fab fragment in the presence of an excess of the paramagnetic hapten I, one obtains a difference spectrum that is due to the protons of some 40-50 amino acids in the combining site region. The unpaired electron on the hapten produces a broadening of proton resonances at distances within a radius of 17Å.[11,12]

2. _Amino Acid Deuteration._ The hybridoma ANO2 can be adapted to growth on medium with a low concentration of fetal calf serum, supplemented with specifically deuterated amino acids. We have found that it is possible to achieve >90% incorporation of specifically deuterated tyrosine and other essential amino acids in the antibody molecule. Under these circumstances, the difference spectra yield the proton signals from amino acid protons which have not been replaced by deuterium. Using this approach we have identified about 75% of the amino acids in the combining site region.[11,12]

3. _Heavy Chain-Light Chain Recombinations._ It is possible to separate and then recombine the heavy and light chains of a Fab fragment, so as to obtain a Fab fragment with full combining site activity. By recombining heavy and light chains from hybridomas grown on different amino acids, and then obtaining NMR difference spectra, it is possible to determine whether individual proton signals arise from the heavy chain, or from the light chains.[13]

4. _Distance Determinations by Paramagnetic Broadening of Proton Signals._ The unpaired electron on the nitoxide group of the paramagnetic hapten broadens proton signals up to distances of the order of 17Å. When the paramagnetic hapten is present in solution in less than saturating concentrations, proton signals from the combining site region undergo intermediate broadening. When the paramagnetic hapten exchange rate is large enough, the observed difference spectra can be analyzed so as to yield information on the distances between specific protons and the unpaired electron.[14]

5. _Nuclear Magnetization Transfer._ A number of diamagnetic analogues of I can be prepared, including the product derived from I by simply adding a hydrogen atom to the NO group to produce the hydroxylamine. Nuclear magnetization transfer between protons of the hapten, and protons in the combining sites can then be used to establish which types of amino acids are in direct contact with the diamagnetic form of the hapten. Such studies are in progress in this laboratory.

## CONCLUSIONS AND PREDICTIONS

From the foregoing discussion we believe it safe to conclude that NMR can provide a reliable "fingerprint" of the combining site of a monoclonal anti-spin label antibody, a fingerprint that depends on both the amino acid composition and structure of the combining site. The combination of theoretical computer modeling and this fingerprint information should lead to a reliable model of the antibody combining site structure. Based on the amino acid sequence of the IgG from ANO2 determined by Mei Whittaker and M. Bond (to be published), M. Levitt at the Weizmann Institute has calculated a "theoretical" model of this protein, a model that we are now comparing with our NMR data.

What kinds of questions can this line of work hope to answer in the immediate future? Perhaps the simplest question to answer will be the structural basis of the maturation of the immune response due to somatic cell mutations. That is, by an examination of the NMR fingerprints of a series of monoclonal antibodies with progressively increasing affinity for a spin label hapten due to one or a small number of changes in amino acid composition in the variable regions, we may hope to determine whether such changes in affinity are due to structural changes localized to the immediate vicinity of the point mutation(s), or whether such alternatives are responsible for more global effects, such as slight realignments of heavy and light chains, and one domain relative to the other. In the former case, the NMR fingerprint changes would be localized to a few signals, whereas in the latter case many resonance signals might undergo small alterations, corresponding to small but significant changes in the entire combining site region.

At the present time, we cannot even speculate as to how the NMR combining site fingerprints will compare for two anti spin label antibodies that employ different germ line genes, and combinations of these genes. If, as is likely, all antibodies that bind our spin label hapten utilize a tryptophan in stacking interaction with the nitrophenyl ring, we should be able to use magnetization transfer experiments to monitor the precision with which the geometry of this stacking interaction is maintained, even when different germ line genes are used for constructing the hapten combining site. A real test of our "understanding" of combining site structure will come hen we attempt to modify the properties of this combining site using recombinant DNA techniques so as to achieve novel properties, such as enzymatic activity.

## REFERENCES

1. K. R. Shoemaker, P. S. Kim, D. N. Brems, S. Marqusee, E. J. York, I. M. Chaiken, J. M. Stewart, and R. L. Baldwin. Proc. Nat. Acad. Sci. USA 82, 2349-2353 (1985).
2. W. Gilbert. Science 228, 823-824 (1985) and references therein.
3. G. M. Griffith, C. Beretz, M. Karartinen and C. Milstein. Nature 312, 271-275 (1984).
4. G. Kohler and C. Milstein. Nature 256, 495- (1975).
5. D. R. Davies and H. Metzger. Ann. Rev. Immun. 1, 87-117 (1983).
6. L. M. Amzel and R. J. Poljak. Ann. Rev. Biochem. 48, 961-997 (1979).
7. R. A. Dwek, S. Wain-Hobson, D. Dower, P. Gettins, B. Sutton, J. Perkins and D. Givol. Nature 266, 31-37 (1977).
8. A. M. Goetze and J. H. Richards. Biochem. 17, 1733-1739 (1978).
9. T. Honjo. Ann. Rev. Immun. 1, 499 (1983).
10. K. Balakrishnan, F. J. Hsu, D. G. Hafeman and H. M. McConnell, BBA 721, 30-38 (1982).
11. J. Anglister, T. Frey and H. M. McConnell. Biochem. 23, 1138-1142 (1984).

12.  T. Frey, J. Anglister and H. M. McConnell.  Biochem. 23, 6470–6474
      (1984).
13.  J. Anglister, T. Frey and H. M. McConnell.  Nature 315, 65–67 (1985).
14.  J. Anglister, T. Frey and H. M. McConnell.  Biochem. 23, 5372–5375
      (1984).

ACKNOWLEDGEMENTS

    This work has benefited from collaborations with Dr. Martha Bond,
Professor Michael Levitt, and Mr. Dan Leahy.  These collaborations will be
described in future publications.  This work is supported by ONR Contract
N00014-83-K-0349 and National Institutes of Health Grant 5R01 AI13587-08.

# NMR APPROACHES TO THE CHARACTERIZATION OF THE

# INTERACTION OF METAL IONS WITH PROTEINS

Thomas C. Williams, Judith G. Shelling and Brian D. Sykes

MRC Group in Protein Structure and Function and the
Department of Biochemistry
University of Alberta
Edmonton, Alberta, Canada T6G 2H7

A general interest of our laboratory is the structure, function and biological role of calcium-binding proteins. Calcium ions are very important in the regulation of a wide variety of biological processes. One such process is contractility. The contraction of mammalian skeletal and cardiac muscle is regulated by the level of calcium ions present and the interaction of calcium ions with several proteins. This occurs in the following fashion. The nerve impulse releases calcium ions from the sarcoplasmic reticulum membrane which surrounds the muscle fibers. The increased intracellular calcium level then results in the interaction of calcium with the calcium-specific sites of the thin filament protein, troponin-C. This turns on the muscle. The calcium then migrates to parvalbumin, a soluble protein whose affinity for calcium ions is very high. Since this turns the contraction off, parvalbumin is referred to as a soluble relaxing factor. Eventually, the calcium is pumped back into the sarcoplasmic reticulum by the SR $Ca^{+2}$ ATPase where it is bound in high concentration to the protein calsequestrin. This process thus involves the interaction of calcium with at least five proteins or membrane channels with varying affinities for calcium.

Two of the proteins mentioned above, troponin-C and parvalbumin, are recognized as part of a large superfamily of calcium-binding proteins. Included in this superfamily are the parvalbumins, troponin-Cs, calmodulins, myosin light chains, intestinal calcium-binding proteins, and the S-100s. This categorization followed Kretsinger and Nockolds' (1973) elucidation of the X-ray crystal structure of parvalbumin pI 4.25 from carp muscle. This structure revealed that each of the two bound calcium ions were chelated in a helix-loop-helix calcium-binding domain. Because this type of metal-binding site is formed from a contiguous section of the polypeptide chain, it was immediately possible to recognize this motif in the sequences of a wide variety of other proteins (for a recent review, see Gariepy and Hodges, 1983). This calcium-binding structure has since been seen in the X-ray structures of the bovine intestinal calcium-binding protein (Szebenyi et al., 1981), turkey skeletal troponin-C (Herzberg and James, 1985), chicken skeletal troponin-C (Sundaralingam et al., 1985), and calmodulin (Babu et al., 1985).

In an attempt to understand the function of these proteins, we have made extensive use of a variety of NMR methods (including $^1H$, $^{13}C$, $^{113}Cd$, and laser photo-CIDNP $^1H$ techniques) to study these calcium-binding proteins in solution: carp, rat, and pike parvalbumins (Lee and Sykes, 1983; Corson et al., 1983; Williams et al., 1984; Lee et al., 1985); rabbit skeletal, bovine cardiac and pike troponin-Cs (Hincke et al., 1981a,b; McCubbin et al., 1982); porcine intestinal calcium-binding protein (Shelling et al., 1983, 1985); bovine brain calmodulin (Hincke et al, 1981b); bovine brain S-100b (Mani et al., 1983); and calsequestrin (Aaron et al., 1984). In addition to these naturally occurring proteins, we have also studied a variety of synthetic peptide analogues of the helix-loop-helix domain (Gariepy et al., 1983, 1985). One particular focus of our work has been the use of the lanthanide(III) series of metal ions as calcium analogues (Corson et al., 1983; Gariepy et al., 1983; Lee and Sykes, 1983; Lee et al., 1985; Shelling et al., 1983, 1985; Williams et al., 1984). These metal ions are of interest for two reasons: first, their interactions with calcium-binding proteins are visible in an NMR spectroscopic sense; and second, they provide a series of metals differing only in ionic radius, a very useful probe of metal-binding sites.

Dealing with all of the above subjects is, of course, beyond the scope of this article. Instead we will focus on the seemingly simple topic of using NMR to characterize the manner in which calcium interacts with these proteins. By that we mean the measurement of the number of metals bound, the affinities of the various sites, and the degree of interaction (if any) between the sites. In principle, this is no different than the study of the interaction of any ligand with a protein. We will further restrict ourselves to typical calcium-binding proteins of the helix-loop-helix type.

We shall now explore in some detail the advantages and limitations of NMR as a tool in the study of metal-binding in this class of proteins.

(1) Although direct observation of the metal ion using $^{43}$Ca NMR techniques is possible, such studies are very difficult in general. $^{113}$Cd NMR studies of cadmium as a calcium analogue are much easier, however, and have proved very useful (for a recent review of $^{43}$Ca and $^{113}$Cd NMR studies of calcium binding proteins see Vogel et al., 1983). But, cadmium(II) is significantly different from calcium(II) in the bioinorganic sense. Therefore, even though calcium competition studies using $^{113}$Cd NMR are possible, we will restrict ourselves to the NMR spectrum of the protein.

(2) The affinity of these proteins for calcium is very high, dissociation constants, $K_D$, typically falling in the range of $10^{-5}$ to $10^{-10}$ M. [In this article we will use $K_D$'s for dissociation constants and $\beta$'s or $K_A$'s for association constants.] Because these values are far less than the concentrations of the protein which are possible to study by NMR, the affinity would be difficult to determine from a titration curve. This we can see in Figure 1 where the theoretical fractional intensity of the calcium-protein complex is plotted versus the amount of calcium added (assuming one-to-one binding) for a typical protein concentration and values of $K_D$ between $10^{-5}$ and $10^{-8}$M. Once the value of $K_D$ is less than $10^{-5}$M, it becomes hard to determine $K_D$ from a metal-ion titration. High affinities will also result in NMR spectra in the slow exchange limit. This, more often than not, is an advantage since it means that separate NMR spectra of the apo protein, the partially liganded protein, and the fully metal saturated protein can potentially be observed during the titration.

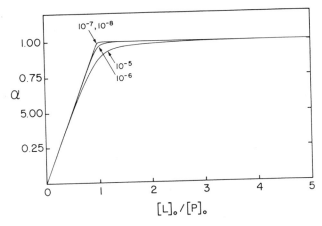

Figure 1: Theoretical plot of the fractional intensity of an NMR resonance corresponding to the metal-protein complex as a function of added metal ion (P+M $\rightleftharpoons$ PM) for a total protein concentration of 500 μM and values of $K_D$ = $10^{-5}$ (bottom curve), $10^{-6}$, $10^{-7}$ and $10^{-8}$M (top curve).

(3) Normally, the protein under study will bind two or more calcium ions. Even for the simple case of n=2, this means that four species are possible, with either intrinsically equal or unequal affinities and with or without interaction between the sites. The following scheme illustrates the equilibria involved in the co-existence of the four forms of a typical two-site calcium-binding protein:

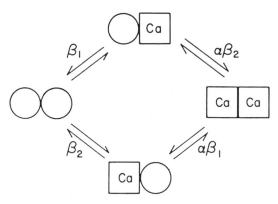

where $\beta_1$ and $\beta_2$ are the intrinsic association constants for the two sites, and $a$ is the degree of cooperativity ($a$ >1 for positive cooperativity). In this regard it is salient to note the paper by

Ferguson-Miller and Koppenol (1981) who remind us of the difference and relationships between the intrinsic constants written for the mechanism shown above and the macroscopic constants determined by fitting the data to the equation

$$P + M \xrightleftharpoons{\quad K_{A1} \quad} PM + M \xrightleftharpoons{\quad K_{A2} \quad} PM_2$$

where $K_{A1}$ and $K_{A2}$ are the macroscopic association constants, and are related to the microscopic constants by

$$K_{A1} = \beta_1 + \beta_2$$

$$K_{A1} + K_{A2} = a \cdot \beta_1 \cdot \beta_2$$

(4) Although not associated exclusively with the study of calcium-binding proteins, two additional limitations which apply to spectroscopic methods in general deserve attention.

(i) If the sensitivity of the spectroscopic probe to metal-binding at different sites is not known, then the spectroscopic changes are difficult to analyze since they may not directly reflect the number of metal-ions bound to the protein (Garabek and Gergely, 1983). In this instance, NMR has a very great advantage over most other spectroscopic tools because the resolution possible normally means that separate NMR resonances can be observed for each of the intermediates involved in the titration.

(ii) Although the total concentration of added metal-ion is usually known, the concentration of free metal-ion is frequently an unknown. This is not a trivial problem; most available mathematical treatments are derived in terms of the free metal-ion concentration. Even for the simplest reaction

$$P + M \xrightleftharpoons{\quad K_D \quad} PM$$

the concentration of the metal-bound form involves solving a quadratic

$$[PM] = \frac{\left(P_0 + M_0 + K_D\right) - \left[\left(P_0 + M_0 + K_D\right)^2 - 4 P_0 M_0\right]^{1/2}}{2}$$

where $P_0$ is the total protein concentration, $M_0$ is the total metal concentration, and $K_D$ is the dissociation constant.

To include the interaction of a second metal-ion, extension to

$$P + M \xrightleftharpoons{K_{D1}} PM + M \xrightleftharpoons{K_{D2}} PM_2$$

involves the solution to a cubic equation:

```
C3=A3-4*A2
C2=A3^2-4*A2*A3*-2*X2*A3
C1=2*X2*X1*A3-X2*A3^2-A2*A3^2-X1*A3^2-A3*X1^2
C0=X1*X2*A3^2
P=C2/C3
Q=C1/C3
R=C0/C3
A=(1/3)*(3*Q-P^2)
B=(1/27)*(2*P^3-9*P*Q+27*R)
Theta=ACS(-(B/2)/SQR(-A^3)/27))
[PM]=2*SQR(-A/3)*COS(Theta/3+240)-P/3
```

where A2 (=$K_{D1}$) is the first macroscopic dissociation constant, A3 (=$K_{D2}$) is the second macroscopic dissociation constant X1 = [M] total, and X2 = [P] total.  While non-linear least squares fitting to these analytical solutions are possible (see Figure 2), the more general problems involve iterative computer simulations.

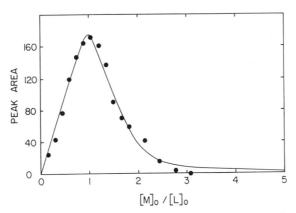

Figure 2:  A plot of the area of a lanthanide shifted [1]H NMR resonance observed during the titration of porcine intestinal calcium-binding protein with ytterbium(III).  This data was fit to the equation P + M $\rightleftharpoons$ PM + M $\rightleftharpoons$ PM$_2$ and yielded a value of $5.0(+/-1.6) \times 10^{-5}$M for the second dissociation constant.  The first dissociation constant, being $<10^{-7}$M, was too small to be determined accurately (from Shelling et al. 1985).

Having laid the above ground rules, we would like to present two examples of the use of NMR to study metal binding to a protein. The first involves the interaction of calcium with the porcine intestinal calcium binding protein (pICaBP), the second involves the interaction of lutetium with the calcium form of rat parvalbumin. Two strategies for addressing the above mentioned problems, and the particular advantages of NMR are demonstrated. Both examples utilize high resolution [1]H NMR to monitor the spectrum of the protein during the titration. The first examples involves competition between the protein and another chelator; the second example involves competition between different metal ions.

## Interaction of Calcium with pICaBP

When the calcium titration of apo pICaBP is followed by [1]H NMR, the observed spectral changes are in the slow exchange limit (Shelling et al, 1983). A plot of the intensity of a clearly resolved aromatic [1]H NMR resonance as a function of added calcium is shown in Figure 3. If one neglects the intensity changes associated with non-specific or weak third site binding following the addition of two equivalents of calcium, the spectroscopic changes between zero to two equivalents of calcium are linear. This immediately implies either that the two known calcium sites on the protein have identical affinities or that the metal ion binding

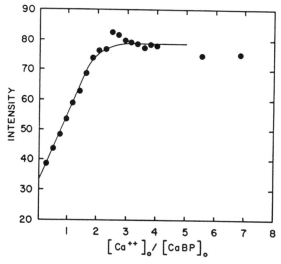

Figure 3: [1]H NMR monitored calcium titration of apo pICaBP. Plotted is the area of a resolved aromatic resonance corresponding to the $PCa_2$ species versus total added calcium (from Shelling et al. 1983).

occurs with complete positive cooperativity. The former situation is consistent with known data but unexpected since the structures and formal charges of the two metal-ion domains are shown to be different in the X-ray structure (Szenbenyi et al., 1981). The N-terminal site is a pseudo EF domain (Kretsinger and Nockolds, 1973); the C-terminal site is a typical EF domain.

To resolve this situation as well as to more accurately determine the affinities, we monitored the titration of the protein with calcium in the presence of the competing calcium chelator EDTA whose [1]H NMR spectrum could also be followed. In this way, the affinity determination became relative to EDTA and not absolute, and the degree of cooperativity could also be evaluated. This experiment was analyzed by modifying the formalism of Garabek and Gergely (1983) to obtain expressions for the fractional change in the NMR resonances of the protein and of the EDTA in terms of the following mechanism:

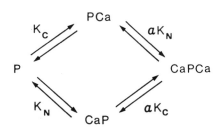

$$E + Ca \xrightleftharpoons{K_E} ECa$$

where the PCa complex has the calcium in the C-terminal site, the CaP complex has the metal in the N-terminal site, ECa is the EDTA complex, and $K_C$, $K_N$ and $K_E$ are the association constants for the C-terminal site, N-terminal site, and EDTA, respectively. The fractional change of the protein and EDTA resonances are given by

$$\frac{A_P^{Obs}}{A_P^{Max}} = \frac{(\beta_C K_C + \beta_N K_N)[M] + a K_C K_N [M]^2}{1 + (K_C + K_N)[M] + a K_C K_N [M]^2}$$

$$\frac{A_E^{Obs}}{A_E^{Max}} = \frac{K_E[M]}{1 + K_E[M]}$$

where $\beta_N$ and $\beta_C$ are the ratios of the spectroscopic changes observed for CaP and PCa, respectively, to that observed for CaPCa. One can then plot the fractional change observed for the protein versus the fractional change observed for the EDTA for various values of the constants $K_N$, $K_C$, $K_E$ (known), $\beta_N$, and $\beta_C$ (see Figure 4). In this method, knowledge of the total concentrations of the protein, EDTA, and metal is not required. Shown in Figure 4 is the series of fits for equal intrinsic $K_N = K_C$, and for values of $a$ = 0.2, 0.5, 1.0, 2.0, 5.0 and 10. The data best fit a non-cooperative model with independent equal sites with a $K_N$ twice that of EDTA under these conditions [$K_E$ = $5 \times 10^6$ M$^{-1}$ (Shelling and Sykes, 1985)].

The extraordinary capability of high-field spectrometers to resolve minute differences in the magnetic microenvironments of nuclei has made the observation of individual protons in macromolecular systems commonplace. This unique attribute of $^1$H NMR spectroscopy is well-illustrated by more than 25 non-overlapping resonances in the 300-MHz spectrum of rat parvalbumin ($M_r$ 12,000), each resonance being uniquely

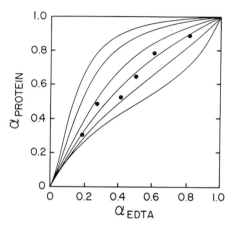

Figure 4:  Plots of the fractional change in the $^1$H NMR spectrum of pICaBP versus fractional change in the $^1$H NMR spectrum of EDTA for various amounts of added calcium.  The points represent actual data (after Shelling and Sykes, 1985), the solid lines represent theoretical curves for $K_E = 5 \times 10^6 M^{-1}$, $K_N = K_C = 1 \times 10^7 M^{-1}$, $\beta_N = \beta_C = 0.5$, and $a = 0.2$, 0.5, 1.0, 2.0, 5.0 and 10 (bottom to top).

assignable to one, two, or at most three magnetically equivalent (or pseudo equivalent) protons.  As judged by numerous spectroscopic techniques, parvalbumins adopt a highly-ordered conformation in solution. However, only NMR methods have probed their tertiary structure in sufficient detail to allow their solution conformation to be correlated directly with the well-defined structure of crystalline carp parvalbumin (Lee and Sykes, 1983).  Several of these well-resolved resonances are extremely informative probes of the subtle conformational changes induced by metal-ion exchange at parvalbumin's two high-affinity Mg(II):Ca(II) sites.  So selective is their sensitivity to this type of exchange that not only are initial, intermediate, and final metal-bound forms readily detected but the sequential conversion of one metal form to another can also easily be quantitated, yielding relative values of stability constants for the two different metals at each of parvalbumin's metal-binding sites.

For example, during the Lu(III) titration of the Ca(II) form of rat parvalbumin, the resonance of the ortho protons of Phe 47 experiences two consecutive, well-defined changes; by contrast, the triplet resonances of the meta and para protons of Phe 29 are virtually unaffected. This is due both to this lanthanide's ability to selectively displace the EF-site calcium ion and to the inherent differences in the sensitivities of each [1]H NMR resonance as a probe of metal-ion exchange.

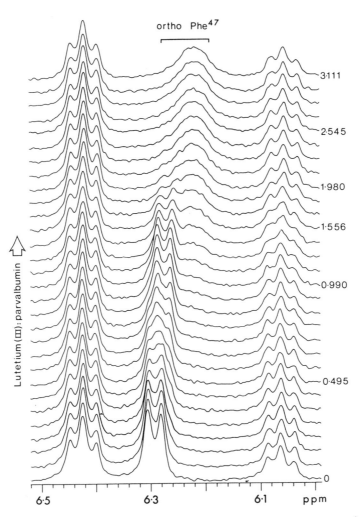

Figure 5. Partial aromatic region (6.5 ppm to 6.0 ppm) of the [1]H NMR spectrum of rat parvalbumin: changes induced by Ca(II):Lu(III) exchange. Several of the metal:parvalbumin ratios are shown at the right of the stacked plot. The doublet resonance has been assigned to the ortho protons of Phe 47 (relative area=2); the triplet resonance at 6.43 ppm (relative area=2) and the triplet resonances at 6.1 ppm (relative area=1) were not affected and have been assigned tentatively to the meta and para protons of Phe 29, respectively.

As seen in Figure 5, the well resolved doublet resonance of the Ca(II) form of the protein (6.30 ppm) steadily decreased in intensity as Lu(III) was added to the sample. An intermediate doublet of nearly identical linewidth emerged at 6.28 ppm and rose to a maximum intensity at one:one Lu(III):parvalbumin; this doublet resonance was assigned to Phe 47 of the mixed-metal:parvalbumin complex in which the EF-site Ca(II) ion had been selectively displaced by Lu(III). As the titration progressed, a much broader resonance appeared further upfield at 6.23 ppm; this resonance was attributed to the ortho protons of Phe 47 in the fully loaded Lu(III) form of rat parvalbumin. The relative proportions of each form of parvalbumin were determined from lineshape analyses of the Phe 47 resonance and plotted versus added Lu(III) (Figure 6). Iterative curve fitting of these three data sets yielded the following stability constants for the Lu(III)-parvalbumin complex relative to the Ca(II)-parvalbumin complex:

$$\beta_{LU:CD} = 1\cdot2 \times 10^2 \qquad \beta_{LU:EF} = 2\cdot5 \times 10^3$$

The absolute values for the Lu(III) stability constants

$$\beta_{LU:CD} = 2\cdot0 \times 10^{10} M^{-1} \qquad \beta_{LU:EF} = 2\cdot3 \times 10^{11} M^{-1}$$

were calculated from the absolute values for the Ca(II) stability constants. The Ca(II) stability constants had themselves been calculated from the relative stability constants determined by Mg(II):Ca(II) exchange and the absolute values for the Mg(II) stability constants determined directly by Mg(II) titration of the apo protein (Williams et al., 1985).

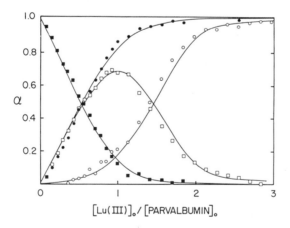

Figure 6: Lu(III) titration of the Ca(II)-form of rat parvalbumin. Curve-analyzed areas of the ortho proton resonance of Phe 47 and the $\epsilon$-CH$_3$ singlet resonance of an unassigned methionine are plotted vs. the ratio Lu(III):parvalbumin. Phe 47, Ca(II)$_2$-form ( ■ ); Phe 47, Ca(II):Lu(III)-form ( □ ); Phe 47, sum of the Lu(III):Ca(II)- and Lu(III)$_2$-forms ( O ); Met, sum of the Ca(II):Lu(III)- and Lu(III)$_2$-forms ( ● ) (adapted from Williams et al., 1985).

# REFERENCES

Aaron, B. B., Oikawa, K., Reithmeier, R. A. F., and Sykes, B. D., 1984, J. Biol. Chem. 259:11876.

Babu, Y. S., Sack, J. S., Greenhough, T. J., Bugg, C. E., Means, A. R., and Cook, W. J., 1985, Nat. 315:37.

Corson, D. C., Williams, T. C., and Sykes, B. D., 1983, Biochem. 23:5882.

Ferguson-Miller, S., and Koppenol., W. H., 1981, TIBS 6:IV.

Gariepy, J., and Hodges, R. S., 1983, FEBS Letts. 160:1.

Gariepy, J., Sykes, B. D., and Hodges, R. H., 1983, Biochem. 22:1765.

Gariepy, J., Kay, L. E., Kuntz, I. D., Sykes, B. D., and Hodges, R. H., 1985, Biochem. 24:544.

Grabarek, Z., and Gergely, J., 1983, J. Biol. Chem. 258:14103.

Herzberg, O., and James, M. N. G., 1985, Nat. 313:653.

Hincke, M. T., Sykes, B. D., and Kay, C. M., 1981a, Biochem. 20:3286.

Hincke, M. T., Sykes, B. D., and Kay, C. M., 1981b, Biochem. 20:4185.

Kretzinger, R. H., and Nockolds, C. E., 1973, J. Biol. Chem. 248:3313.

Lee, L., and Sykes, B.D., 1983, Biochem. 22:4366.

Lee, L., Corson, D. C., and Sykes, B. D., 1985, Biophys. J. 47:139.

Mani, R. S., Shelling, J. G., Sykes, B. D., and Kay, C. M., 1983, Biochem. 22:1734.

McCubbin, W. D., Oikawa, K., Sykes, B. D., and Kay, C. M., 1982, Biochem. 21:5948.

Shelling, J. G., Sykes, B. D., O'Neil, J. D. J., and Hofmann, T., 1983, Biochem. 22:2649.

Shelling, J. G., Hoffman, T., and Sykes, B. D., 1985, Biochem. 24:2332.

Shelling, J. G., and Sykes, D. B., 1985, J. Biol. Chem. 260:00000.

Sundaralingam, M., Bergstrom, R., Strasberg, G., Rao, S. T., and Roychowdbury, P., 1985, Science 227:945.

Szebenyi, D. M. E., Obendorf, S. K., and Moffat, K., 1981, Nat. 294:327.

Vogel, H. J., Drakenburg, T., and Forsen, S., in: NMR of Newly Accessible Nuclei, P. Laszlo, ed., Academic Press, N.Y. 157 (1983).

Williams, T. C., Corson, D. C., and Sykes, B. D., 1984, J. Amer. Chem. Soc. 106:5698.

Williams, T. C., Corson, D. C., Oikawa, K., McCubbin, W. D., Key, C. M., and Sykes, B. D., Biochem. submitted.

# VOLUME SELECTION STRATEGIES FOR IN VIVO BIOLOGICAL SPECTROSCOPY

R. J. Ordidge, A. Connelly, R. E. Gordon, J. A. B. Lohman

Oxford Research Systems Limited, Abingdon, England

## INTRODUCTION

In addition to the inherently low sensitivity of the NMR technique and low metabolite concentration, a major problem of in vivo spectroscopy has been the accurate assignment of the acquired spectrum to a specific region within the sample. Surface coils have provided one method of limiting the field of view of an NMR spectrometer, although frequently in the past in an ill-defined manner. Improvements in the use of surface coils have resulted from the introduction of multipulse techniques, the incorporation of imaging capabilities in biological spectrometers, and the use of multiple RF coils in conjunction with "depth pulses". For most RF coil designs localization can be achieved also by the use of selective excitation in the presence of magnetic field gradients. These techniques offer complementary advantages and often can be combined to suit a particular application. There follows a brief description of several methods which use these basic volume selection techniques in various combinations.

## SURFACE COILS

A major innovation for in vivo spectroscopic studies was the introduction of surface coils.[1] These coils can be designed to provide adequate sensitivity and offer several advantages in comparison to solenoidal and saddle-shaped coils. Their size and shape are not controlled by the dimensions of the whole sample but rather by the location and size of the region under investigation. In contrast to solenoids or saddle-shaped coils that aim to produce a uniform $B_1$ field across the sample, the surface coils generate a non-uniform $B_1$ field. For a circular coil, the $B_1$ field reduces with increasing distance away from the plane of the coil. In similar fashion the signal received from successive elemental volumes also diminishes. Normally, the pulse width can be set to give a 90° pulse to an approximately disc shaped region lying immediately in front of the coil of thickness roughly equal to the coil radius. Consequently, signal is received only from a tightly localized volume close to the surface of the sample. Setting the pulse width to give a 180° pulse to this region would mean that the relative contribution of signal from the tissues lying further from the coil would be enhanced. In principle then, surface coils could be used to investigate deep-seated regions. In practice, however, this 180° condition is sometimes difficult to obtain and the regions distant from the coil that contribute most of the signal are rather widely distributed.

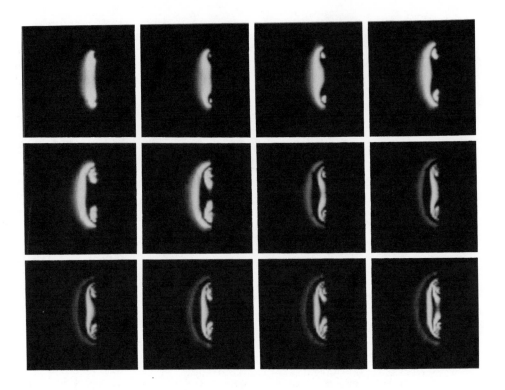

Figure 1

Proton images of a thin planar water phantom placed across the diameter of a surface coil and orthogonal to the plane of the coil.
The images are 64 x 64, took 1 minute to acquire at 80.29 MHz and
show the changes in signal distribution with increasing pulse
length.  Pulse width increases from left to right and then from top
to bottom starting with 74 µs and increasing in 75 µs increments.
The complexity of the coil response increases with increasing pulse
width.

The non-uniform response of the coil is illustrated in Figure 1, [1]H
images are presented which show the spatial response of a surface coil for a
pulse duration which is incremented in linear steps.  If the coil is placed
close to a sample that is spatially homogeneous then, despite the non-
uniform response of the coil, a spectrum will still be obtained that accurately reflects the chemical composition of the sample.  The heterogeneous
nature of intact biological samples dictates that particular attention must
be paid to optimizing the operating conditions of this type of rf coil.  In
Figure 2, [31]P spectra of the head are presented which illustrate the alterations produced by varying the pulse width applied to the coil.  The [31]P
spectra shown were obtained with simple pulse-acquire sequences.[2]

MULTIPLE PULSE TECHNIQUES

In coping with the problems set by the inhomogeneous nature of the rf
field produced by the surface coil, a set of pulse sequences has been
devised that eliminate some of the artefacts that can be introduced and also
improve the spatial resolution that is obtainable with these coils.  Localization of spectra can be achieved to a limited degree by the use of depth
pulse schemes in conjunction with separate transmit and receiver coils.[3,4]
In these sequences, the FID are accumulated in the normal fashion but the

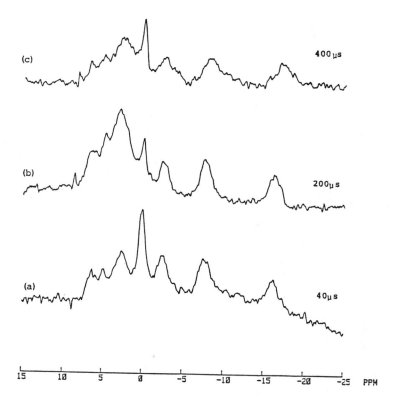

Figure 2

$^{31}$P spectra (256 scans at 2s intervals) obtained at 27.4 MHz with
a 6 cm surface coil placed over the fronto-parietal suture of an
adult. The pulse widths used are as indicated. The assignment
and chemical shifts (PPM ± 0.07) are: sugar phosphate region
(6.7); inorganic phosphate (4.9); phosphodiester region (3.0);
phosphocreatine (0); γ-ATP(-2.5); α-ATP(-7.6); and β-ATP(-15.9).
The 200μs spectrum is largely from brain tissue lying between the
brain and the surface coil. (These spectra were obtained in
collaboration with the Biochemistry Department, Oxford University.)

phase relationship between successive radiofrequency pulses is cycled in a
specific manner. Together with the $B_1$ inhomogeneity, this phase cycling
during the accumulation sequence produces self-cancellation of the NMR
signals derived from certain regions within the "field of view" of the surface coil and can be used to eliminate unwanted signals. In theory it is
easier to shape the localized sensitive volume by-applying part of a depth
pulse sequence with one transmit coil and part with a second transmit coil.
The principles of this method have been described by Bendall.[5] A requirement of the technique is that during application of pulses with one coil,
the other must be detuned. An active means of tuning/detuning is described
in Reference 6. Using a twin surface coil system as illustrated in Figure
3, and by applying a depth pulse scheme of the type:

$$2\theta \ [\underline{+}x]; \left\{ \frac{2x \ 2\theta}{3} + \frac{4\theta}{3} \right\}; \ 2\theta \ [\underline{+}x, \ \underline{+}y] \ -\tau-2\phi[\underline{+}x', \underline{+}y'] \ -2\tau-2\phi[\underline{+}x', \underline{+}y']$$

-τ- Acquire with coil θ

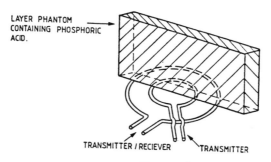

LAYER PHANTOM
CONTAINING PHOSPHORIC
ACID.

TRANSMITTER / RECIEVER        TRANSMITTER

Figure 3

Double surface coil and $H_3PO_4$ slice phantom used to obtain the
images shown in Figure 4.

where $\theta$ signifies pulse applied with the large coil $\theta$ and $\phi$ signifies pulses
applied with the same coil $\phi$, complete localization of the sensitive volume
can be achieved.

The sensitive volume of each coil was imaged at $^{31}P$ frequencies using a
slice phantom of $H_3PO_4$ by means of standard 2DFT imaging procedure. The
results for both individual coils are shown in Figures 4(a) and (b) respectively.

For the complete double coil, magnetic field gradients as used in the
imaging sequence were added to the last two periods in the depth pulse
scheme. (The phase-cycling for the refocusing pulse is unnecessary for a
homogeneous phantom when using pulsed field gradients.) The image of the
sensitive volume in the XY plane is shown in Figure 4(c), which indicates
clearly that it corresponds to the overlap of the 90° signal regions of the
separate coils. Figure 4(d) confirms the result in the XZ plane and demonstrates the expected smaller Z dimension. The extent to which depth pulses
improve the spatial resolution of the surface coil can be seen from results
published by Ng et al.[7] showing $^{31}P$ spectra of rat liver.

Other sequences have been proposed (Cox and Styles,[8] Haase et al.,[9]
Haselgrove et al.,[10] and Shaka et al.[11]) that also make use of the inhomogeneous $B_1$ produced by the surface coil but there has yet to be any detailed
assessment of the usefulness of these methods for in vivo investigations.


SELECTIVE EXCITATION/MAGNETIC FIELD GRADIENTS

The use of imaging has provided a means of determining the field of
view of a surface coil, as demonstrated in Figure 1. The addition of a further selective RF pulse in the presence of a magnetic field gradient to a
standard imaging sequence allows the assignment of the acquired signal to a
particular volume. The full response of a surface coil at a particular
pulse length is represented in Figure 5(a). If the RF pulse and gradient
sequence used to obtain this is preceded by a selective 90° pulse in the
presence of a field gradient, as shown in Figure 6, the result is the selection of the spins in a particular plane and thus the suppression of the
signal from such a plane. The response is shown in Figure 5(b). Subtraction
of the response shown in Figure 5(b) from that of Figure 5(a) gives only the
spins in a disc shaped plane corresponding to those which were excited by
the 90° pulse as shown in Figure 5(c). In an NMR spectroscopy experiment,
the optimum signal-to-noise ratio is obtained from the excited disc when a
selective 180° pre-pulse is applied. Figure 7 shows an example of the $^{31}P$
spectrum obtained from a defined plane within a human brain by application

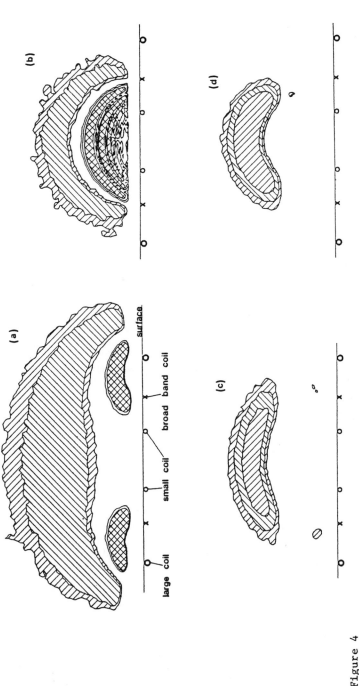

Figure 4

Intensity contours of the surface coil response patterns. The contours displayed are illustrative and are of arbitrary magnitude, with the lowest contour being a little above the noise level.

(a) Image of the large coil sensitive volume in the XY plane with the small coil detuned. The smaller cross-hatched regions correspond to angles close to 270°.

(b) Image of the small coil sensitive volume with the large coil detuned (XY plane). The complicated area close to the surface is the high flux region. The 270°, 450° and 630° signal regions can be discerned (cross-hatched).

(c) Image of the sensitive volume in the XY plane using both coils (see text for the depth pulse scheme).

(d) Image of the sensitive volume as in (c) but in the XZ plane.

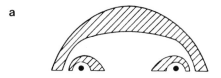

a

**Full response of Surface Coil
in Central Plane.**

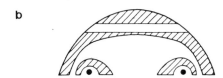

b

**Response minus Selected Plane.**

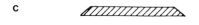

c

**Response of ① minus response
of ② = Selected Plane.**

Figure 5

(a)   Diagram of a 2-dimensional slice through the response pattern
of a surface coil at a particular pulse length.   Shaded areas
indicate regions of 90° and 270° spin nutation, with 270° spin
nutation occurring in the two small areas nearest to the coil.

(b)   A diagram of the surface coil response pattern at the same
pulse length as in Figure 5a following selection of a layer with a
90° selective pulse as shown by Figure 6.

(c)   The selected plane resulting from subtraction of the response
pattern in (b) from that shown in (a).   This plane represents a
cross-sectional slice of the three dimensional disc of material
selected by this procedure.

of this technique.[12]   The $^{31}P$ spectrum of Figure 7(a) was acquired using the
full response of a 10cm surface coil.   A second spectrum was obtained after
application of the plane suppression technique, and subtraction gave the
difference spectrum shown in Figure 7(b).

It is important to realize that the data obtained from the plane of
interest corresponds to that obtained in a simple pulse-acquire experiment.
Consequently, the metabolite concentration can be estimated from the spectra
which are free from $T_2$ effects sometimes observed in spin echo methods.

A new technique which we have called ISIS (Image Selected in Vivo Spectroscopy), offers some further advantages.[13]   Cubic volumes can be selected
by the differencing of NMR signals from eight experiments, which results in
coaddition of NMR data from within the cube, and cancellation of signals
from all external regions.   The technique does not require accurate spin

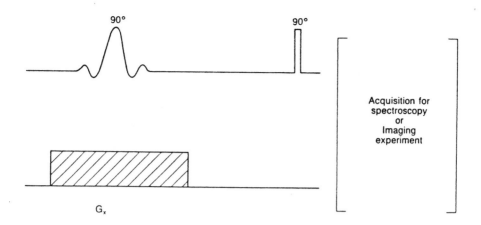

Figure 6

RF and gradient pulse sequence used for plane selection with a
surface coil.  A selective pulse is applied in conjunction with a
magnetic field gradient along the X direction.

nutation angles and can be implemented in combination with RF coils which
show gross RF inhomogeneity, for example, surface coils.  The selected
volume may be easily varied in all its dimensions and may be accurately
positioned and repositioned under computer control by movement of a cursor
over a standard NMR image of the specimen.  Selection is complete after a
single sequence of eight experiments, and the NMR spectrum does not contain
any $T_2$ distortion with only a slight dependence of signal strength upon $T_1$
value.

The method again relies on the principle of selective inversion of the
spin population prior to data accumulation.  Three dimensions of spatial
selection are achieved by incorporation of three selective RF pulses in the
preparation period prior to data accumulation.  Each of the three pulses is
applied in conjunction with a magnetic field gradient, and the gradients are
applied along the three cartesian axes, X, Y and Z, in order to provide
three dimensions of spatial selection.  Eight experiments are required to
localize the spatial distribution of NMR signal to a cube of material, and
the experimental sequence of selective pulses for the eight experiments is
summarized in Table 1.

The RF pulse timing sequence and associated gradient sequence for
experiment 8 is shown in Figure 8.  Each selective RF pulse is amplitude
modulated with a SINC function, and negative RF powers are produced by 180°
phase inversion of the applied carrier frequency.  This gives an excitation
spectrum with an approximately rectangular distribution of frequency components and a spectral width related to the duration of the pulse.  The width
of the cube along any axis may therefore be varied either by adjustment of
the selective RF pulse length, or by adjustment of the size of the respective field gradient.  Let us consider the effect on the spatial distribution
of Z magnetization following each of the experiments in Table 1.  We can
readily see the effect of the pulse train by considering three planes of
spins, corresponding to a plane above the desired cube, a plane below the
cube, and the central plane containing the cube.  Figure 9 shows the three
planes diagramatically, and each plane has been further divided into three
rows and three columns, corresponding to rows either side and including the
cube along the Y axis, and columns either side and including the cube along
the X axis.  The cube to be localized is therefore represented by the center
square of the center plane, and each square we can assume has an equal net
spin magnetization of unity.

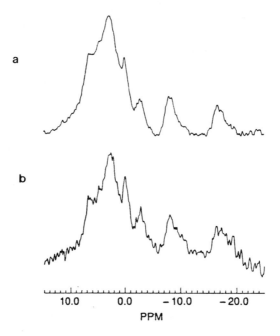

Figure 7

(a) The $^{31}P$ spectrum of a human brain at 27.4MHz acquired using
the full response of a 10cm diameter surface coil positioned over
the fronto-parietal suture. The repetition rate was 2 seconds and
the number of scans 256. Peak assignments are the same as for
Figure 2.

(b) The $^{31}P$ spectrum of a disc-shaped plane within a human brain
obtained using the subtraction method. The vertical scale is
expanded by a factor of two with respect to Figure 7(a).

Table 1

Experimental sequence of selective RF pulses applied during

the preparation period

| Experiment Number | X Selective Pulse | Y Selective Pulse | Z Selective Pulse | Contribution to Total Spectrum |
|---|---|---|---|---|
| 1 | OFF | OFF | OFF | +1 |
| 2 | ON | OFF | OFF | −1 |
| 3 | OFF | ON | OFF | −1 |
| 4 | ON | ON | OFF | +1 |
| 5 | OFF | OFF | ON | −1 |
| 6 | ON | OFF | ON | +1 |
| 7 | OFF | ON | ON | +1 |
| 8 | ON | ON | ON | −1 |

OFF refers to the absence of a selective pulse, and ON refers to the application of a selective pulse of sufficient power to cause 180° nutation.

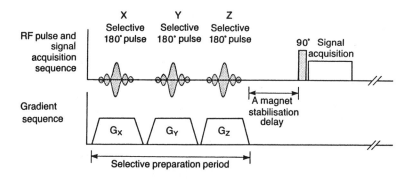

Figure 8

RF pulse and magnetic field gradient sequences for the ISIS experiment. Selective inversion of three orthogonal slices is shown
during the preparation period (i.e., Table 1; experiment 8). All
other experiments in the ISIS sequence may be constructed by omis-
sion of one or more of the selective inversion pulses.


The spin nutation angles for the X, Y and Z selective pulses are
defined as $\alpha$, $\beta$ and $\gamma$, and the measured signal during the subsequent acquisition period has the magnitude and sign of the residual Z magnetization
following the selective preparation pulse train. We can also assume that
any XY components excited by application of the selective pulses dephase
either between pulses or before signal acquisition. The residual Z magnetization is simply the product of the cosines of the individual nutation
angles experienced during the preparation period by the spins in the various
regions of the sample. Figure 9 therefore shows the three dimensional
signal distribution in each of the eight experiments, that will appear upon
investigation by a subsequent nonselective 90° pulse.

In order to achieve the desired localization, a linear combination of
the eight sets of data must be sought in which all signals cancel except in
the selected cube. For the areas in the sample indicated in Figure 9 by
shaded squares the total signal is:

$$(C_1+C_3) + (C_2+C_4)\cos \alpha + (C_5+C_7)\cos \gamma + (C_6+C_8)\cos \alpha .\cos \gamma$$

where $C_i$ denotes the coefficient of the ith experiment in the linear combination of the data from all eight experiments. Expression[1] is zero for all
values of $\alpha$ and $\gamma$ when

$$C_1 = C_4 = C_6 = C_7 = +1$$

and

$$C_2 = C_3 = C_5 = C_8 = -1$$

as indicated in the last column of Table 1.

Inspection shows that with this linear combination of the eight experiments of Figure 9, the signals cancel in all squares except in the one
corresponding to the selected cube. This cancellation occurs independent of
the values of $\alpha$, $\beta$ or $\gamma$ and therefore the residual signal must always come
from the central cube. A further consequence of this cancellation property
is that the technique may be used in combination with RF coils which have a
highly non-uniform RF distribution and intensity, e.g., surface coils. The

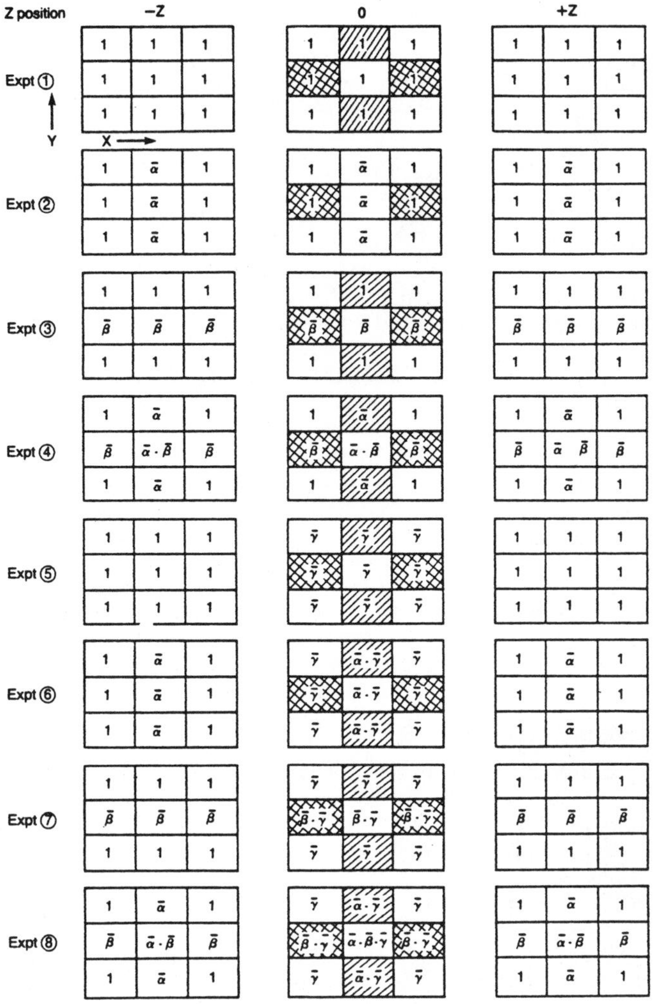

Figure 9

Matrices representing three dimensional space and showing planes of material below, including and above the selected cube. Each plane is further divided into rows and columns on either side and including the volume of interest. The selected cube is therefore the central region of the center plane, and the diagram shows the Z magnetization in the different regions following the preparation periods of the eight experiments of Table 1. $\bar{\alpha}$, $\bar{\beta}$ and $\bar{\gamma}$ represent cos α, cos β and cos γ respectively, and therefore $\bar{\alpha}.\bar{\beta}.\bar{\gamma}$ represents the product of these three cosines.

114

overall signal intensity I, from the linear combination of all eight experiments is given by:

$$I = 1 - \cos \alpha - \cos \beta + \cos \alpha . \cos \beta - \cos \gamma + \cos \alpha . \cos \gamma + \cos \beta . \cos \gamma - \cos \alpha . \cos \beta . \cos \gamma$$

If $\alpha = \beta = \gamma = 180°$ then I = 8, and the overall signal is eight times the signal contribution from the central cube in a single data acquisition, which is equivalent to a signal average of eight performed on the central cube in isolation. The selected volume may be easily moved in three-dimensional space along any direction by either adjustment of the spatial position of the gradient zero-crossing point, or more conveniently, by adjustment of the RF frequency carrier during the respective selective RF pulse. In this manner, the desired location for the selected cube may be encoded as three frequency offsets corresponding to the three spatial axes. A standard NMR image provides spatial information encoded along two orthogonal frequency axes, therefore, the position of the cube can be easily selected by reference to the NMR image.

In Figure 10, an image is reproduced of a cross sectional slice through the lower leg midway between knee and ankle. Figure 10(a) shows the total spectrum of the volume of leg within the field of view of the RF coil. The

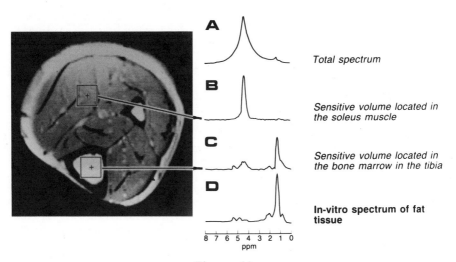

A    Total spectrum

B    Sensitive volume located in the soleus muscle

C    Sensitive volume located in the bone marrow in the tibia

D    **In-vitro spectrum of fat tissue**

8 7 6 5 4 3 2 1 0
ppm

Figure 10

An 80 MHz proton image of a cross sectional slice through the lower leg midway between knee and ankle, with the overall spectrum shown in (A). The ISIS proton spectrum of soleus muscle is shown in (B), and the ISIS proton spectrum of bone marrow in the tibia is shown in (C). Proton resonances arise from fatty acid (-HC=CH-) (I), water (II), fatty acid $(-CH_2-)_n$ (III), and fatty acid ($-CH_3$) (IV). The ISIS spectra are plotted at a scale which is two orders of magnitude larger than that of the total spectrum. The spectrum shown in (D) is a 100 MHz proton spectrum of fat tissue obtained <u>in vitro.</u> (Reproduced by permission from Reference 14.)

spectrum from a cube of material positioned within the soleus muscle is shown in Figure 10(b), and the spectrum in Figure 10(c) was obtained from a cube positioned within the bone marrow of the tibia. The position of the cubes are indicated by boxes superimposed on the standard image. The volume of each cube is $4.1 cm^3$. Approximately 1% of the total signal is derived from material within each of the selected cubes. The overall spectrum A shows only two signals which originate from water (II) and the protons in fatty acid chains (III). In the spectrum of the muscle in Figure 10(b) the latter peak has virtually disappeared. In the bone marrow spectrum of Figure 10(c), the water signal (II) is greatly reduced and several signals are visible from fatty acid chains. These are the protons in unsaturated bonds at 5.4 ppm (I), the protons in saturated bonds between 2.3 and 1.2 ppm (III), and the protons in terminal methyl groups at 0.8 ppm (IV). For comparison, reproduced in Figure 10(d) is the _in vitro_ spectrum of fat tissue from Reference 14.

The ISIS method can also be extended to other nuclei, e.g., to $31P$ NMR spectroscopy on living systems. Proton NMR images are still required to provide spatial information of the specimen in order to select the position of the cube. However, by multiplying the gradient magnitudes for the ISIS technique by the ratio of the magnetogyric constants of hydrogen and the nucleus under investigation, the frequency encoding evaluated by spatial positioning in the proton image, is still valid for localization of the cube for spectroscopic examination of any desired nucleus. Furthermore, the cube is the same size at both resonant frequencies. The only assumptions are that the water signal is on-resonance during the imaging experiment, and for spectroscopy the carrier frequency is centered in the spectrum of the resonant nucleus.

Spatial selection is effectively independent of RF nutation angle, however, S/N ratio obviously deteriorates as the RF pulses vary from either their 180° or 90° conditions. The selective 180° pulses can be generated using an amplitude and phase waveform proposed by Silver et al.[15] This has the tremendous advantage that selective inversion of the spin population occurs over an extremely wide range of RF pulse powers although the pulse length required is quite long. If the non-selective 90° read pulse is also replaced by an adiabatic half-passage pulse,[16] the ISIS method can be implemented to obtain ideal S/N ratio with virtually no dependence upon RF pulse power, making the technique very easy to apply.

Other methods of spatial localization using selective pulses and field gradients have been proposed and demonstrated by Bottomley et al. (DRESS technique), and Aue et al. (VSE method). In the DRESS technique a disc of material is selectively excited parallel to the surface coil by the use of a selective 90° pulse. Signal from this layer is then sampled in the absence of field gradients. Several _in vivo_ phosphorus spectra have been obtained by this method,[17] however, spatial selectivity is limited in two dimensions by the size of the surface coil.

The VSE method[18] has a capability for spatial selection similar to ISIS, however, it relies on the destruction of Z magnetization in all volumes around the desired cube prior to data acquisition. This feature of the technique necessitates very high power radio frequency pulses. Another method of spatial localization is chemical shift imaging,[19] however, this requires a long experimental time, and the final images, which map out the distribution of each chemically shifted resonance, show a strong dependence upon T2 value.

# CONCLUSION

Spatial localization for NMR spectroscopy can be achieved by a large variety of techniques. The problems of sensitivity for nuclei with low metabolic concentrations has meant that surface coils have found widespread application. Recent NMR techniques have therefore concentrated on refining the spatial response of surface coils by the use of multiple RF pulses and magnetic field gradients. The most versatile techniques which allow the operator to actually select the volume of interest, will ultimately prove to be the most useful. Techniques similar to ISIS and VSE should, therefore, find most widespread application in future NMR research in the fields of medicine and biology.

# ACKNOWLEDGEMENTS

The authors would like to thank all members of Oxford Research Systems for their support with hardware and software, and M. R. Bendall for several useful discussions.

# REFERENCES

1. J. J. H. Ackermann, T. H. Grove, G. G. Wong, D. G. Gadian, and G. K. Radda, Nature 283:167 (1980).
2. R. E. Grodon, Phys. Med. Biol. 30, No. 8, 741 (1985).
3. M. R. Bendall and R. E. Gordon, J. Magn. Reson. 53:365 (1983).
4. M. R. Bendall and W. P. Aue, J. Magn. Reson. 54:149 (1983).
5. M. R. Bendall, Chem. Phys. Lett. 99:310 (1983).
6. M. R. Bendall, J. M. McKendry, I. D. Cresshull, and R. J. Ordidge, J. Magn. Reson. 60:473 (1984).
7. T. C. Ng., J. D. Glickson, and M. R. Bendall, J. Magn. Reson. 1:450 (1984).
8. S. J. Cox and P. Styles, J. Magn. Reson. 40:209 (1980).
9. A. Haase, C. Malloy, and G. K. Radda, J. Magn. Reson. 55:164 (1983).
10. J. C. Haselgrove, V. H. Subramanian, J. S. Leigh, L. Gyulai, and B. Chance, Science 220:1170 (1984).
11. A. J. Shaka, J. Keeler, M. B. Smith, and R. Freeman, J. Magn. Reson. 61:175 (1985).
12. R. J. Ordidge, M. R. Bendall, R. E. Gordon, and A. Connelly, "Magnetic Resonance in Biology and Medicine," (Govil, Khetrapal and Saran, Tata, eds) McGraw-Hill, New Delhi, India (1985).
13. R. J. Ordidge, A. Connelly, and J. A. B. Lohman, J. Magn. Reson., to be published.
14. R. E. Gordon, Ph.D. Thesis, Aberdeen University (1975).
15. M. S. Silver, R. I. Joseph, and D. I. Hoult, J. Magn. Reson. 59:349 (1984).
16. T. Farrar and E. Becker, "Pulse and Fourier Transform NMR," Academic Press, London (1971).
17. P. A. Bottomley, L. S. Smith, W. M. Leue, and C. Charles, J. Magn. Reson. 64:347 (1985).
18. S. Muller, W. P. Aue, and J. Seelig, J. Magn. Reson. 63:530 (1985).
19. A. A. Maudsley, S. K. Hilal, W. H. Perman, and H. E. Simon, J. Magn. Reson. 51:147 (1983).

# THE USE OF NUCLEAR MAGNETIC RESONANCE ROTATING FRAME EXPERIMENTS

# FOR ONE DIMENSIONAL DISCRIMINATION OF METABOLITES IN TISSUES

Gerald B. Matson[+], Thomas Schleich[*,+], Michael Garwood[*],
Ronald T. Bogusky[#], and Larry Cowgill[†]

[+]NMR Facility
University of California
Davis, CA 95616

[*]Department of Chemistry
University of California
Santa Cruz, CA 95064

[#]Department of Internal Medicine
School of Medicine
University of California
Davis, CA 95616

[†]Department of Medicine
School of Veterinary Medicine
University of California
Davis, CA 95616

## INTRODUCTION

Over the last decade nuclear magnetic resonance spectroscopy (NMR) has emerged as the premier tool for the non-invasive study of tissue metabolism and its regulation, for examining cellular energetics, for monitoring physiologically relevant metabolic events, and for the assessment of tissue viability (1-11). This emergence to a position of prominence has occurred despite several restrictions inherent to the technique: observation is limited to NMR-active nuclei such as $^1H$, $^{19}F$, $^{31}P$, $^{23}Na$, $^{13}C$, $^{15}N$, and $^{39}K$, present in low molecular weight compounds or ions and existing unbound in the tissue milieu, and for the most part at concentration levels exceeding 0.1 mM. Despite these restrictions, NMR spectroscopy has become an extremely powerful tool by virtue of its ability to measure steady state metabolite levels and elucidate metabolic pathways and controls; to monitor intracellular pH; to assess reaction rates and cellular fluxes using specialized NMR techniques; and to perform these experiments in non-invasive, and hence a non-destructive, manner. The important movement of this research to _in vivo_ experiments in animals has been facilitated by the recent development of wide bore, superconducting NMR magnets.

119

For many in vivo NMR applications the region of interest is still more restricted than the active volume of the surface coil, and a variety of experimental techniques have been developed to further localize or limit the region of tissue giving rise to the NMR spectrum. Magnetic field profiling involves limiting the region over which the magnetic field has sufficient homogeneity to produce high resolution NMR signals (17). A class of experiments termed depth pulse techniques have been developed to take advantage of the nonuniform surface coil $B_1$ field to obtain a greater degree of signal localization than exists with the single pulse surface coil experiment (18), and analogous experiments have followed (19,20). Other localization techniques which can be accomplished with surface coils involve applying time-dependent field gradients or coupling switched magnetic field gradients (21) with selective excitation pulses (22). These techniques are referred to in this article as localization techniques as they yield a single spectrum from a volume more restricted than the active volume of the surface coil.

There is another class of experiments which may be referred to as discrimination experiments which provide a suite of spectra from discrete regions of tissue over the active volume of the NMR probe. Experiments in this latter class are related to imaging experiments with the important distinction that most imaging experiments do not retain the chemical shift information which is essential to spectroscopy. Examples include the spin echo - pulsed field gradient experiment demonstrated by the Chance group (23), and recently introduced experiments such as the utilization of gradients of constant magnitude (24), the use of a correlation type of pulse experiment to achieve chemical shift encoding (25), and spectroscopic imaging by projection reconstruction through inclusion of a frequency dimension (26). Disadvantages of these experiments include the need to achieve rapid gradient switching on the first two types of experiments, and less than optimal sensitivity, and the broadening of the spectral width (which can aggravate resonance offset effects), respectively, on the last two experiments. Still, the advantage of discrimination techniques is that they have the potential of acquiring spectra over a suite of localized regions in a time roughly comparable to that in which a localization experiment acquires one spectrum over a single, localized region.

This review focuses on yet another discrimination experiment developed by Hoult (27) and termed a rotating frame experiment. The rotating frame experiment achieves discrimination on the basis of a gradient in the $B_1$ field, and has the advantage that it can be implemented with surface coils to achieve discrimination in the direction of the surface coil $B_1$ field gradient (28,29). The surface coil rotating frame experiment is executed by collecting data files as a function of an incremented evolution pulse length. Double Fourier transformation of the data yields a suite of spectra termed a metabolite map (29), where each individual spectrum corresponds to metabolites within a section of tissue bounded by $B_1$ isocontour surfaces. The metabolite map thus indicates the topological distribution of metabolites along the direction of the $B_1$ gradient, termed the mapping dimension. For cases in which the desired result is a single section of tissue, certain improvements in the efficiency of the surface coil rotating frame experiment are possible (20). It is shown that these improvements may be viewed as altering the experiment to make it analogous to a depth pulse experiment.

REVIEW OF PERTINENT THEORY

Nuclear Signal Reception and Relaxation

A number of authoritative presentations of NMR theory have appeared in the literature (30-34), and this section highlights aspects of basic NMR theory pertinent to surface coil and rotating frame experiments. The absorption lines in NMR may be thought of as arising from magnetizations composed of nuclei precessing at the same frequency about the external polarizing magnetic field:

$$\Omega = \gamma(1-\delta)B_0.$$ (1)

The frequency of the particlar absorption line is given by $\Omega$, $\gamma$ is the nuclear gyromagnetic ratio for the nucleus under consideration, $\delta$ is the chemical shift for the nuclei in question, and $B_0$ is the external magnetic field. Spin couplings and other interactions are neglected in this simple review. The existence of nuclei in electronically distinct environments (i.e., chemically distinct) gives rise to absorption lines at different frequencies according to changes in the value of the chemical shift, $\delta$. The Fourier transform NMR experiment provides an RF pulse which tips or nutates the sample magnetizations away form their initial orientation along the z axis, which is defined by the direction of the external magnetic field. Following the application of the RF pulse, magnetization components within the plane perpendicular to the direction of the external field (the transverse plane) are detected by the NMR spectrometer. The degree of magnetization tipping is proportional to the strength of the rotating magnetic field produced by the RF, and to the duration of the RF pulse. As shown in Figure 1, the surface coil $B_1$ field is non-uniform, so the degree of nutation away from the z axis is spatially dependent:

$$\theta_i = \gamma B_{1i} t.$$ (2)

Here $\theta_i$ is the angle of nutation away from the direction of the external magnetic field at sample position i, $B_{1i}$ represents the strength of the rotating magnetic field perpendicular to the external field at the same sample position, $\gamma$ is the gyromagnetic ratio, and t is the duration of the RF pulse. The quantity $(1-\delta)$ is omitted from Equation 2 as the chemical shift, $\delta$, is always a very small number. For a single resonance line with magnetization $M_z$ aligned along the external magnetic field, the magnetization $M_s$ detected immediately following the tipping pulse is given by:

$$M_{si} = M_{zi}\sin\theta_i.$$ (3)

Again, the subscript i indicates that the magnetizations and the nutations are spatially dependent. The magnitude of the NMR signal would appear to be optimized by a nutation angle of $90^\circ$, and indeed this is the case for data accumulated with long repetition (or interpulse) times. However, signal intensity optimization with a surface coil clearly cannot be accomplished throughout the sample by a single pulse experiment. The detected magnetization $M_s$ decays with time, and the spectrometer collects the voltage induced in the NMR probe by $M_s$ as a function of the time. This signal, called a free induction decay or FlD, provides the magnitude and frequency of $M_s$, while the width of the resonance line is determined by the rapidity with which $M_s$ decays. Usually, the FlD is subjected to Fourier transformation to provide a spectral display of the resonance lines present.

The magnetization component along the external field, $M_z$, is altered by the application of the RF pulse. The z-component magnetization is usually assumed to grow back in an exponential fashion towards its thermal equilibrium value according to:

$$M_0 - M_z(T) = [M_0 - M_z(0)]\exp(-T_1/T),$$ (4)

The ability to apply NMR spectroscopic techniques to _in vivo_ experiments on animals has also been enhanced by the introduction of surface coils by Ackerman et al. (12). Because of their external placement, surface coils relieve the necessity of enclosing the entire body within an NMR probe. Since these coils are spatially selective, they also act to provide localization of the experiment in that only signals from sample regions in proximity to the surface coil (the active volume of the surface coil) are observed. Other surface coil advantages include the fact that, unlike a whole body NMR probe, the surface coil can be designed and optimized for the region or volume of tissue of interest. The excellent sensitivity of the surface coil derives in part from its good filling factor, which arises because of its proximity to the region to be examined. Finally, the localization afforded by surface coils also eases homogeneity constraints on the polarizing magnetic field, as only the region sensitive to the surface coil, rather than the complete body, is required to be in a region of homogeneous magnetic field.

Surface coils are not without their disadvantages; foremost among them is the poor $B_1$ field homogeneity associated with surface coils. A plot indicating the $B_1$ field gradient through a display of contour lines at constant $B_1$ field strength for a surface coil is provided in Figure 1. Successive isocontour lines as one proceeds away from the coil indicate regions of progressively weaker $B_1$ field strength. This figure shows that the $B_1$ isocontours are curved surfaces, such that successive isocontour surfaces define tissue volumes that have been compared to onion peels. In single pulse experiments the non-uniform field results in a diversity of magnetization tip angles throughout the sample, resulting in loss of signal and creating difficulties in quantifying the effects of $T_1$ discrimination (13). However, as discussed later, composite pulse schemes have the potential to create a uniform tip angle throughout the active volume, thus ameliorating the adverse effects arising from the $B_1$ field gradient (14-16).

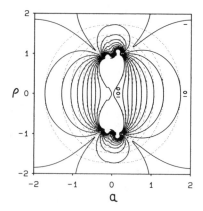

Fig. 1.    Calculated $B_1$ field (transverse plane component) isocontour lines generated by a two-turn surface coil. The radius of the second turn is 0.9 times that of the first turn, and its position is .25 of the large turn radius distal to the sample. The radial coordinate, rho, and the axial coordinate, a, are expressed in units of the large coil radius. The solid and dashed lines represent isocontours in planes parallel and perpendicular to the direction of the $B_0$ field, respectively. The calculated relative $B_1$ magnitudes are indicated, with successive isocontours incremented by units of 10. Taken from ref. 29.

where $M_O$ represents the equilibrium z-component magnetization, the time following application of the RF pulse is denoted by T, $M_z(0)$ and $M_z(T)$ represent the z-component magnetizations at times zero and T following the RF pulse, respectively, and $T_1$ is the longitudinal or spin lattice relaxation time for the z-component magnetization. Because of the low sensitivity of the NMR experiment, spectral accumulation is normally accomplished by scanning repetitively to take advantage of the increased signal-to-noise which occurs according to the square root of the number of accumulations. Straightforward application of theory (35) shows that the optimal signal collection efficiency occurs when the interpulse time is made short compared to $T_1$ and the nutation angle is adjusted according to:

$$\cos \theta = \exp (-T_r/T_1) \quad , \tag{5}$$

where $\theta$ is the nutation angle, and the interpulse time (the time between successive applications of the RF tipping pulse) is denoted by $T_r$.

Unfortunately, it is often difficult to assess with accuracy the relative metabolite levels from NMR data taken under conditions of optimal signal collection efficiency i.e., with a repetition time short compared to $T_1$. When long repitition times are utilized ($5T_1$), the sample magnetizations reach their equilibrium values prior to the tipping pulse, so that the quantity $M_{zi}$ in Equation 3 can be replaced by $M_{oi}$:

$$M_{si} = M_{oi} \sin \theta_i \quad . \tag{6}$$

Under conditions of uniform tipping, the resulting spectrum provides resonance areas proportional to the component thermal equilibrium magnetizations, and thus proportional to the relative number of nuclei observed. Experiments are often performed under these conditions in order to facilitate the reliable determination of relative metabolite levels. The drawback is that the experimental run time necessary to achieve acceptable signal-to-noise is considerably lengthened. On the other hand, under conditions of optimal signal collection efficiency (repetition time shorter than $T_1$) the resonance areas depend upon the component $T_1$ values as well as the number of nuclei, so that resonances arising from nuclei with long $T_1$ values have signal areas suppressed compared to resonance areas of short $T_1$ nuclei. An example of severe $T_1$ discrimination obtained with an NMR probe producing a relatively uniform $B_1$ field is shown in Figure 2. When both the nutation angle and the component $T_1$ values are known, the relative resonance areas can be corrected for the effects of $T_1$ discrimination. In principle, this holds true even for single pulse experiments performed with surface coils, although the spatial variation of the $B_1$ field must be known so that the nutation angle can be determined from Equation 2. The sample volumes associated with the different $B_1$ values must also be known, since the sensitivity of the coil to receiving transverse magnetization components is proportional to the $B_1$ magnitude. In practice, correction for $T_1$ discrimination in single pulse surface coil experiments is difficult, and cannot be accomplished at all when the metabolite levels or their $T_1$ values are also spatially dependent.

Under conditions of optimal signal collection efficiency, the effects of $T_1$ discrimination may be thought of as altering the signal intensity profile (signal intensity as a function of position) in single pulse surface coil experiments. The spatially dependent tipping angle conspires with the component $T_1$'s of the individual magnetizations to give signal intensity profiles which are dependent on experimental run parameters (RF pulse duration and repetition time). In general, the

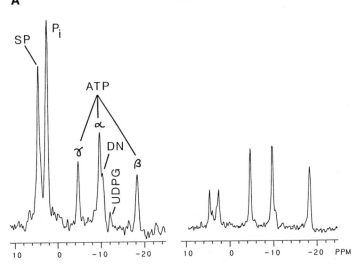

A          B

Fig. 2.    $^{31}$P- NMR spectra of rabbit lenses in organ culture acquired using (A) long (35 sec) and (B) short (.38 sec) repetition times. The spectra were scaled to one another by the beta-ATP resonance. Indicated in the figure are resonances from sugar phosphates (SP), inorganic phosphate (Pi), adenosine triphosphate resonances (ATP), dinucleotides (DN), and uridinediphosphoglucose (UDPG). Taken from ref. 36.

intensity maps show that the majority of the signal is received from sample located well within a coil radius of the surface coil center (37). Because metabolites with different $T_1$ values will have different signal intensity profiles, careful choice of spectrometer parameters, and prudence in interpretation are necessary in surface coil experiments.

In summary, the spatial dependence of the surface coil $B_1$ field creates nonuniform tipping over the sample volume, reducing the sensitivity of the experiment, and making it difficult to correct for effects of $T_1$ discrimination. These difficulties would be alleviated if uniform tipping over the sample volume could be achieved, and in the last section it is demonstrated that composite pulse schemes have the potential to accomplish this, and a preliminary pulse scheme is provided.

## The Rotating Frame Experiment with Surface Coils

The nutation of the sample magnetization away from its equilibrium orientation is accomplished by the component of the rotating magnetic field (produced by the RF pulse) that is perpendicular to the direction of the external magnetic field. This component, which has been designated $B_1$, is readily calculated for a circular surface coil (12,37). As shown in Figure 1, the $B_1$ field magnitude diminishes markedly with distance from the surface coil. Although the previous discussion has focused on the disadvantages associated with the spatial dependence of the surface coil $B_1$ field, a spatially dependent $B_1$ field is essential for the execution of a class of metabolite mapping experiments based on the rotating frame experiment (27). In effect, the rotating frame experiment operates by monitoring the magnetization nutational rate about the $B_1$ field. In practice, the experiment is performed by acquiring data sets at increasing, equally incremented values of the RF pulse duration, termed the evolution pulse. Fourier transformation of successive free induction decays (FIDs) yields a spectral data set containing resonance intensities which oscillate in an approximately sinusoidal fashion as a function of RF pulse duration. The frequency of this amplitude modulation depends upon the spatial location of the nucleus giving rise to the resonance signal. Thus, NMR active nuclei spatially disposed proximal to the coil in a large $(B_1)$ field give rise to a higher frequency of signal modulation than those located more distally, i.e., the frequency is dictated by the value of the spatially dependent $B_{1i}$ term. A standard two-dimensional Fourier transformation of the FID data set (34) produces a two-dimensional spectrum containing a separation of the component spectra according to their spatially dependent $B_1$ nutational frequencies, yielding a metabolite map of the tissue. The basic concepts of the metabolite mapping experiment are illustrated in Figures 3A, B.

In more quantitative terms the FID signal intensity from a particular sample region of a single resonance line resulting from an evolution pulse of length $t_1$ is given by (29):

$$S(t_1, t_2) \propto B_{1i} \sin (\Omega_1 t_1) \exp ( i\Omega t_2 - t_2/T_2) , \qquad (7)$$

where $t_1$ and $t_1$ are the evolution and detection periods, $\Omega_1$ and $\Omega$ are the nuclear nutational and precessional frequencies about the $B_1$ and $B_0$ fields, respectively, and any relaxation effects during the evolution pulse are ignored. $T_2$ is the experimental transverse relaxation time of the resonance line. From this equation it is apparent that if the evolution pulse width is incremented in an increasing fashion the signal amplitude from successive FIDs arising from a particular region oscillates sinusoidally as a function of $t_1$. The amplitude oscillation occurs with a frequency dictated by the spatially dependent $B_{1i}$ field strength, while each FID retains the chemical-shift information in $t_2$. Thus, the Fourier transform of $S(t_1, t_2)$ with respect to $t_2$ and $t_1$ results in a two-dimensional spectrum comprising the metabolite map. One axis of the metabolite map represents chemical shift , while the other represents the nutational frequency about $B_1$ $(\Omega_1)$. However, knowledge of the $B_1$ field allows the $\Omega_1$ dimension, termed the mapping dimension, to be identified

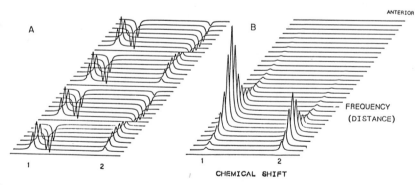

Fig. 3. Panel A: Simulated spectral set produced by Fourier transformation of hypothetical FIDs obtained through constant incrementation of the evolution pulse. The peak amplitudes vary in approximate sinusoidal fashion with evolution pulse duration, with the modulation for resonance 1 being double that of resonance 2. Panel B: Hypothetical two-dimensional NMR spectrum of Fourier transformation with respect to the pulse duration of the data set contained in panel A. Note that resonance 1 appears at higher frequency than resonance 2 along the frequency (distance) axis.

with sample volumes as outlined by particular $B_1$ isocontours (surfaces of constant $B_1$ magnitude). The coil is positioned anterior to the sample.

Figure 4 illustrates the metabolite map resulting from a one-dimensional rotating frame experiment applied to a phantom containing seven small capillary tubes spaced at equal intervals and centered on the axis of the surface coil. Each tube is filled with a small amount of sample, such that it represents a "point" source located on the axial coordinate. Because the surface coil $B_1$ field decrease is nearly linear along the axis of the coil (at least for dimensions well within one coil radius), the spectra in this case represent near linear mapping of the capillary tube positions from the center of the coil. The decreasing amplitude of signal from successive capillary tubes reflect the reciprocity of surface coils giving decreased signal reception proportional to the diminished $B_1$ strength. The actual resolution of the experiment is determined by the initial evolution pulse duration and number of evolution pulse increments (29). Advantages of the experiment include the fact that it is accomplished without the use of pulsed magnetic field gradients, and it retains the advantages inherent in surface coil experiments for _in vivo_ NMR studies.

Despite its attractive features, there are several potential problems with the rotating frame metabolite mapping experiment. Because the mapping dimension corresponds to successive $B_1$ isocontours, the mapping is non-linear with distance from the coil. Each spectrum of the metabolite map represents metabolites contained within a slice of tissue as outlined by successive $B_1$ isocontours, i.e., the sample volumes are curved about the coil. Intensity corrections to take into account not only the diminished coil sensitivity with decreasing $B_1$ field strength, but also the spatially dependent change in slice volume, as well as corrections for $T_1$ discrimination, must be applied in order to obtain relative metabolite concentrations. If the experiment is executed with short repetition time to achieve optimal signal collection efficiency, $T_1$ discrimination effects occur which manifest themselves through smearing in the mapping dimension, leading to a degradation in resolution as illustrated in Figure 5A. While such effects can be avoided by increasing the repetition time to $5T_1$, as shown in Figure 5B, such a procedure severely lengthens the experimental run time. Figures 6A, B illustrate the results of a more efficient approach which consists of applying a saturating burst of RF, i.e., a preparation pulse, prior to the application of the evolution pulse.

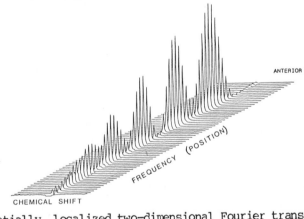

ANTERIOR

FREQUENCY (POSITION)

CHEMICAL SHIFT

Fig. 4. Spatially localized two-dimensional Fourier transform spectrum of 7 capillary tubes (1.5 mm diam.) containing 85% $H_3 PO_4$ spaced 4.4 mm apart along the surface coil axis. A two turn surface coil as described in Fig. 1 was used, with the large turn diameter of 4 cm. Taken from ref. 29.

126

A short delay between the preparation and evolution pulses allows the component magnetizations to partially regain their thermal equilibrium values. This technique maintains good experimental efficiency while avoiding the $T_1$ discrimination effect which leads to smearing. This experiment also allows the determination of spatially resolved metabolite $T_1$ values by the collection of metabolite maps with different delay times between the preparation and evolution pulses. The method is illustrated below.

A final, potential problem is that unless the nuclear nutational frequencies about the $B_1$ field are large compared to the frequency separations of the resonance lines from the carrier position, resonance offset artifacts can occur producing distortions in the metabolite positions in the mapping experiment. Composite pulse sequences have the potential to reverse this effect, as well as to provide additional benefits to the rotating frame experiment, and additional discussion of the advantages to be gained through incorporation of composite pulses is presented in the last section.

## Resolution and Run Time Considerations

For purposes of this initial discussion, we assume a sample of uniform metabolite concentration, an NMR probe which has uniform sensitivity over the sample, and a discrimination technique which selects out a suite of identical volumes in different parts of the sample. While these last criteria are not met rigorously for the surface coil rotating frame experiment, these criteria are approximately satisfied for adjacent volumes giving rise to sequential spectra in the metabolite map as long as the rotating frame experiment is accomplished at high resolution in the mapping dimension. It is well established that the signal-to-noise (S/N) is proportional to the number of spins being observed, and improves with the square root of the number of scans. Under the above criteria, the S/N ratio for a particular delineated volume will be linear with the size of the volume, leading to the result that the run time for acceptable S/N improves with the square of the delineated volume. That is, doubling the size of the delineated volume decreases the experimental run time by a factor of four (or halving the resolution in a three dimensional imaging

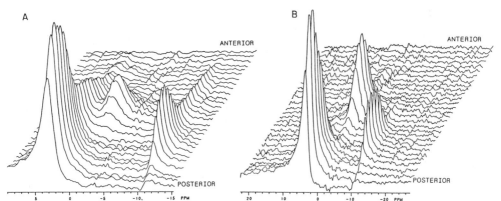

Fig. 5.    Spatially localized two-dimensional Fourier transform spectrum (metabolite map) of phosphorus metabolites contained in a human globe phantom. The anterior pole of the phantom was placed at the center of the coil. Panel A illustrates the smearing effect obtained by the use of a short repetition time relative to the metabolite $T_1$ values, and Panel B shows the disappearance of the smearing artifact upon lengthening the repetition time to a value long compared to $T_1$. Taken from ref. 29.

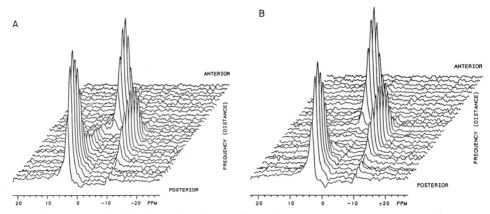

Fig. 6.    Spatially localized two-dimensional spectrum (metabolite map) of
the phantom used in the previous figure, but demonstrating the ability
of the preparation pulse described in the text to eliminate the
smearing artifact.    Panel A, which shows $T_1$ smearing, has no
preparation pulse, while Panel B demonstrates the elimination of the
smearing by including the preparation pulse sequence in the experiment.
Taken from ref. 29.

experiment decreases the run time by a factor of sixty four).

If the adjacent, delineated volumes are of small dimensions in the
mapping dimension, then the experiment may be said to be a high resolution
mapping experiment. The S/N of a high resolution mapping experiment may be
improved by adding the signals from adjacent volumes together, thus
simulating a lower resolution mapping experiment. However, the S/N
improves only with the square root of the number of added volumes, leading
to the result that adding signals from n adjacent or contiguous volumes
acquired in a high resolution mapping experiment still requires an
experimental run time of n times the lower resolution experiment to achieve
the same S/N. The point to be made is that the price paid for an
experiment accomplished with an unnecessarily high degree of resolution is
a large increase in the experimental run time. In general, for a rotating
frame experiment accomplished with N different evolution pulse lengths with
initial duration T, the resolution in nutational frequency is $1/NT$.
Translation from nutational frequency to tissue location can be
accomplished through knowledge of the $B_1$ gradient over the sample.

EX VIVO APPLICATIONS

The enucleated bovine globe is chosen to illustrate ex vivo
applications of the rotating frame experiment. The existence of discrete
ocular tissues within the globe makes it particularly suitable for
exploiting the one-dimensional discrimination provided by the rotating
frame experiment. The architecture of the bovine globe is indicated in
Figure 7 by way of a proton NMR image. The lens tissue, which is the
ocular tissue of greatest interest to us, is clearly evident in the proton
image. Figure 8 shows a tracing of the bovine globe proton image with
superimposed $B_1$ field isocontour lines of a two turn, circular surface
coil. This figure illustrates the variation of the $B_1$ field over the tissue
volume.

A $^{31}$P NMR spectrum obtained by use of a 3.8 cm diameter, two
turn, circular surface coil of an intact bovine globe is shown in Figure 9.
To obtain this spectrum the RF pulse duration was varied until a maximum in

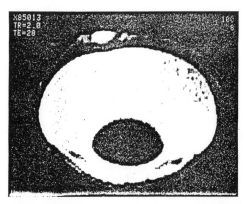

Fig. 7.  Proton image (sagittal view) of an enucleated bovine globe. The size and shape of the lens and its location within the globe are clearly evident. The image was made at the University of California at San Francisco Radiologic Imaging Laboratory on a 0.35 Tesla instrument with the assistance of Dr. L. Crooks and Mr. T. Bereito.

the signal-to-noise of the ATP resonances was obtained. The ATP resonances were chosen since the lens is known to have a high ATP content and occupies a significant volume of the globe. A negligible contribution from both aqueous humor (38,39) and virteous (39) to the intact globe spectrum is expected because of the low total phosphate levels including the absence of ATP. Resonances arising from sugar phosphate (SP), inorganic phosphate ($P_i$), GPC, ATP, dinucleotides (DN), uridinediphosphoglucose (UDPG), and an unknown resonance at 6.3 ppm are evident (13). ADP is apparent as a shoulder on the upfield side of the $\alpha$ -ATP resonance.

The question of individual ocular tissue contributions to the overall spectrum arises; this can be addressed by resorting to successive surgical ablation. When the bovine globe is rendered aphakic by surgical removal of the lens, the original ATP signal intensity (average of the $\alpha$ , $\beta$, and $\gamma$ resonances) is reduced by 71% as shown in Figure 9B; a substantial portion of the initial SP + $P_i$ contribution (54%) remains. Crucial to the success of this experiment is the insertion of a lens phantom filled with

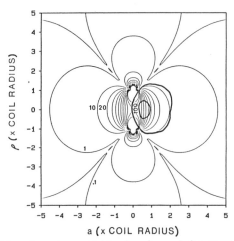

Fig. 8.  Outline tracing of the bovine globe proton image shown in Figure 7 with superimposed, calculated $B_1$ isocontours for a 3.8 cm diameter (large turn) two turn surface coil as in Figure 1. Only the lens outline is indicated within the globe.

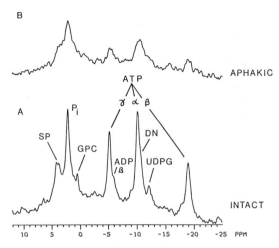

Fig. 9.     $^{31}$P  NMR  spectra  of  an  (A)  intact  and  (B)  aphakic bovine
globe, obtained with a 3.8 cm diameter surface coil as described in the
previous  figure.    A  glass  lens  phantom containing 120  mM  NaCl  was
inserted  into the lens cavity  and   the globe sutured to obtain spectrum
B.   Taken from ref. 13.


120 mM NaCl in the lens cavity  of  the globe prior to closure by suturing.
This  not only facilitates shimming of  the  aphakic globe, but also  helps
to  insure  dimensional  stability,  and  affords  a  means to preserve the
dielectric  and  conductivity  characteristics  of the tissue  sample.    The
latter are important factors  affecting  probe  tuning, and need to be kept
constant in order to keep from altering the S/N of the acquired spectrum.

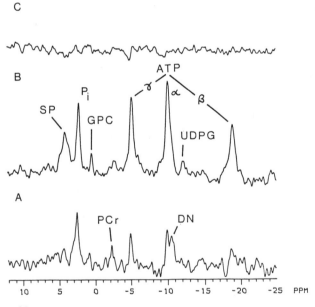

Fig. 10.     $^{31}$P  NMR   difference  spectra  representing  (A) cornea,  (B)
lens,  and (C) iris phosphorus metabolite contributions to  the  bovine
globe  spectrum.    Spectra were   obtained   by   subtraction of  the
appropriate surgically altered globe spectrum from the spectrum of  the
intact globe.  Taken from ref. 13.


130

Difference spectra representing individual tissue contributions acquired when the surface coil experiment is optimized for the lens compartment of the bovine globe are shown in Figure 10. The bovine iris contributes no detectable phosphorus containing metabolites (Figure 10C). Negligible contributions from both aqueous humor and vitreous to the intact globe spectrum are expected as noted above. The remaining signal arises from other ocular tissues such as the retina and choroid. The effect of surgical trauma on the phosphorus metabolite levels of bovine ocular tissue was shown to be small, during the time required to perform the above experiments, by pseudosurgery controls (13).

The significance of the rotating frame experiment is that it provides a means of assessing the metabolite concentrations of the various globe tissues without invasive surgery. As noted in the theory section, execution of the experiment with short repetition time leads to smearing in the mapping dimension due to $T_1$ discrimination effects. Our approach to circumvent the adverse effects of $T_1$ discrimination-induced smearing and still achieve reasonable signal collection efficiency is to apply a preparation pulse to eliminate all z-component magnetizations, followed by a delay, $D_1$, to allow for partial recovery of the magnetizations along the z axis prior to application of the evolution pulse. Our preparation pulse consists of a phase-cycling pulse sequence along each of the orthogonal axes of the rotating frame (40), thus effectively saturating all sample magnetizations.

Rotating frame experiments were performed on a Nicolet Magnetics spectrometer equipped with a 4.7 T widebore magnet, a Nicolet 293A' pulse programmer, and a Nicolet 1180 computer system. Data reduction was accomplished using a Nicolet 1280 computer system. Typical spectrometer parameters were: pulse width, variable; 2000 data points per FID; sweep width $\pm$ 4000 Hz (quadrature phase detection); repetition time, variable. The pulse sequence utilized was:

Low power, $[P1(x'),P1(y'),P1(-x'),P1(-y')]_2$, D1, high power, $P2(t_1)$, acquire.

$$(8)$$

The P1 pulse controls the saturating field of the preparation pulse, and is typically between 60 and 80 ms in length. D1 is the delay to allow for partial recovery from saturation, and $P2(t_1)$ is the evolution pulse with incremented duration $t_1$. Prior to placing the bovine glove in the globe holder, a capillary tube containing 1.0 M methylenediphosphonic acid (MDPA) was placed in the optic nerve to serve as a position marker. This compound exhibits a single resonance signal at 17.13 ppm, well outside the range of phosphorus-metabolite resonances usually encountered. The anterior pole of the globe is located at point 0,0 of the coil. Spectral accumulations (with a phase cycling saturation preparation pulse) were initiated within 4 hours of enucleation (29). Throughout the course of the 9 hour experiment, $0.5^0$ C air was blown over the globe to stabilize metabolite levels. The resulting two-dimensional spectral data set which represents a one-dimensional mapping of phosphorus-containing metabolites in the globe from posterior to anterior is shown in Figure 11. The most prominent resonances occur in slices containing the lens region. The phosphorus metabolite contributions noted above are apparent. A contour plot representation, which allows visualization of the SP region of the metabilite map, is shown in Figure 12. Of particular interest are the fluctuating amplitudes of the GPC and UDPG resonances which may signify differential contributions from lens anatomical regions (epithelium, cortex, and nucleus). $P_1$ is not present to any significant extent in the vitreous, but is abundant in the retina and choroid (13). Thus the SP +

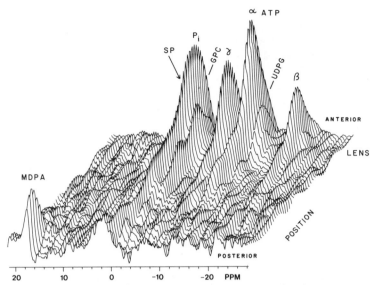

Fig. 11.    Metabolite map of the phosphorus metabolites present in an
enucleated bovine globe, taken with the surface coil described in Fig.
8. The anterior pole of the globe was placed at the coil center. A
capillary tube containing 1.0 M methylenediphosphonic acid (MDPA) was
placed in the optic nerve to serve as a position marker. Taken from
ref. 29.

$P_i$ contributions which appear beyond the lens region and before the
posterior pole in the metabolite map must arise from these latter tissues
which extend around the globe in an approximately hemispherical fashion.
Other posterior metabolite contributions include DN, and nucleoside
triphosphates (NTP). The resonances originating in the posterior of the
globe are poorly resolved and a pronounced reduction in signal intensities
occurs due to the lower $B_1$ field in this region. The anomalous phasing
present in the MDPA resonance is indicative of resonance off-set at the
globe posterior, the region of weakest $B_1$ field strength. As a result,
the MDPA resonances in the two-dimensional Fourier transformed spectrum
appear at higher frequencies (or shorter axial distances) than dictated by
the capillary's actual position in the sample. Resonance off-set effects
could be eliminated by the use of higher power RF pulses.

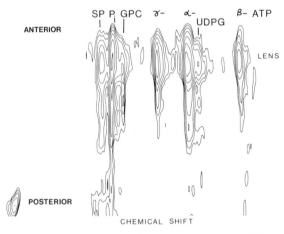

Fig. 12.    Contour plot representation of the metabolite map for the bovine
globe shown in Fig. 11. Taken from ref. 29.

132

An analogous spatial localization experiment utilizing the $^{23}$Na nucleus was performed on the enucleated bovine globe. In the eye, the lens has an approximately 8-fold lower Na$^+$ concentration than either the aqueous humor or vitreous, which are disposed anteriorly and posterior, respectively, to the lens (41). Interest in the Na$^+$ ion emerges from the fact that its increase in the lens is associated with the development of cataracts.

The one-dimensional $^{23}$Na$^+$ map of the bovine globe (42) is shown in Figure 13. The total time for this experiment was 6 minutes in contrast to the phosphorus metabolite map which takes considerably longer. As expected the lens region of the map is characterized by significantly lower Na$^+$ concentration. If the globe is allowed to "run down", changes in the Na$^+$ map are observed. The rapidity of the measurement makes it feasible for a variety of metabolic studies.

The use of a phase cycled saturating (preparation) pulse, followed by a delay prior to the application of the evolution pulse, forms the basis for the determination of spatially localized metabolite $T_1$ values. Such an experiment becomes feasible with $^{23}$Na$^+$ because of the short time required to generate a series of metabolite maps, each acquired with a different delay time between the preparation and evolution pulses. Spatially localized $T_1$ values can be determined from peak amplitudes in individual slices of the metabolite maps acquired with different delay times following the customary procedures employed in the evaluation of $T_1$ by saturation recovery.

A set of $^{23}$Na$^+$ ion metabolite maps of the bovine globe were acquired with different delay times between the preparation and evolution pulses to permit the assessment of $T_1$ values for Na$^+$ in the aqueous, lens, and vitreous of the eye. The $T_1$ values for Na$^+$ in aqueous, the lens, and the vitreous were found to be 45, 29, and 49 msec, respectively.

IN VIVO APPLICATIONS

The rat kidney is chosen to illustrate in vivo applications of the rotating frame experiment. Phosphorus-31 NMR spectroscopy has been

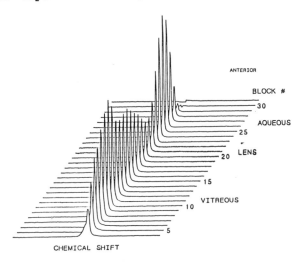

Fig. 13. Metabolite map showing the distribution of NMR-visible $^{23}$Na ions in an enucleated bovine globe.

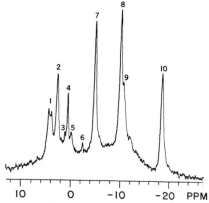

Fig 14.    $^{31}$P NMR spectrum of an _in vivo_  mouse kidney recorded
at 146 MHz using an elliptical, two turn surface coil. The
spectrum took 30 minutes to acquire. The resonance assignments
are: (1), SP; (2), Pi; (3), urine phosphate; (4), phosphodiesters;
(5), unidentified; (6) PCr; (7), gamma-ATP; (8), alpha-ATP; (9),
beta-ATP. Taken from ref 50.

utilized for the study of renal metabolism in both isolated perfused
(43-46) and intact kidneys (47-49). Emphasis has been directed principally
to the evaluation of high-energy phosphate metabolism and pH regulation in
renal tissue. Here we illustrate the utilization of rotating frame
experiments for $^{31}$P and $^{23}$Na NMR spectroscopy for the _in vivo_ study of
renal function in rats utilizing conventional high field NMR
spectrometers (50).

The basic strategy adopted (50) is to expose the kidney of an
anesthetized mouse or rat by means of a flank incision. The kidney is
supported outside the peritoneal cavity by insulated copper foil positioned
between the kidney and the external abdominal wall. The exposed kidney is
draped with plastic film to prevent drying. The animal is secured to a
non-metallic stage such that its kidney is positioned beneath a two-turn
elliptical surface coil.

Figure 14 depticts the $^{31}$P NMR spectrum of an _in vivo_  Swiss-Webster
mouse kidney obtained at 146 MHz by use of an elliptical surface coil (50).

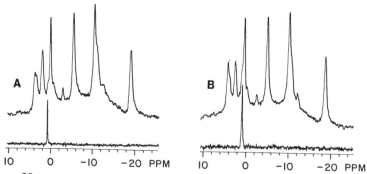

Fig. 15.    $^{31}$P NMR spectra of an _in vivo_ mouse kidney and bladder
urine. Kidney spectra (upper spectra, A and B) were acquired as in
Fig 14. Urine spectra (lower spectra, A and B) were acquired from ca.
1 ml of urine contained in a glass phantom placed adjacent to the
surface coil. Panel A: Before oral phosphate load; Panel B: Five hours
after oral phosphate load. Taken from ref. 50.

134

The spectrum reveals a phosphorus metabolite profile typical of intact tissue. Of particular interest is the assignment of resonance 3 to urine phoshate (50). This assignment was confirmed by comparing the in vivo mouse $^{31}$P NMR spectrum with the corresponding spectrum of its urine (Figure 15A). In addition, five hours after oral phosphate load the kidney spectrum of the mouse kidney was again compared to the $^{31}$P NMR spectrum of the accumulated urine (Figure 15B). The concentration of phosphate in urine changes from 37 mg/dl to 86 mg/dl, paralleling the change in intensity of the urine spectra. Thus, the urine phosphate resonance in the intact kidney spectrum increases with phosphaturia.

The application of the rotating frame experiment with surface coils for the spatial localization of phosphorus metabolites and the visualization of Na$^+$ within an intact organ under in vivo conditions was examined in the rat kidney employing the basic methodology described above (51). Experiments were performed on a Nicolet Magnetics spectrometer equipped with an Oxford Instruments 4.7 Tesla widebore magnet, a Nicolet 293A' pulse programmer and a Nicolet 1180 computer. Typical spectrometer parameters were: Pulse width, variable; 2000 data points per FID; sweep width +/-4000 Hz (Quadrature Phase Detection); repetition time, 2.2 sec for phosphorus and 0.3 for sodium. The number of data sets taken were either 16 or 18, yielding 8 or 9 actual slices through the sample. Because the data was zero-filled once or twice the number of individual spectra comprising a complete map were variable.

Male Sprague-Dawley rats (350-400 gms) were obtained from Simonson's Breeding Laboratories, San Jose, CA. Control rats were fed Purina$^R$ rat chow (0.4% sodium in the whole diet) and water ad libitum. A group of rats were made hypokalemic by feeding them a diet low in potassium for 14 days (0.1% potassium and containing 1% sodium in the whole diet). These rats also received 1 mg deoxycorticosterone acetate (DOCA) daily by subcutaneous injection. In addition, a solution of 0.9% NaCl was given to them as drinking water. Three days prior to the NMR study the saline drinking water was replaced by tap water. Thus, at the time of study sodium intakes of the potassium-depleted and control rats were approximately the same. Under these conditions serum potassium concentrations fell from $5.26 \pm 0.19$ (SEM) to $2.21 \pm 0.16$ mEq per liter (n=12) after 14 days of depletion (p=0.001 by students 't' test). Another group of rats was made acidotic by feeding them 1.5% NH$_4$Cl plus 0.2 M sucrose in their drinking water for seven days.

The rats were anesthetized with a single intraperitoneal injection of Inactin$^R$ (100 mg/kg body weight). The left flank of each rat was shaved and the left kidney exposed through a flank incision. The incision was loosely closed around the pedicle of the exteriorized kidney with a single ligature through the skin. Copper Faraday shielding was placed beneath the kidney to diminish resonance signals from the abdominal wall and the kidney was covered with Saran Wrap$^R$ to prevent drying. The rat was secured with tape to the plexiglass support of the NMR probe and the exteriorized kidney positioned next to the two-turn surface coil. Ambient temperature within the probe was maintained at 38$^o$ by heated air to keep the rat's body temperature constant.

Different regions within the kidney were identified from photographs of serial sections of kidney obtained with a microtome. The photographs were then converted into digitized computer images and superimposed on computer simulations of the B$_1$ field profiles of the surface coil used in the in vivo rat experiments (Figure 16).

The slices giving rise to the spectra in a metabolite map are depicted

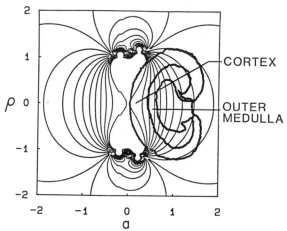

Fig. 16.    Calculated $B_1$ field isocontour lines generated by a two-turn surface coil with superimposed digitized saggital section of kidney. The large diameter of the coil is 2.2 cm and the second turn (dia. 2.0 cm) is 0.3 cm away from the first turn. The radial (p) and axial (a) coordinates are expressed in units of the large-coil radius. Taken form ref. 51.

in Figure 16. This figure also indicates that the slices further from the coil are larger, thus partially cancelling the decreased sensitivity of the coil which occurs proportional to the diminished $B_1$ field strength. The data have been taken under conditions of $T_1$ discrimination, so the relative levels of different metabolites within a slice do not follow directly from peak areas.    Figure 16 also indicates a disadvantage of the rotating-frame experiment implemented here, wherein the slices extend back to the coil, so that slices penetrating interior regions of the kidney also contain some contamination from more exterior regions. Because the thickness of the slice narrows as it approaches the coil, the contamination is not large. An indication of the level of contamination is provided below.

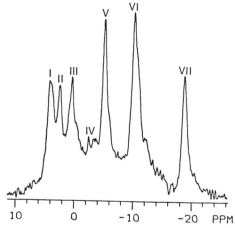

Fig. 17.    Phosphorus metabolites present in the _in vivo_ rat kidney. I: Sugar-phosphates and adenosine monophosphate; II: Inorganic phosphate; III: Glyceroylphosphorylcholine (GPC) plus urinary phosphate; IV: Phosphocreatine; V: Gamma-phosphate of ATP; VI: Alpha-Phosphate of ATP; VII: Beta-phosphate of ATP. This spectrum of _in vivo_ rat kidney was obtained using the surface coil of Fig. 16. Taken from ref. 51.

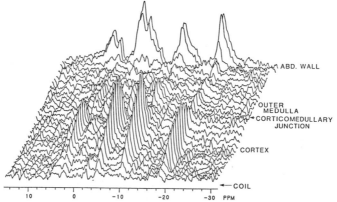

Fig. 18.    Phosphorus metabolite map of exteriorized kidney from normal
rats.  The phosphorus containing metabolites of in vivo rat kidney in
the  cortex and outer medulla are shown in the figure.  Identified also
are the corticomedullary junction  and  the  abdominal wall of the rat.
The  map demonstrates that the cortex contains the greatest  amount  of
ATP in the kidney.  Taken from ref. 51.

Phosphorus containing metabolite  resonances observable in the in vivo
rat kidney are shown in Figure 17 and a phosphorus metabolite map of normal
rat kidney is shown in Figure 18.   The  results  show that the metabolite
mapping  technique, although uncorrected for the fall in $B_1$ field  strength
along the axial distance from the  coil,  can readily identify the presence
of  two discrete anatomical regions within the in vivo kidney.   Figure  18
shows  resonances  immediately  adjacent  to  the  surface  coil  which are
contained  in  a homogeneous region that corresponds to the cortex of  the
kidney.  Adjacent to the cortex is another  anatomical region that contains
relatively  lower ATP levels than the cortex.  This region  corresponds  to
the outer  medulla of kidney.   The  metabolite  map  of  kidney  shows a
separation  between  the cortex and outer medulla at  the  corticomedullary
junction.  At the junction the  content  of ATP and inorganic phosphate are
lower than  in either adjacent region.  In fact, the levels indicated at the

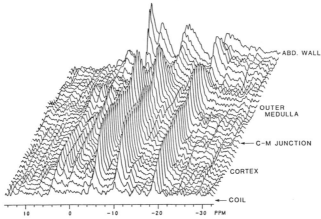

Fig. 19.    Phosphorus metabaolite map of kidney from potassium-depleted and
DOCA  treated rats.  The spectra show a decrease in inorganic phosphate
content of the cortex in treated  rats  compared to untreated controls.
The spectra also reveal an increase in ATP content of the outer medulla
in kidneys of treated rats  when  compared  to controls.  Identified in
the figure is the cortex, corticomedullary junction (C-M Junction), the
outer medulla and the abdominal wall of the rat.  Taken from ref. 51.

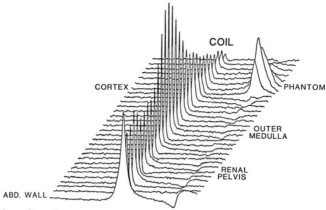

Fig. 20. Distribution of sodium present in the in vivo rat kidney. The figure shows that the highest content of sodium in the kidney can be found in the outer medulla. Identified in the figure is a resonance intensity standard containing 1M NaCl plus dysprosium tripolyphosphate. This standard is marked as PHANTOM in the figure. Also identified are the sodium resonances present in the cortex, outer medulla, renal pelvis and abdominal wall. Taken from ref. 51.

junction in the metabolite map may actually be dominated by cortex contamination because the slice through the corticomedullary junction also extends back through the cortex. These low levels provide an estimate of contamination by the cortex on inner slices. The highest contents of ATP and inorganic phosphate in kidney are present in the cortex with relatively lower levels appearing in the region of the outer medulla. The difference in ATP content between cortex and medulla confirms a previous report of ATP content of kidney obtained using standard invasive techniques (52). ATP resonances in the region of the inner medulla and papilla could not be detected at the present level of sensitivity. The spectra show that the tissue content of phosphocreatine is located largely in the cortex while glyceroylphosphorylcholine was found to be higher in the outer medulla than in the cortex. This observation confirms a previous NMR measurement of glyceroylphosphorylcholine in kidney tissue (53). The intracellular pH, determined from the chemical shift of inorganic phosphate, in the renal cortex and outer medulla of control rats was found to be $7.37 \pm 0.02$ (n=4). A map of the sodium ion distribution within kidney was also obtained. The

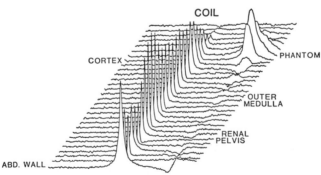

Fig 21. Sodium content of regions of kidney in potassium-depleted and DOCA treated rats. This figure shows the sodium content of the outer medulla of treated rats is less than in untreated controls despite similar sodium intakes at the time of experiment (compare to Figure 20). Taken from ref. 51.

results show that in control kidneys sodium is concentrated to its highest levels in the outer medulla (Figure 19).

The phosphorus metabolite map from DOCA treated and potassium-depleted rats is strikingly different from that of control rat kidney. (Figure 20). The proportion of ATP present in the outer medulla versus the cortex in these kidneys was greatly increased when compared to the proportion of ATP in outer medulla versus the cortex in untreated controls. Also observed was a decrease in tissue inorganic phosphate relative to the ATP content of cortex in kidneys from potassium-depleted rats. Inorganic phosphate content in the region of the outer medulla was not decreased relative to the ATP content in these kidneys. The cortex probably contributes to the resonance signals present in the region of the outer medulla; however, the level of contribution is probably small because the inorganic phosphate levels demonstrate two distinct and easily recognized anatomical regions present in these kidneys. Intracellular pH of cortex and medulla in kidney from potassium-depleted rats was 7.15 $\pm$ 0.02 (n=4) while systemic pH was 7.61 $\pm$ 0.04 and serum bicarbonate was 38 $\pm$ 0.04 mEq/l (n=4). The spectra demonstrate that levels of glyceroylphosphorylcholine present in the outer medulla are increased in these kidneys when compared to untreated controls. This confirms a previous study that reported an increase in glyceroylphosphorylcholine synthesis in the medulla of potassium-depleted rat kidney (54). Resonances from regions furthest from the coil may have large contributions from the cortex; therefore, no interpretation of metabolic events occurring in inner medulla and papilla of these kidneys can be made. The absolute sodium content of outer medulla is lower in kidneys of potassium-depleted rats than that of control kidneys (Figure 21). This observation may be related to the well known renal sodium concentrating defect that occurs during potassium depletion.

The phosphorus metabolite map of kidney form $NH_4Cl$-fed rats was also different from controls (Figure 22). Kidneys from $NH_4Cl$-fed rats show an increase in ATP content in the region of the outer medulla when compared to untreated control kidneys. Intracellular pH of the renal cortex was 7.24 $\pm$ 0.05 while the pH of the outer medulla was 6.95 $\pm$ 0.03 (n=3). A map of the sodium resonances present in kidney of $NH_4Cl$ fed rats was not different from controls (not shown).

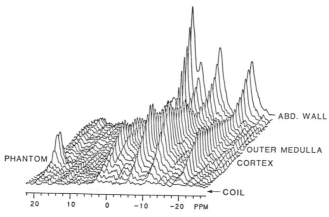

Fig. 22. Phosphorus metabolite map of kidney from $NH_4Cl$-fed rats. The spectra show an increase in ATP content of the outer medulla of kidney when compared to normal controls. The spectra also show a phantom containing methylenediphosphonic acid placed on the cortical surface of the kidney. Taken from ref. 51.

## In Vivo Summary

An important goal for the biological application of nuclear nuclear magnetic resonance is to be able to obtain spectra from known regions of tissue. The one-dimensional metabolite mapping experiments presented here represent an important first step towards that goal. The metabolite maps obtained using NMR rotating frame experiments were accomplished with surface coils. These experiments retain the advantages of high sensitivity inherent with surface coils for in vivo studies and are accomplished without recourse to switched field gradients. In addition, they are capable of high resolution in the mapping dimension. In present experiments with the in vivo rat kidney the anatomical structures observed in the mapping dimension were verified by superimposing photographs of successive slices through the kidney to computer simulations of the $B_1$ field profiles of the coil used to obtain the spectra. Surface coil rotating frame experiments have been employed previously to profile the phosphorus metabolites of phantoms (28,29) and the enucleated bovine globe (29). Here we have reviewed in vivo applications of this technique to measure pH, ATP and sodium content in the kidney of a rat and illustrate its utilization to follow alterations as a result of potassium-depletion and chronic metabolic acidosis (51).

## EXTENSIONS AND FUTURE DIRECTIONS

### Rotating Frame Experiment Modifications

One of the disadvantages of the rotating frame experiment as described in this article is that the experiment nutates magnetizations in a plane containing the z axis, while the spectrometer collects only the transverse components of these magnetizations. Thus, the experiment is not collecting the data at optimal efficiency. The section below on composite pulses makes the point that, if the nutated magnetizations could be transferred to the transverse plane for data collection, the run time of the experiment would be improved by a factor of two (27). Here we indicate that if only a single tissue region is of interest, as opposed to the complete map, then some increase in efficiency is possible without resorting to composite pulses.

In general, the nutational frequency resolution, in Hertz, of a rotating frame experiment performed with N different evolution pulse lengths of inital duration T is 1/NT. Translation from nutational frequency to tissue location is accomplished through use of the calculated $B_1$ isocontours over the sample. The desired resolution of the experiment thus sets the length of the longest evolution pulse, NT. The length of the initial evolution pulse, T, must be short enough to capture the highest nutational frequency, or Nyquist frequency in the mapping dimension, as given by 1/2T. Even when only a limited region of tissue is of interest, the entire volume of tissue seen by the surface coil must be taken into consideration in order to choose proper values of N and T, so that signals from unwanted regions do not aliase into the region of interest.

When the end result is to be a single spectrum from a particular region of the tissue, then the values of N and T may be re-adjusted slightly to maximise the number of times that the magnetizations corresponding to the center of the region of interest would be nutated through an integer multiple of 180 degrees by the evolution pulse. It can be shown that the data files in which the center magnetizations are nutated a multiple of 180 degrees would not be utilized in the workup of the desired spectrum; thus, these files may be omitted from the data set to improve the data collection efficiency of the experiment.

In its limit, this version of the rotating frame now consists of applying evolution pulses to nutate the magnetizations in the region of interest through 90 degrees, 270 degrees, 450 degrees, etc. Moreover, the data sets from sequential evolution pulse lengths are alternately added and subtracted, and the frequency width of the region of interest is governed by the number of different evolution pulses used. In this version, the rotating frame experiment has some of the characteristics of a depth pulse experiment (18). Additional details of this approach have been recently reported (20).

Fourier transformation of the data in the mapping dimension leads to a representation of the data in terms of multiples of the resolution frequency, $1/NT$, discussed above. This may prove restrictive if the center of the region of interest is not centered about a multiple of $1/NT$, or if the width of the region of interest in Hertz is not a multiple of $1/NT$. Some additional flexibility in the presentation of the data can be obtained through use of what we term a Fourier series window (FSW) function to process the data in the mapping dimension (20). To understand the FSW approach, we first consider a line in the spectrum resulting from the Fourier transformation of a data file in the chemical shift $(t_2)$ dimension. From the viewpoint of the Fourier transform approach, this spectral line resulting from the $n^{th}$ evolution pulse may be written as:

$$S(nT) = \sum_k M(\Omega_k) \sin(\Omega_k nT),\qquad(9)$$

where $S(nT)$ represents the spectral line, and $M(\Omega_k)$ represents the signal magnitude associated with the nuclear spins which nutate about the $B_1$ field with frequency $\Omega_k$. Included in $M(\Omega_k)$ are such effects as coil reciprocity, slice volume metabolite concentration, and degree of $T_1$ discrimination. The set of frequencies are given by

$$\Omega_k = 2\pi k/T; \quad k = 1 \text{ to } (N+1)/2,\qquad(10)$$

where it is assumed that N is odd. In the usual data workup, the data are Fourier transformed in the mapping $(t_1)$ dimension to recover the $M(\Omega_k)$ associated with the nutational frequencies $\Omega_k$. In the FSW approach, signal associated with $\Omega$ from $\Omega_1$ to $\Omega_2$ is selected according to

$$S(\Omega_1, \Omega_2) = \sum_n (CnT)S(nT),\qquad(11)$$

where the window coefficients are calculated from the equation

$$C(nT) = [2/n\pi][\cos(\Omega_1 nT) - \cos(\Omega_2 nT)],\qquad(12)$$

and the region from $\Omega_1$ to $\Omega_2$ represents the region of interest, so that the sum in Equation 11 picks out the contributions over just this frequency region. In practice it is the FIDs that are used in Equation 11, so that Fourier transformation of the sum in the $t_2$ dimension results in the metabolite spectrum over this (nutational) frequency region of interest. Repeated use of Equations 11 and 12 allows a single data set to be utilized for examination of multiple regions of tissue. While the FSW approach removes the restriction on representing the mapping dimension in terms of the frequencies $\Omega_k$, the resolution of the experiment is still given by $1/NT$.

The concept of omitting unnecessary evolution pulse lengths for improved data collection efficiency may be utilized with the FSW approach. The window coefficients $C(nT)$ corresponding to the region of interest may be calculated before the experimental data is collected, and the data sets corresponding to zero or very small values of the coefficients C(nT) simply omitted to improve the collection efficiency without degrading the resolution of the experiment in the mapping dimension. Additional information on these approaches is provided by reference 20.

## Implementation of Composite Pulses

Although the $B_1$ field inhomogeneity of surface coils is a prerequisite for accomplishing the rotating frame experiment, the inhomogeneity makes it difficult to perform experiments which require uniform nutation of the sample magnetizations. For instance, single pulse experiments with surface coils would be improved if the sample magnetizations could be nutated through 60 degrees throughout the sample. Composite pulses, which are a series of closely spaced, individual pulses, have the potential to create uniform magnetization nutations even when applied with a non-uniform $B_1$ field. Quite a variety of composite pulses have been developed recently to overcome the effects of $B_1$ inhomogeneity (14-16). An example of a composite pulse creating an approximately 60 degree rotation is shown in Figure 23, where the composite pulse sequence is:

$$P(45,-y')P(90,x')P(100,y')P(45,x')P(210,-y')P(40,-x'). \qquad (13)$$

The notation indicates that the first pulse is nominally a 45 degree pulse applied along the negative direction of the y' axis in the rotating frame.

As discussed previously in this review, the rotating frame experiment could be improved in efficiency if the nutated magnetizations could be rotated back into the transverse plane before data acquisition (27). The rotation would have to be equivalent to a rotation of the y'z plane into the x'y' plane in order to preserve the relative positions of the nutated magnetizations. We term such a rotation a faithful 90 degree rotation since it corresponds to a 90 degree rotation about a single axis for all of the sample magnetizations.

Our approach to this rotation has been to develop a modification of the 90 degree pulse developed by Levitt (14). While Levitt's pulse sequence performs properly for the z-component magnetizations, it disperses the transverse components. However, a simple modification of the Levitt sequence consisting of adding a 90 degree pulse about the negative y' axis transforms the sequence into one which produces a reasonably faithful 90 degree rotation over a moderate range of $B_1$ inhomogeneity. The basic sequence is thus

$$P(45,-y')P(90,-x')P(90,y')P(45,x')P90,-y'). \qquad (14)$$

Concatonation schemes (15) can be applied to improve the effectiveness of this basic sequence. Thus, the rapid development seen recently in pulses to produce uniform rotations even when applied with a non-uniform $B_1$ field makes it likely that these pulse schemes will be applied to the rotating frame experiment to improve its efficiency in run time by a factor of two.

## Localized Observation of Magnetization Perturbations

The rotating frame experiments described so far are executed with an evolution pulse applied with the sample magnetizations initially aligned along the direction of the external field. Thus, any preparation that leaves the magnetizations along the external field may be used as the starting point of the rotating frame experiment. Perhaps the simplest

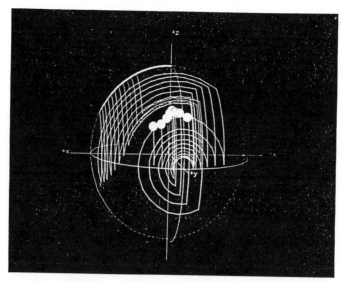

Fig. 23.    Computer graphics display showing the result of a composite
pulse scheme for generating a tipping pulse of ca. $60^0$ in an
inhomogeneous $B_1$ field.  The    lines    represent    the trajectory of
individual  magnetization vector tips on the surface of a unit  sphere.
The initial pulse spreads the magnetization  vectors out from along the
z axis into the x'z plane.  The rest of the pulse sequence collects the
vectors close to the y'z  plane  with  a  nearly uniform tipping angle.
The  tips of the final vector positions are filled circles for ease  of
identification.  The composite pulse sequence is described in the text.

example  to  consider  is  the    rotating    frame  longitudinal  relaxation
experiment described earlier in which the metabolite maps are generated   as
a function of the delay period between the preparation and evolution pulses
in  Equation  8.   This experiment represents a  recovery  from  saturation
experiment, so the  peaks  in  the  different  maps  can  be  analyzed as a
function  of  the delay  period  to generate  localized $T_1$ values.  This  is
the experiment  described  earlier to  obtain localized $T_1$ values of sodium
at different sections of the bovine globe.

    The inversion recovery technique  is a more efficient  way  to collect
$T_1$ information,  and  one  can  envision an  improved  experiment  using  a
composite inverting pulse as the preparation  pulse, and the resulting maps
generated as a function of the delay time become the data set for localized
$T_1$  by  the  inversion  recovery  technique.  A  related  experiment  is  a
localized  saturation  transfer  experiment,  in which the preparation  pulse
is  a  selective  saturation  pulse.  The  generation  of two maps with the
frequency  of  the  saturating  irradiation  placed  on the  resonance  to be
saturated,  and at a control  position,  respectively,  allows the maps to be
analyzed  to  show  localized saturation transfer.  In  fact,  preliminary
saturation transfer experiments of  this  type  have been performed by the
authors to show regional differences of saturation transfer in phantoms and
in tissue.

    Additional experiments are  suitable  for  utilization in place of the preparation pulse of the rotating frame experiment. Although the rotating frame experiment has been discussed in terms of initial magnetization preparation along the z-axis, a trivial modification in the data processing would allow the processing of experiments that prepared the magnetizations along an axis in the transverse plane. Thus, a spin echo experiment could be used for the magnetization preparation, presumably with composite pulses to compensate for the $B_1$ inhomogeneity of the surface coil. The evolution pulse would be applied at the time of the echo to obtain localized $T_2$ values, or, with the addition of pulsed magnetic gradients, even localized molecular diffusion (55). Other preparation experiments may be envisioned in which the sample magnetizations are perturbed in a particular way, and regional differences in the response to the perturbation sampled through the rotating frame experiment.

Summary

    The rotating frame experiment utilizing surface coils is a simple discrimination experiment that requires no special spectrometer capabilities such as RF pulse shaping or magnetic field gradient switching. As shown in this review, the technique can produce metabolite maps with high resolution in the mapping dimension to provide one-dimensional information on the topological distribution of metabolites in tissue. Modifications of the experiment are discussed to improve its data collection efficiency, or to observe regional differences in variables other than metabolite concentration or chemical shift position, such as relaxation or saturation transfer.

    Perhaps the single greatest disadvantage to the technique is the fact that the slices are bounded by the surface coil $B_1$ isocontours, giving them an onion peel shape. One technique to reduce the extent of the slice is to incorporate two coils of different diameters into the experiment (56), to acheive results similar to those that have been demonstrated for depth pulses (57). Another approach could be to include volume selection in directions other than the mapping dimension through gradient switching experiments. The experiment would then be a combined volume selection and rotating frame experiment with the volume selection along two directions performed through some combination of selective irradiation in the presence of a magnetic field gradient. Other combinations are possible as well.

    The power of the rotating frame experiment, combined with its ease of execution and ability to be combined with other experiments, probably ensures that the surface coil version of the rotating frame experiment will be an important tool in the arsenal of NMR spectroscopy techniques utilized by the in vivo NMR spectroscopist for some time to come.

Acknowledgements: This review is based on a number of recent publications (13,20,29,36,50,51), as well as on work carried out in the laboratories of the authors. We thank Galo Acosta for his computer-generated slots of surface coil B1 isocontours, and James Willis for his contributions in some of the eye globe NMR experiments. The work reported here was supported in part by grants from the United States Public Health Service to T.S. (EY 04033) and to R.T.B. (AM 31531).

REFERENCES

1.  C.T. Burt, S.M Cohen, and M. Barany, Analysis of intact tissue with $^{31}$P NMR, Ann. Rev. Biophys, Bioengr. 8: 1-25 (1979).
2.  D.G. Gadian, G.K. Radda, R.E. Richards, and P.J. Seeley, $^{31}$P NMR in living tissue: The road from a promising to an important tool in

biology, in: "Biological Applications of Magnetic Resonance", R.G. Shulman, ed., Academic Press, New York, pp. 463-535 (1979).

3. T. Glonek, Applications of $^{31}$P NMR to biological systems with emphasis on intact tissue determinations, in: "Phosphorus Chemistry Directed Toward Biology", W.J. Stec, ed., Pergamon Press, Oxford, pp. 157-174 (1980).

4. D.P. Hollis, Phosphorus NMR of cells tissues, and organelles, in: "Biological Magnetic Resonance", L.J. Berliner and J. Ruben, ed., Plenum Press, New York, pp. 1-44 (1980).

5. I.K. O'Neill and C.P. Richards, Biological $^{31}$P NMR spectroscopy, Ann Reports NMR Spect. 10A: 134-236 (1980).

6. T. Glonek, C.T. Burt, and M. Barany, NMR analysis of intact tissue including several examples of normal and diseased human muscle determinations, in: "NMR in Medicine", R. Demadian, ed., Springer-Verlag, pp. 121-159 (1981).

7. A.I. Scott and R.L. Baxter, Applications of $^{13}$C NMR to metabolic studies, Ann. Rev. Biophys. Bioengr. 10: 151-174 (1981).

8. D.G. Gadian, "Nuclear magnetic resonance and its application to living systems", Clarendon Press, Oxford (1982).

9. R.A. Iles, A.N. Stevens, and J.R. Griffiths, NMR studies of metabolites in living tissue, Prog. NMR Spect. 15: 49-200 (1982).

10. D.G. Gadian, Whole organ metabolism studied by NMR, Ann. Rev. Biophys. Bioengr. 12: 69-89 (1983).

11. M. Barany and T. Glonek, Identification of diseased states by phosphorus-31 NMR, in: "Phosphorus-31 NMR, principles and applications", D.G. Gorenstein, ed., Academic Press, New York, pp. 511-546 (1984).

12. J.J.H. Ackerman, T.H. Grove, G.G. Wong, D.G. Gadian, and G.K. Radda, Mapping of metabolites by $^{31}$P NMR using surface coils, Nature 283: 167-170 (1980).

13. T. Schleich, G.B. Matson, J.A. Willis, G. Acosta, C. Serdahl, P. Campbell, and M. Garwood, Surface coil phosphorus-31 NMR studies of the intact eye, Exp. Eye Res. 40: 343-355 (1985).

14. M.H. Levitt, Symmetrical composite pulse sequences for NMR population inversion. I. Compensation of radiofrequency field inhomogeneity, J. Magn. Reson. 50: 95-110 (1982).

15. M.H. Levitt and R.R. Ernst, Composite pulses constructed by a recursive expansion procedure, J. Magn. Reson. 55: 247-254 (1983); A.J. Shaka and R. Freeman, Spatially selective radiofrequency pulses, J. Magn. Reson. 59: 169-176 (1984).

16. R. Tycko, H.M. Cho, E. Schneider, and A. Pines, Composite pulses without phase distortion, J. Magn. Reson. 61: 90-101 (1985); R. Tyko, Broadband population inversion, Phys. Rev. Lett. 51: 775-777 (1983).

17. P.E. Hanley, and R.E. Gordon, The use of high-order gradients to vary the spatial extent of $B_0$ homogeneity in a high resolution NMR experiment, J. Magn. Reson. 45: 520-524 (1981); R.E. Gordon, P.E. Hanley, and D. Shaw, Topical magnetic resonance, Prog. NMR Spect. 15: 1-47 (1982).

18. M.R. Bendall and D.T. Pegg, Theoretical description of depth pulse sequences, on and off resonance, including improvements and extensions thereof, Magn. Reson. Med. 2: 91-113 (1985); M.R. Bendall, Elimination of high-flux signals near surface coils and field gradient sample localization using depth pulses, J. Magn. Reson. 59: 406-429 (1984); M.R. Bendall, Surface coils and depth resolution using the spatial variation of radiofrequency field, in: "Biomedical Magnetic Resonance", T.L. James and A.R. Margulis, ed., Radiology Research and Education Foundation, San Francisco, pp. 99-126 (1984).

19. A.J. Shaka, J. Keeler, M.B. Smith, and R. Freeman, Spatial localization of NMR signals in an inhomogeneous radiofrequency field, J. Magn. Reson. 61: 175-180 (1985); R. Tycko and A. Pines, Spatial localization

of NMR signals by narrowband inversion, J. Magn Reson. 60: 156-160 (1984).

20. M. Garwood, T. Schleich, B.D. Ross, G.B. Matson, and W.D. Winters, A modified rotating frame experiment based on a Fourier series window function: application to in vivo spatially localized NMR spectroscopy, J. Magn. Reson. (in press).

21. K.N. Scott, Localization techniques for nonproton imaging or nuclear magnetic resonance spectroscopy in vivo, in: "Biomedical Magnetic Resonance", T.L. James and A.R. Margulis, ed., Radiology Education and Research Foundation, San Francisco, pp. 79-97 (1984).

22. P.A. Bottomley, T.B. Foster, and R.D. Darrow, Depth-resolved surface-coil spectroscopy (DRESS) for in vivo $^1$H, $^{31}$P, and $^{13}$C NMR, J. Magn. Reson. 59: 338-342 (1984).

23. J.C. Haselgrove, V.H. Subramanian, J.S. Leigh Jr., L. Gyulai, and B. Chance, In vivo one-dimensional imaging of phosphorus metabolites by phosphorus-31 nuclear magnetic resonance, Science 220: 1170-1173 (1983).

24. Y. Manassen and G. Navon, A constant gradient experiment for chemical-shift imaging, J. Magn. Reson. 61: 363-370 (1985).

25. J.F. Martin and C.G. Wade, Chemical-shift encoding in NMR images, J. Magn Reson. 61: 153-157 (1985).

26. P.C. Lauterbur, D.N. Levin, and R.B. Marr, Theory and simulation of NMR spectroscopic imaging and field plotting by projection reconstruction involving an intrinsic frequency dimension, J. Magn. Reson. 59: 536-541 (1984).

27. D.I. Hoult, Rotating frame zeugmatography, J. Magn. Reson. 33: 183-197 (1979).

28. A. Haase, C. Malloy, and G.K. Radda, Spatial localization of high resolution $^{31}$P spectra with a surface coil, J. Magn. Reson. 55: 164-169 (1983).

29. M. Garwood, T. Schleich, G.B. Matson, and G. Acosta, Spatial localization of tissue metabolites by phosphorus-31 NMR rotating-frame zeugmatography, J. Magn. Reson. 60: 268-279 (1984).

30. T.C. Farrar and E.D. Becker, "Pulse and Fourier transform NMR", Academic Press, New York (1971).

31. E.D. Becker, "High resolution NMR, theory and chemical applications", 2$^{nd}$ edition, Academic Press, New York (1980).

32. M.L. Martin, J.-J. Delpuech, and G.J. Martin, "Practical NMR spectroscopy", Heyden, Philadelphia (1980).

33. E. Fukushima and S.B.W. Roeder, "Experimental pulse NMR, a nuts and bolts approach", Addison-Wesley, Reading (1981).

34. O. Jardetzky and G.C.K. Roberts, "NMR in molecular biology", Academic Press, New York (1981).

35. E.D. Becker, J.A. Ferretti, and P.B. Gambhir, Selection of optimum parameters for pulse Fourier transform nuclear magnetic resonance, Anal. Chem. 51: 1413-1420 (1979).

36. T. Schleich, J.A. Willis, and G.B. Matson, Longitudinal ($T_1$) relaxation times of phosphorus-metabolites in the bovine and rabbit lens, Exp. Eye Res. 29: 455-468 (1984).

37. A. Haase, W. Hanicke, and J. Frahm, The influence of experimental parameters in surface coil NMR, J. Magn. Reson. 56: 401-412 (1984); J.L. Evelhoch, M.G. Crowley, and J.J.H. Ackerman, Signal-to-noise optimization and observed volume localization with circular surface coils, J. Magn. Reson. 56: 110-124 (1984).

38. J.H. Prince and E. Eglitis, The crystalline Lens, in: "The Rabbit in Eye Research", J.H. Prince, ed., Charles C. Thomas, Springfield, p. 362 (1964).

39. H. Davson, The intraocular Fluids. The Intraocular Pressure, in: "The eye", 2$^{nd}$ Ed., Vol. 1, Vegetative Physiology and Biochemistry, H. Davson, ed., Academic Press, London, p. 147 (1969).

40. G.B. Matson, T. Schleich, C. Serdahl, G. Acosta, and J.A. Willis, Measurement of longitudinal relaxation times using surface coils, J. Magn. Reson. 56: 200-206 (1984).

41. H. Davson, "The Physiology of the Eye", 3$^{rd}$ Ed., Academic Press, New York, p. 73 (1972).

42. M. Garwood, T. Schleich, G.B. Matson, and G. Acosta, (manuscript in preparation).

43. P.A. Sher, P.J. Bore, J. Papatheofanis, and G.K. Radda, Nondestructive measurement of metabolites and tissue pH in the kidney by $^{31}$P nuclear magnetic resonance, Brit. J. Path. 60: 632-641 (1979).

44. G.K. Radda, J.J.H. Ackerman, P. Bore, P. Sehr, G.G. Wong, B.D. Ross, Y. Green, S. Bartlett, and M. Lowry, $^{31}$P NMR studies on kidney intracellular pH in acute renal acidosis, Int. J. Biochem. 12: 277-281 (1980).

45. J.J.H. Ackerman, M. Lowry, G.K. Radda, B.D. Ross, and G.G. Wong, The role of intrarenal pH in regulation of ammoniagenesis: $^{31}$P NMR studies of the isolated perfused rat kidney, J. Physiol. 319: 65-79 (1981).

46. G.G. Wong and B.D. Ross, Application of phosphorus nuclear magnetic resonance to problems of renal physiology and metabolism, Mineral Electrolyte Metab. 9: 282-289 (1983).

47. R.S. Balaban, D.G. Gadian, and G.K. Radda, Phosphorus nuclear magnetic resonance study of the rat kidney in vivo, Kidney Int. 20: 575-579 (1981).

48. A.P. Koretsky, S. Wang, J. Murphy-Boesch, M.P. Klein, T.L. James, and M.W. Weiner, $^{31}$P NMR spectroscopy of rat organs, in situ, using chronically implanted radiofrequency coils, Proc. Natl. Acad. Sci. USA 80: 7491-7495 (1983).

49. N.J. Siegel, M.J. Avison, H.F. Reilly, J.R. Alger, and R.G. Shulman, Enhanced recovery of renal ATP with postischemic infusion of ATP-MgCl determined by $^{31}$P NMR, Amer. J. Physiol. 245: F530-F534 (1983).

50. L.D. Cowgill, G.B. Matson, and R.T. Bogusky, Application of $^{31}$P nuclear magnetic resonance to the study of renal phosphate excretion in vivo, in: Biochemical aspects of kidney function, R. Dzurik, ed., Nijhoff, Boston, and Avicenum, Prague (in press).

51. R.T. Bogusky, M. Garwood, G.B. Matson, G. Acosta, L.D. Cowgill, and T. Schleich, Localization of phosphorus metabolites and sodium ions in the rat kidney, Magn. Reson. Med. (in press).

52. B.K. Urbaitis and R.H. Kessler, Concentration of adenine nucleotide compounds in renal cortex and medulla, Nephron. 6: 217-234 (1969).

53. R.S. Balaban, D.G. Gadian, G.K. Radda, and G.G. Wong, An NMR chamber for the study of aerobic suspensions of cells and organelles, J. Analyt. Biochem. 116: 450-455 (1981).

54. F.G. Tobak, N.G. Ordonez, S.L. Bortz, and B.H. Spargo, Zonal changes in renal structure and phospholipid metabolism in potassium-deficient rats, Lab. Invest. 34: 115-124 (1976).

55. M.I. Hrovat, C.O. Britt, T.C. Moore, and C.G. Wade, An alternating pulsed magnetic field gradient apparatus for NMR self-diffusion measurements, J. Magn. Reson. 49: 411-418 (1982).

56. P. Styles, C.A. Scott, and G.K. Radda; A method for localizing high-resolution NMR spectra from human subjects, Magn. Reson. Med. 2: 402-409 (1985).

57. M.R. Bendall, Portable NMR sample localization method using inhomogeneous RF irradiation coils, Chem. Phys. Lett. 99: 310-315 (1983).

PROTON-NMR OF NUCLEI, CELL AND INTACT TISSUE IN NORMAL AND ABNORMAL STATES:
SIGNIFICANCE OF RELAXATION TIMES AS CORRELATED WITH OTHER NON-INVASIVE
BIOPHYSICAL PROBES

C. Nicolini*, A. Martelli**, L. Robbiano**, C. Casieri[+],
C. Nuccetelli[+], F. De Luca[+], B.C. De Simone[+], and
and B. Maraviglia[++]

*Chair of Biophysics and **Institute of Pharmacology
University of Genova School of Medicine, Italy
[+]Departimento di Fisica, Universita´ di Roma "La Sapienza"
00185 Roma, Italy

INTRODUCTION

In vivo Proton NMR imaging is becoming an increasingly popular tool in
diagnostic medicine for its non-invasive nature and for its high resolution
(1,2). In most clinical applications the 3-D reconstructed human images are
based on local measurements of Tl and T2 proton relaxation times. Increases
in these relaxation times in tumors (3) have been attributed to a change in
the water concentration at the cytoplasmic and/or extracellular level (4) or
to a change in the physical state of water (3,5). Similarly, during the
cell cycle the variations in Tl, i.e., its shortening during the Gl-S transcription (6), have been correlated with cellular changes in water concentration (7). More importantly, it has been found (7) that prior to mitosis
an increase in relaxation times of water protons preceeds by 4 hours the
increase in water concentration, suggesting that a change in the physical
state of water may preceed cell division.

The essential role of water molecules in life processes is indeed well
known since the early times (3,8,10) - where also the percentage of water in
tumors was shown to be higher than that of the corresponding host tissues
(10). However, no real insights exist yet as to the structure, physical
states and function of this simple molecule in cells and tissues (cytoplasmic, nuclear and extracellular) nor in the wide range of functional states
of mammalian cells, namely differentiation, proliferation and transformation. Ideally one should separate nuclei from cytoplasm, cellular from
extracellular material, and determine the role of each component in any
given tissue in changes in relaxation times. By doing this and by using
known experimental systems to induce in rat liver either normal cell proliferation, differentiation or cancer, we may then answer yet unanswered
questions under controlled situations. Furthermore the molecular nature of
the changes can be best estimated by correlating the evaluation of Tl and T2
proton relaxation times with the physical state of water and with the structure of related macromolecules, as determined by other independent non-
invasive biophysical probes (11-16) on the same samples.

Finally, what is the nature of hepatocytes proliferation? Focal, as in
the chemically-induced preneolastic nodules, or uniformly diffuse over the
liver? Can we discriminate between a resting (G0) cell and a normally

cycling cell (in the pre-replicative Gl phase or in the replicative
S phase), and between them and a cell either in a preneoplastic curable
stage or in a neoplastic "non-curable" stage? Are the changes in terms of
both free and bound water at tissue, cellular and nuclear levels similar or
do they occur in opposite directions? Answers to these critical issues are
hereby attempted.

MATERIALS AND METHODS

Chemicals and Diets

Diethylnitrosamine (DEN), 2-acetylaminofluorene (2AAF), phenobarbital
sodium salt (PB), CCl and glutaraldehyde were obtained from E. merck,
Darmstadt, West Germany. 0.02% 2AAF or 0.05% PB was incorporated in a standard diet by Nossan (Italy).

Rats

Random-bred male albino Sprague-Dawley rats (200-250) were used. The
animals were exposed to the following treatments.

a) Normal untreated rats used as control, where all liver cells are in
a non-proliferating G0 phase.

b) Rats killed 5 hr after partial hepatectomy (i.e. removal 2/3 of the
liver), where about 40% of the liver cells have entered a GI proliferating
phase.

c) Rats killed 20 hr after partial hepatectomy (i.e. removal 2/3 of the
lvier), where about 40% of the liver cells have now entered the S phase (DNA
replication).

d) Rats killed during the 7th week of chemical treatment to induce
cancer, where several hepatocytes form preneoplastic nodules (islands) of
hepatocytes in a pre-cancer stage.

e) Rats killed during the 16th week of chemical treatment to induce
cancer, where in some instances several heptocytes are now tumor (neoplastic) cells.

Preneoplastic and Neoplastic Nodules Induction

The rats were injected i.p. with a single carcinogenic does of DEN (200
mg/kg, dissolved in 0.9% NaCl solution). Two weeks later, the selection
procedure described by Solt and Farber (17) was appled by feeding the rats
with a diet containing 0.02% 2AAF (acetylaminofluorene) for two weeks. In
the middle of this selection period the animals received a necrogenic dose
of $CCl_4$ (2 ml/kg, v/v, in corn oil). Thereafter all rats were given a basal
diet for one week, then they were fed with a diet containing 0.05% phenobarbital (PB) which is a tumor promoter. Rats were sacrificed both during
the 7th week and about the 16th week after DEN administration.

Histological sections from the right hepatic lobe of four rats induced
with the Solt and Farber procedure have been prepared; only one liver showed
evident neoplastic alterations. The livers of the other three animals
showed more undefined regressive phenomena with focal degradation and parvi-
cellular infiltrations.

## Analysis of Proportion of γ-GT-Positive Hepatocytes

Hepatocytes were analyzed for γ-GT activity by the histochemical technique developed by Rutenburg et al. (18), according to Leishes et al. (19), with some minor modifications. In brief, the cultures were washed twice with cold Merchant's solution (0.14 M NaCl: 1.47 mM $KH_2PO_4$: 2.7 mM KCl: 8.1 mM $Na_2HPO_4$: 0.53 mM $Na_2EDTA$; pH 7.5), and the cells fixed in methanol for 20 min. A section of the plastic air-dried culture dish bottom was cut out and immediately incubated (at 25°C) in a freshly prepared solution containing the synthetic substrate N-(γ-L--glutamyl)-4-methoxy-2-naphtylamide and fast blue butyl(4-hydroxybutyl)nitrosamine as a coupling agent. The incubation time was 10 min, because preliminary assays revealed that shorter or longer time yields either less active cells or more intense background, respectively. Following incubation, the slides were rinsed in 0.9% NaCl solution for 2 min and then transferred to a 0.1 M solution of cupric sulfate for 2 min. After another saline rinse, the slides were immediately analyzed for γ-GT activity by phase-contrast light microscopy. Slides were scanned at random, and the number of cells exhibiting an orange-red stain (γ-GT-positive) were computed as a percentage of the total number of cells observed in each field. A total of 1000 cells were analyzed in each preparation.

## Cell, Nuclei and "in toto" Liver Isolation

Hepatocytes were isolated from the rat livers by collagenase perfusion according to Williams (20). Cells, that were greater than 80% viable, were immediately fixed in Krebs-Ringer phosphate buffer (pH 7.3) containing 2% glutaraldehyde at 37°C for about 3 hr.

The nuclei were obtained from hepatocytes by purification performed by 5 min incubation in dissociation medium (0.075 M NaCl, 0.024 M $Na_2EDTA$; pH 7.5) including 0.75% (v/v) Triton X-100, followed by centrifugation for 5 min at 150xg dat 4°C. The treatment was repeated and finally the nuclei were washed with Merchant's solution (0.14 M NaCl, 1.47 mM $KH_2 PO_4$, 2.7 mM KCL, 8.1 mM $Na_2HPO_4$, 0.53 mM $Na_2EDTA$; pH 7.5) again centrifuged and fixed with Krebs-Ringer phosphate buffer with 2% glutaraldehyde.

For NMR image, at each time point studied, rats were sacrificed, and liver was excised and fixed in Krebs-Ringer phosphate buffer containing 2% glutaraldehyde.

## Experimental Evaluation of Free Induction and Relaxation Times

Measurement of the free induction decay (FID) is the basic way in which the magnitude and other characteristics of the total magnetization M are determined. The FID resulting from sequences of two or more pulses is used in the determination of relaxation times T1 and T2 in a Bruker Spectrometer Model SXP100 and 0,15 Tesla.

For measuring T1 over a wide range of values the 180°, τ, 90° sequence is employed where τ is the time between the two magnetic pulses. A free induction signal results, the initial height of which is proportional to the magnitude of M. If the system is now allowed to return to equilibrium by waiting at least five times T1 and the 180°, τ, 90° sequence repeated for a different value of τ, the decay rate of M can be established as indicated in Fig. 1.

In practice, considering the direct relationship between the magnetization M and the induced signal A in the rf coil of the spectrometer, the final equation can be recast into the form

$$(A_\tau - A_\infty) = \ln 2A_\infty - \tau/T1,$$

where $A_\tau$ is the initial amplitude of the FID following the 90° pulse at time $\tau$, and $A_\infty$ is the limiting value of $A_\tau$ for a very long interval between the 180° and 90° pulses. T1 is determined from the slope of a plot of $\ln (A_\infty - A_\tau/2A_\infty$ versus $\tau$.

It can be seen from the equation that when $A_\tau = 0$ $\tau$ = T1 ln2 = 0.69T1. Thus T1 can be found from the pulse separation resulting in zero free induction signal following the 90° pulse. While useful for a rough measurement, this procedure is, however, inadequate for accurate determination of T1.

The spin-echo method is utilized to measure the transverse relaxation T2. The method consists of the application of a 90°, $\tau$, 180° sequence and

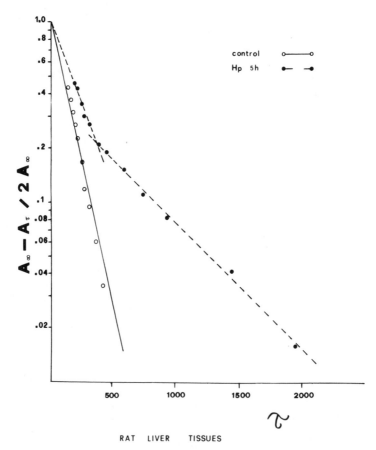

RAT LIVER TISSUES

Fig. 1. Normalized free induction NMR signal as function of
the time (milliseconds) between the 180 and 90
degree magnetic pulse, for that liver tissue before
(0---0) and 5 hours after partial hepatectomy
(●---●).

the observation at a time $2\tau$ of a free induction "echo." The echo amplitude depends on T2, and this quantity is determined from a plot of peak echo amplitude as a function of $\tau$. As in the measurement of T1 it is necessary to carry out the pulse sequence for each value of $\tau$ and to wait between pulse sequences an adequate time (at least five times T1) for restoration of equilibrium.

## Determination of the Percentage of Water

Following the NMR measurements, the culture cells were transfered to tared dishes and initial weights determined. The dishes with cells were then placed in an oven at 65°C. The dishes were reweighed at 24 hour intervals until a constant weight was determined.

## Higher Order Chromatin-DNA Structure Determination

The tertiary and quaternary chromatin-DNA structure has been determined as previously described by three parallel and independent biophysical methods, namely circular intensity differential scattering of isolated nuclei (13), scanning and flow cytometry following differential staining for DNA of intact cells either with Feulgen reaction (absorbance measurements) or with Acridine-Orange (green fluorescence emission) (11,12). An ACTA Image Analyzer and Phybe Flow Cytometer were respectively used in the last two measurements.

## Electric Properties of Nuclei

The complex dielectric constant was measured on a Network Analyzer in the 500 - 2,000 Hz range, as previously described (15).


RESULTS

In order to conduct a correlated study between NMR relaxation times and other biophysical characterizations, which require a prior mild fixation (i.e., image analysis of Feulgen-stained for Acridine-Orange stained hepatocytes) and to allow a parallel or sequential analysis on the same samples, the effect of the mildest fixative (2% glutaraldehyde) has been explored.

As it has long been known (11-15), nuclear-DNA morphometry (11) of the fixed and Feulgen-stained rat liver tissues reveals the existence of either one (G0) or two (G0 and G1) homogeneous populations, respectively prior to or after partial hepatectomy. The same data are obtained by fluorescence cytometry on single hepatocytes isolated from the same tissue and Acridine-Orange stained for nuclear-DNA (12): namely after partial hepatectomy, either with or without fixation with 2% gluteraldehyde, a large portion of the isolated rat liver cells appears in the G1 (higher green fluorescence and larger nuclear area, with a parallel lack of DNA synthesis) and the balance in the control G0 state (11,12).

Comfortingly (see Tables 1 and 2 and Fig. 1) when comparing the same tissues in different functional states (the regenerating liver with the resting control G0) the major features of the NMR relaxation times and water content remain unaltered before and after fixation, namely:

- the presence of resting tissue of only one population (G0);

- the appearance in the regenerating tissue of two subpopulations (G0 and G1), the second (G1) being with quite larger T1 and T2 with respect to the first (G0);

Table 1.  Water content, in percentage for nuclei, cells and
         tissues, either fixed and unfixed.  The standard
         deviation over 2-3 measurements is given in
         parenthesis.

| TREATMENT | Fixed° | | | Unfixed | | |
|---|---|---|---|---|---|---|
| | Tissue | Cells | Nuclei | Tissue | Cells | Nuclei |
| Control | 71.7% | 82.9% | 93.8% | 68.9% | 81.7% | 95.6% |
| | (2.12) | (1.90) | (1.13) | (1.40) | (0.36) | (0.67) |
| HP5h | 68.9% | 85.9% | 93.9% | 73.1% | 85.1% | 96.3% |
| | (1.42) | (3.04) | (2.33) | (0.85) | (1.41) | (0.4) |
| Preneoplastic nodules | 70.3 | 83.4 | - | 69.0 | 84.0 | - |

°Samples are fixed with 2% glutaraldehyde in Kreb's solution for 3
days.


Table 2.  Relaxation times (in milleseconds) Tl and T2 for resting,
         cycling and chemically-transformed liver tissue, either
         fixed or unfixed.

| Sample | Viable Unfixed Tissue | | | | Fixed Tissue | | | |
|---|---|---|---|---|---|---|---|---|
| | T1 | | T2 | | T1 | | T2 | |
| | short | long | short | long | short | long | short | long |
| Control | 226 | - | 19 | - | 167 | - | 11 | - |
| Cycling (S phase) | 380 | 404 | 27 | 35 | 262 | 361 | 22 | 28 |


    - the increase in water content and hydration at cellular level, but
not at the level of intact nuclei;

    - the magnitude of spin-spin relaxation time T2 is quite less pro-
nounced than that for the spin-lactice relaxation time Tl.

    We have noticed, however, that the increase in Tl for the new Gl
subpopulation (with respect to the control G0) is much higher in the unfixed
tissue than in the fixed counterpart.  This is compatible with the marked
water increase in the unfixed tissue compared to its fixed counterpart;
suggesting that a change in the physical state of water rather than a mere
change in hydration may be also responsible for the difference in relaxation
times Tl.

    The complexity of the changes resulting at the various levels from
induced cell proliferation and induced neoplastic and preneoplastic transformation is apparent in Tables 3-5 and in Figs. 1-5.  In general, within
any given functional state, the increase in relaxation time Tl is linearly
related to the increase in hydration (gm water/gm dry mass), going from
tissues to cells and nuclei (Table 3).

Table 3. T1 relaxation times, water content and hydration
per fixed tissue, cell and nucleus isolated from
rat liver in G0 and G1 phase.

| | | T1(ms) | | % $H_2O$ | | gm $H_2O$/dry mass | |
|---|---|---|---|---|---|---|---|
| | | G0 | G1 | G0 | G1 | G0 | G1 |
| Tissues | (I) | 167 | 244 | 71.7 | 68.9 | 2.5 | 2.2 |
| | (II) | – | 371 | | | | |
| Cells | (I) | 352 | 406 | 82.9 | 85.9 | 4.8 | 6.1 |
| | (II) | – | 716 | | | | |
| Nuclei | (I) | 908 | 583 | 93.8 | 93.9 | 15.1 | 15.3 |
| | (II) | – | – | | | | |

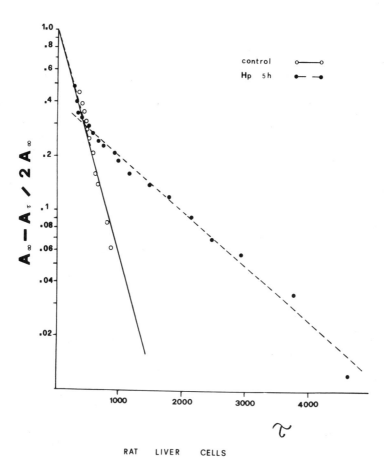

RAT   LIVER   CELLS

Fig. 2.   As Figure 1, but for the isolated cells.

Table 4.　Relaxation times (in milliseconds) Tl of
gluteraldehyde fixed tissues, cells and nuclei
from rat liver before and after partial
hepatectomy, and after either seven weeks
(preneoplastic nodules) or 16 weeks (hepatoma)
after administration of a chemical carcinogen.
Mean and standard deviations are computed from
independent measurements on two to four different
samples. The relaxation times are computed by
linear regressions of the experimental data, which
yield correlation coefficients equal or larger
than 0.99.

|  |  | Tissues | Cells | Nuclei |
|---|---|---|---|---|
| Control | (I) | 167±3.5 | 352±70 | 908±83 |
|  | (II) | absent | absent | absent |
| Cycling | (I) | 244±46 | 406±7 |  |
|  |  |  |  | 583±94 |
| (G1) | (II) | 371±58 | 747±382 |  |
| Cycling | (I) | 292±61 | 357±69 |  |
| (S) | (II) | 372±131 | 470±1 |  |
| Preneoplastic | (I) | 254±131 |  |  |
|  |  |  | 300-2500(**) | 180-179(++) |
|  | (II) | 254±24 |  |  |
| Hepatoma | (I) | 239 |  |  |
|  | (II) | 373 |  |  |

(**) From one (most) to two different Tl, depending on the
number of $\gamma$-GT labelled preneoplastic cells (see Table 7).
(++) From two to three different Tl, depending on the number
of $\gamma$-GT labelled preneoplastic cells (see Figure 5).

If we compare resting with proliferating rat liver at the various
levels (either fixed or unfixed) a similar increase in water content and
hydration becomes apparent, which is of cytoplasmic (mostly) and
extracellular (partly) origin - since the nuclei display an invariant
hydration (Table 3). During the G0-G1 transition the dramatic decrease in
Tl at nuclear level is then due only to a change in the physical state of
water, namely a redistribution in large number of water molecules from free
to bound (Tables 3 and 4 and Fig. 3). This exactly parallels both the
increase in water tightly bound (to all macromolecules) per unit nuclei and
the increase in bound water per unit (Table 5), independently determined by
complex impedence measurements on the same nuclei (15). The latter change
in bound water per unit DNA at the nuclear level is probably caused by the
change in the tertiary-quartenary chromatin-DNA structure, namely in the
number of the chromatin-DNA primary binding sites for Acridine-Orange probed
by scanning cytometry (Table 6) and in the degree of DNA superpacking probed
by viscoelastometry (14).

At the same time (Table 3), for the cytoplasmic changes taking place
during the G0-G1 transition, the increased hydration apparent at the
cellular level (about 27%) does not explain the sizeable increase in Tl
(about 100%), which implies a significant redistribution of water molecules
from bound to free. Similar alteration in Tl relaxation time occurs during
further progression into the cell cycle (S phase) and for neoplastic
transformation at the level of intact tissue (Fig. 4 and Table 4). The

observed increase in Tl – observed only for the one liver sample displaying clear neoplastic alterations by classical histology – is in agreement with previous reports of the increased water concentration in cancer tissues.

For the preneoplastic tissue – typically containing nodules of different size and number – the picture is rather complex and, while the intact tissue displays also a second population of larger Tl (Table 4), at cellular level (Table 7 and Figs. 5-6) there appears to exist a linear correlation between the percentage of $\gamma$-GT labeled preneoplastic cells and the magnitude of the mean "preneoplastic" Tl with respect to the control.

For the nuclei isolated from the preneoplastic nodules up to three relaxation times are detectable (Figs. 5-6), similar or lower than the control and compatible with an increase in bound water per nuclei as determined on the same nuclei by complex dielectric constant measurements in the EM frequency range of 500-2000 Hz (Table 5). For all nuclear pellets (both from preneoplastic and S phase cells) an increase in nuclear water bound to all macromolecules parallels a slight decrease in water content for the same nuclei, which in turn display a parallel decrease in Tl relaxation time.

Conversely, the dielectrically derived volumetric fraction of tightly bound water per unit DNA (computed subtracting for the large amount of water bound to RNA and proteins) goes in the opposite directions for S nuclei and

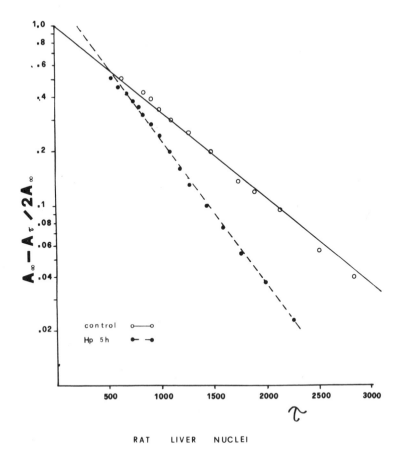

RAT   LIVER   NUCLEI

Fig. 3.   As Figure 1, but for the isolated nuclei.

Table 5. Electric properties of intact nuclei determined by complex impedence measurements. The percentage error in these derived parameters are less than 1%.

| | Normality (mM) | P | F | TD/VD | WT | WF | T |
|---|---|---|---|---|---|---|---|
| G0 | 99 | 48. | 491 | 0,24 | 961. | 910. | 9.6 |
| S | 104 | 74. | 776 | 0,38 | 940. | 899. | 14. |
| Preneoplastic Nodules | 91 | 68. | 470 | 0,12 | 950. | 900. | 11.2 |

TD/VD = volumetric percentage of strongly bound water per unit DNA.
P(ml/l) = volumetric fraction of biopolymers (RNA, DNA and proteins) and of bound water per nuclear pellet.
WT(ml/l) = bound and free water.
F(MHz) = relaxation frequency of loosely bound water molecules; a measure of the nuclear microviscosity.
WF(ml/l) = free water.
T (ml/l) = volumetric fraction of total tightly bound water per nuclear pellet given by (P-M)/2.5, where M is the volumetric fraction of all macromolecules (DNA+RNA+Protein) biochemically determined.

Table 6. Structural and electric properties of nuclei versus chromatin-DNA structure in situ.

| | r | CIDS | TD/VD |
|---|---|---|---|
| G0 | 0,24 | high | 0,22 |
| G1 | 0,38 | low | 0,38 |
| S | 0,44 | absent | |
| Preneoplastic Nodules | 0,12 | very high | 0,12 |
| Hepatoma | 0,10 | very high | - |

r = number of available primary binding sites for chromatin-DNA in situ, as measured by scanning cytometry of Acridine-Orange stained cells (12).
CIDS = Circular Intensity Differential Scattering of intact nuclei and native chromatin, as measured by spectropolarimetry outside the absorption band (13).
TD/VD = bound water per unit DNA, as determined by complex impedence measurements (14).

for preneoplastic nuclei (shown in ref. 15), respectively increasing (0.49) and decreasing (0.12) with respect to G0; exactly what is expected from the molar ratios of bound dye per unit DNA, for G0, G1, S and preneoplastic nuclei (Table 6).

The very high water content in nuclei (about 95.6% by weight) is also confirmed by the electric measurements about 96.1% by volume), considering

that the average density of nuclear biopolymers (RNA+DNA+proteins) is about
1.36 gm/ml.


DISCUSSION

The increase in water content appears to be confined to the level of
cells and intact tissues, particularly at the cytoplasmic level rather than
the extracellular level, while it is practically absent at the nucelar
level.  The fact that similar values are obtained for T1, T2 and for
structural parameters of the chromatin, in presence or absence of
glutaraldehyde, confirms that it is possible to use such a fixative to
preserve the integrity of the samples for a rather long time.

At the nuclear level (Tables 4-6) the structure of the biopolymers such
as chromatin appears to determine changes in the physical state of water
causing changes in the relaxation of the magnetization vector.  This
confirms previous findings on the effect of spermine, a known inducer of
chromatin condensation, which appears to cause an increase in the T1 of
synchronized S phase cells without any alteration in the percentage of water

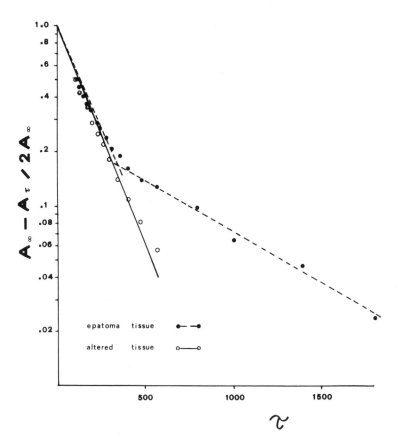

Fig. 4.   As Figure 1, but for liver tissue 16 weeks after
          the chemical induction of cancer.  True hepatoma
          (●--●) and merely altered liver tissue (0---0).
          See Material and Methods for further details.

(7). G0 quiescent hepatocytes initiated by a chemical carcinogen to form preneoplastic focal islands appear to have structural properties at the level of water bound to chromatin-DNA completely different (17,16) from normal cycling hepatocytes (either in G1 or S phase) or from hepatoma cells. These unique properties are, however, not apparent by proton NMR at any level including the nuclear level, where only redistribution of DNA-bound and free water appear uniquely associated with changes in the microviscosity and the diffusion of the ionic environment (in perfect agreement wiht the known unique change in pitch and radius in the chromatin-DNA superhelix). These unique properties unfortunately are not reflected at the nuclear level, nor at the extracellular tissue level, where a similar increase in total bound water (and then decreased T1 for nuclei) or a similar increase in tissue hydration (and then increased T1 for tissues) characterize normal proliferation, preneoplastic and neoplastic transformation.  Such a

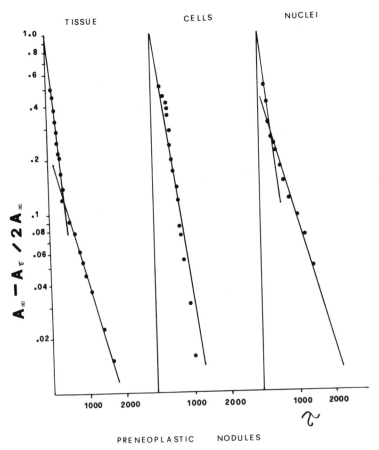

PRENEOPLASTIC   NODULES

Fig. 5.  As Figure 1, but for intact tissue (left) and corresponding isolated cells (center) and nuclei (right) taken from rat liver seven weeks after preneoplastic nodules induction (the percentage of γGT-labeled cells is 7%).

biophysical study conducted at various levels of spatial resolution is useful not only to clarify the fundamental mechanisms which control cell proliferation and neoplastic transformation, but gives also an idea of the limits and the significance of images acquired through proton NMR tomography and may give an idea of new possible avenues to explore for enhancing the value of the expensive tools. The discriminatory power among different functional states and among different pathologies is very high at the DNa level and it may be possible to recognize a preneoplastic state from a normal resting or cycling state for early treatment of the preneoplastic state.

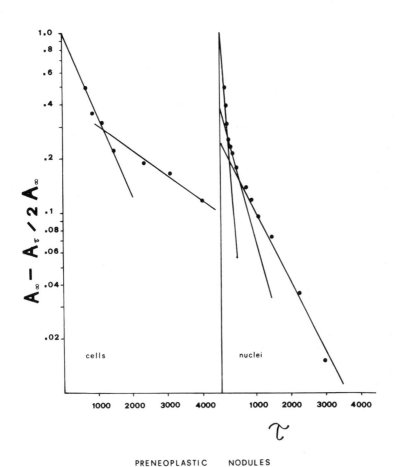

PRENEOPLASTIC    NODULES

Fig. 6.  As Figure 4 (center), but nuclei (right) and cells (left) from rat liver tissue with the preneoplastic nodules - clearly visible - of larger size and number of yielding a percentage of γ-GT labeled hepatocytes of 22%. In the case of nuclei (left), the best-fitted three relaxation times are respectively 180, 435 (normal G1-like) and 695 (normal G0-like) milliseconds. IN the case of "preneoplastic" cells (right) the two relaxation times are respectively 980 and 2500 milliseconds.

Table 7. Ratio among the average relaxation times T1 apparent in gluteraldehyde-fixed cells isolated from rat liver tissue control T1(C) with respect to the one T1(N) containing pre-neoplastic nodules of increasing size, as measured by γ-GT staining (see Materials and Methods).

| T1(N)/T1(C) | γ-GT |
|---|---|
| 1.0 | 5 |
| 1.0 | 7 |
| 1.2 | 12 |
| 5.5 | 22 |

## ACKNOWLEDGEMENTS

This work has been supported by grants from the Ministery of Public Education (National Project "Biophysical Control of Cell Growth") and from the National Research Council (Finalized project "Oncology" contract number CN84.00702.44).

## REFERENCES

1. T. Budinger and P. Lauterbur, Nuclear magnetic resonance technology for medical studies, Science 226:288 (1984).
2. L. Kaufman, A. Margulis, and L. Crooks, "Nuclear Magnetic Resonance Imaging in Medicine," Igaku-Shoin, New York, (1981).
3. R. Damadian, Tumor detection by nuclear magnetic resonance, Science 171:1151 (1971).
4. J. E. Downing, W. M. Christopherson, and W. L. Broghamer, Nuclear water content during carcinogenesis, Cancer 15:1176 (1962).
5. C. Hazelwood, D.C. Chang, D. Medina, G. Cleveland, and B.L. Nichols, Distinction between the preneoplastic and neoplastic state of murine mammary glands, Proc. Natl. Acad. Sci. USA 69:1478 (1972).
6. P. T. Beall, C. F. Hazelwood, and P. N. Rao, Nuclear magnetic resonance patterns of intracellular water as a function of HeLa cell cycle, Science 192:904-907 (1976).
7. P. N. Rao, C. F. Hazelwood, and P. T. Beall, Cell cycle phase-specific changes in relaxation times and water content in HeLa cells, in: "Cell Growth," C. Nicolini, ed., Plenum Publishing Corporation, New York (1982).
8. W. Cramer, J. Physio. 50:322 (1961).
9. R. C. Mellors, A. Kupfer, and A. Hollender, Quantitative cytology and cytophatology. I. Measurement of the thickness, the volume, the hydrous mass and the anhydrous mass of living cells by interference microscopy, Cancer 6:372 (1953).
10. H. D. McEween and F. L. Haven, Cancer Res. 1:148 (1941).
11. M. Grattarola, P. Carlo, R. Viviani, and C. Nicolini, Early effects of chemical carcinogens as compared to induced cell proliferation. II. Automated image analysis, Bas. Appl. Histochem. 26:153 (1982).

12. P. Miller, W. Linden, and C. Nicolini, Biophysical studies of chromatin in situ and isolated after rat partial hepatectomy, Z. Naturforsch. 340:442 (1979).
13. C. Nicolini and F. Kendall, Differential light-scattering in native chromatin: Corrections and inferences combining melting and dye-bindning studies: two-order superhelical model, Physiol. Chem. Phys. 9:265 (1977).
14. C. Nicolini, P. Carlo, A. Martelli, R. Finollo, F. A. Bignone, E. Patrone, V. Trefiletti, and G. Brambilla, Viscoelastic properties of native DNA from intact nuclei of mammalian cells. Higher-order DNA packing and cell function, J. Mol. Biol. 161:155 (1982).
15. C. Nicolini, Chromatin, Nuclei and Water: Alterations and Mechanisms for Chemically-induced Carcinogenesis, in: "Chemical Carcinogenesis," C. Nicolini, ed., Plenum Publishing Corporation, New York (1982).
16. C. Nicolini, "Biophysics and Cancer," Plenum Publishing Corporation, New York (1985).
17. O. Solt and E. Farber, New principle for the analysis of chemical carcinogenesis, Nature 263:701 (1976).
18. A. M. Rutenburg, H. Kim, J. W. Fischbein, J. S. Hanker, H. L. Wasserkrug, and A.M. Seligman, Histochemical and ultrastructural demonstration of $\gamma$-glutamyltranspeptidase activity, J. Histochem. Cytochem. 17:517 (1969).
19. B. A. Lashes, K. Ogawa, E. Roberts and E. Farber, Gamma-glutamyltrans-peptidase, a positive marker for cultured rat liver cells derived from putative premalignant and malignant lesions, J. Natl. Cancer Inst. 60:1009 (1978).
20. G. M. Williams, Further improvements in the hepatocyte primary culture DNA repair test for carcinogens: detection of carcinogenic biphenyl derivatives, Cancer Letter 4:69 (1978).
21. R. Dickerson, H. Drew, B. Conner, R. Wing, A. Fratini, and M. Kopa, The anatomy of A-, B-, and Z-DNA, Science 216:475 (1982).

# TOWARDS NMR SPECTROSCOPY IN VIVO:   THE USE OF MODELS

C. Andrea Boicelli▲●, Angela M. Baldassarri▲, Marcello
Giomini■, and Anna Maria Giuliani*

▲CNR, Instituto San Raffaele, Milano
●Instituto di Anatomia Umana Normale, Bologna
■Dipartimento di Chimica, Universita La Sapienza, Roma
*CNR - ITSE, Area della Ricerca, Montelibretti (Roma)

## INTRODUCTION

In recent years the use of NMR for clinical purposes has been increasing.  Magnetic resonance imaging has great diagnostic potential, despite
the many problems and drawbacks involved in its practice (1).  More contro-
versial is the possibility to exploit NMR spectroscopy as a diagnostic tool
in clinical practice.  Its applications seem to be restricted to the study
of phosphorus containing metabolites (2), in particular to muscle energetics
and to the viability of organs.  However, some very recent research, based
on $^1$H (3) and $^{13}$C (4,5) NMR, opens new fields in the applications of in vivo
NMR to clinical problems.

We feel, however, that at present the most fruitful approach to medical
NMR spectroscopy is through models, starting from very simple systems like
membrane models, going to intact tissues, to perfused organs, and finally to
living animals.

## THE TECHNIQUE

Nuclear magnetic resonance spectroscopy provides two kinds of information:  high resolution NMR affords insight into the chemical properties of
highly mobile molecular species and low resolution (high power) NMR explores
the dynamic properties of bulk matter.

This and the following chapter deal essentially with low resolution
NMR, with the parameters $T_1$ and $T_2$ (the relaxation times) which describe
the evolution of the magnetization towards equilibrium and with their use in
the study of tissues and living systems.  In another part of this book the
applications of high resolution NMR spectroscopy and the information it
affords on metabolites and small molecules are reported; certain large biopolymers or bonded chemical species, however, cannot be detected in the tissues even when they are abundant constituents of the living matter.  Low
resolution NMR, can give a description of the motional properties of the
components of a sample and of their compartmentation.  Thus high and low
resolution NMR should be considered as complementary sources of information
for tissue characterization.  The determination of the so-called relaxation

times is experimentally difficult (6,7) and errors and artifacts are frequent. The use of a high resolution NMR spectrometer can lead to an incorrect evaluation of $T_1$ and $T_2$ because of a too narrow passband, or an r.f. power insufficient to completely invert all spins spread over a large spectral width, or a too long receiver dead time. However, the use of a high power NMR spectrometer can also lead to wrong evaluations of the relaxation times, since very often the full magnetization decay cannot be described because the sampling rate is inadequate or the dead time of the electronics (even when very short, in the range of $\mu s$) is long compared to the fastest components of the magnetization decay.

Other sources of error are the mismatch and the detuning of the instruments or an incorrect phase relationship between transmitter and receiver (7) which lead to large deviations of the measured relaxation times from the real ones in favourable cases or to a meaningless behaviour of the magnetization in the worst cases. Values of the relaxation times in error by as much as 30% for $T_1$ and 50% for $T_2$ (7) may also derive from a wrong choice of the operator selectable parameters, even when the most reliable pulse sequences—inversion—recovery for $T_1$ (IR) and Carr-Purcell-Meiboom-Gill (CPMG) for $T_2$ – are employed (6).

Other critical factors are the shape of the sample which can modify the filling factor of the receiver coil (7) and the handling and storage of the samples (7,8) especially when tissues are considered. When measuring the relaxation times, it is strongly advisable to reduce to a minimum the manipulation of the tissue and to avoid non-fresh, irregularly shaped specimens.

The major drawback in the correct evaluation of the relaxation times, is, however, theoretical. The concept of $T_1$ and $T_2$, and the methods for their determination come directly from the Bloch equations. The postulates, on which these equations are based, hold only for low viscosity, very dilute solutions of non-interacting spin systems and this is certainly not the case with tissues or animals. Thus, extrapolation of the concept of $T_1$ and $T_2$ to tissues is not simple (10) and the parameters describing the time evolution of the magnetization are only time constants resembling $T_1$ and $T_2$. Nevertheless, the operational meaning and significance of the experimental parameters can be retained and used.

MODELS

The reverse micelles as membrane models and their spectroscopic behaviour.

Small unilamellar liposomes are considered the best model of the microenvironment of living cells (12), though they yield poor information on the internal cell compartment, since the inside—outside exchange phenomena average the properties over the whole system.

The problem can be circumvented, and information on the endocellular compartment gathered, by the study of reverse micelles (13), where the intercompartmental exchange phenomena are much slower, and can in practice be neglected if techniques having an appropriate time scale are used. Suitable techniques, in this respect are i.r. and NMR spectroscopies, which have the advantage of being non-invasive, since the information directly comes from the nuclei (NMR) or atomic groups (i.r.) present in the system, and no extraneous probe is needed.

One of the crucial points for the understanding of the function of cellular membranes is to clarify the state of the water in their vicinity, since the properties of this "vicinal" water are distinctly different from those of bulk water (14).

The water pool of reverse micelles (RM) is a good model of such "vicinal" water, since it is expected to be highly organized because of the small dimensions of the micellar cavity (ca. 15–20 nm diameter). The water molecules should be involved in strong interactions with one another and with the polar heads of phospholipids. Indeed, the amount of water present in the internal compartment of RM affects the dynamic behaviour of the phosphate groups. The $^{31}P$ longitudinal relaxation time of RM of egg yolk phosphatidylcholine (EPC) in benzene (50 mg/ml) increases linearly with the value of $w_o$ (i.e. the number of water molecules per polar head) up to a value of the parameter of ca. 25, and remains essentially constant for larger values of $w_o$.

Additional information of great interest on the micellar water comes from the i.r. spectra in the region of the OH stretching vibration (4000 – 3000 $cm^{-1}$). This band, in the spectra obtained for RM of EPC in benzene, prepared with increasing amounts of water and recorded against benzene as reference, can be instrumentally deconvoluted in Gaussian components and the important spectral parameters, frequency, bandwidth and molar extinction coefficient, can be obtained for each component (16). The relevant data are reported in Table 1, taken from Ref. 16. the presence of several spectral components has been interpreted as due to water populations with different degree of organization.

More than one type of endomicellar water is evidenced also by proton NMR. The $^1H-T_1$ of water has been measured by the IR method for RM of EPC in benzenze ($w_o$ = 30) and the plot of the magnetization decay cannot be fitted by a single exponential (13). Two values of the longitudinal relaxation time have been derived from the experimental data, corresponding to water populations with different motional characteristics (Table 2). Both populations have a much shorter $T_1$ than pure water ($T_1$ = 3.7 $\pm$ 0.21$_s$ (17)), indicating a smaller degree of motional freedom.

The experimental results suggest that the endomicellar water is organized in layers around the polar heads of phospholipids which constitute the micellar wall. Each layer is characterized by an individual correlation time, $\tau_c$, which depends on the geometrical constraints and intermolecular interactions to which the molecules are exposed. The number of populations, in slow exchange with each other, that can be detected depends on the time window of the experimental technique; thus the faster i.r. technique detects more populations than the slower NMR spectroscopy. It should, however, be

Table 1. I.r. parameters of the Gaussian components of the OH stretching band for RM of EPC in benzene. The values of $\nu$ and $\Delta\nu_{1/2}$ are given $\pm$ half width.

| Band | $\nu$ ($cm^{-1}$) | $\Delta\nu_{1/2}$ ($cm^{-1}$) | $\varepsilon . 10^3$ ($cm^2 mol^{-1}$) |
|------|------|------|------|
| A[a] | 3250 $\pm$ 20 | 400 $\pm$ 20 | 57 $\pm$ 5 |
| B[b] | 3450 $\pm$ 20 | 300 $\pm$ 20 | 83 $\pm$ 5 |
| C[c] | 3590 $\pm$ 20 | 180 $\pm$ 20 | 32 $\pm$ 2 |

a) more structured or "polymeric water; b) water with intermediate degree of organization or "oligomeric"; c) water involved in weakest interaction or "free."

Table 2. NMR relaxation parameters of the water protons in RM of EPC in benzene.

| Water Population | $T_1$ (s)[a] | $x$[a] |
|---|---|---|
| I (more structured) | 0.31 ± 0.02 | 0.35 ± 0.05 |
| II (less structured) | 0.53 ± 0.02 | 0.65 ± 0.05 |

a) $T_1$ and the fractional population x are given ± half dispersion.

always kept in mind that each population might comprise several groups of molecules, with different motional properties, in fast interchange.

Intracellular pH is another parameter of paramount importance, whose value is easily deduced from the [31]P chemical shift of the inorganic phosphate $P_i$ resonance (18). However, when phosphate buffers are isolated in RM of EPC, no [31]P resonance is detected separate from that of the phospholipid phosphorus in the pH region between 4 and 8, and the only signal observed has a constant chemical shift (19). On the other hand, the [31]P-$T_1$ changes with the buffer pH following a titration curve and the apparent pK obtained from the plot (pK = 6.85 ± 0.05) is in agreement with literature values. This result suggests that the availability of protons in the vicinity of cell membranes, where many important biological processes take place, might be different from what is expected on the basis of the pH deduced from the $P_i$ chemical shift inside the cell.

Low molecular weight species, like small peptides and electrolytes, are always present inside the cells and may considerably affect the properties of "vicinal" water and of the membrane phospholipids. The inclusion of such small molecules inside RM and observation of their effects on some physico-chemical properties of the endomicellar water and of the phospholipids polar heads may help to clarify their mode of action in the cells. Aminoacids and peptides build up their hydration shell competing with the phospholipids for water molecules. Ions, on the other hand, might have more complex interactions with the chemical species present in the inner region of RM: the concentration effects (solvation, mainly) and the nature of the ion should be considered together with a screening effect in the aqueous layer near the micellar wall and with specific binding to the charged groups of the phospholipids.

The perturbations induced by the presence of the aminoacids or oligopeptides in the internal cavity of RM are easily detectable in their i.r. spectra: the three populations of the micellar water are perturbed such that, in some cases, one of them disappears (20).

The relaxation behaviour of the water protons also exhibits dramatic changes. The presence of the perturbing species alters the equilibrium between the two water populations as evidenced by NMR: in particular, any variation in the number of individuals in the more structured water layer I modifies their dynamic characteristics. The mean free path of the molecules is affected and the relaxation rate is modified accordingly. $T_1$ (I) has indeed been found to be a linear function of the fractional water population $x_I$ in the I layer and to obey the relationship (taken from Ref. 13; $T_1$ in seconds):

$$T_1 (I) = 0.532 - 0.006 \ x_I \qquad (1)$$

While aminoacids and peptides influence essentially the micellar water organization, electrolytes may also modify the phosphate group characteristics, because of their interactions with the phospholipids polar heads. The aqueous solutions of many electrolytes (chlorides and nitrates of several cations) have been isolated inside RM; sodium, potassium, calcium and magnesium have been studied more extensively because of their biological relevance.

$^{31}$P-NMR spectra and longitudinal relaxation times show that divalent cations interact more efficiently than monovalent ions with the phosphate group (Figs. 1 and 2).

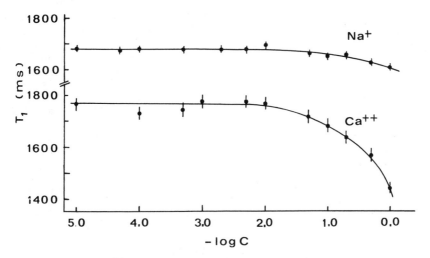

Fig. 1.   $^{31}$P-$T_1$ of reverse micelles of EPC in benzene as a function of the electrolyte concentration in the water pool.   ($B_0$ = 4.7 T, T = 301 K, C in mol.L$^{-1}$).

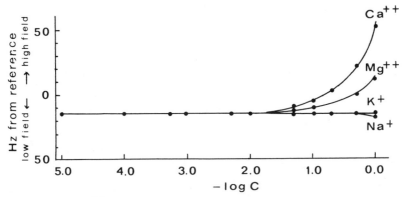

Fig. 2.   $^{31}$P chemical shift of reverse micelles of EPC in benzene as a function of the electrolyte concentration in the aqueous pool ($B_0$ = 4.7 T, T = 301 K, C in mol.L$^{-1}$, external reference 85% aqueous $H_3PO_4$).

The decrease of $T_1$ at increasing electrolyte concentrations suggests, according to the results described above (16), that the cations remove water molecules from the first hydration layer of phospholipids, causing a closer packing of the phosphocholine moieties and a change in the overall organization of the endomicellar water (21). It should be kept in mind that the water in the first hydration layer of the phospholipids need not necessarily coincide with either "A" or "I" water populations evidenced by infrared and proton NMR, respectively. This change in the hydration of phospholipds is supported by changes in the i.r. spectra: the fraction of the three water populations, as derived by deconvolution of the OH stretching band, is markedly affected by the electrolyte concentration. This data is given in Table 3 (taken from Ref. 22).

Table 3.  Dependence of the fractional water populations in RM of EPC on the concentration of a secluded electrolyte. (The electrolyte is KCl; the estimated error on the populations is ± 2).

| Electrolyte concentration (M) | Water population "A" | "B" | "C" |
|---|---|---|---|
| $1 . 10^{-4}$ | 40 | 2 | 58 |
| $5 . 10^{-4}$ | 41 | 16 | 43 |
| $5 . 10^{-2}$ | 38 | 28 | 34 |
| $1 . 10^{-1}$ | 36 | 27 | 37 |
| $5 . 10^{-1}$ | 46 | 54 | – |
| $1 . 10^{\circ}$ | 69 | 31 | – |

Also the dynamic parameters of the water are affected by the presence of the electrolytes in the water pool of RM: in Table 4 the [1]H longitudinal relaxation time of the more organized water population I is reported for several electrolytes at different concentrations.

The infrared spectral data indicate that the amount of the "A" water increases at high ionic concentration: this may be due both to a progressively larger portion of water being engaged in the hydration layer of the ions and to an increase in the fraction of oriented water near the micellar wall resulting from a conformational change of the phosphocholine group. It has indeed been found that the binding of ions to phosphatidylcholine multibilayer vesicles induces a progressive change in the orientation of the phosphocholine group from parallel towards perpendicular to the vesicle surface, resulting in an increased fraction of oriented water (23).

The proton relaxation data (Table 4) show a decrease in the mobility of the more highly organized water population I. This population is in fact an ensemble of populations, with different dynamic properties, in fast exchange on the NMR time scale: an increase of one of the faster relaxing populations could lead to the observed decrease of $T_1$ and match well the i.r. findings described above.

It emerges from the reported results that many parameters have great influence in determining the NMR responses of the simple model systems considered.

The importance of these factors is even more critical when dealing with the more complex living systems, and careful consideration should be given to them if meaningful results are to be obtained and significant conclusions reached.

Table 4.  Effect of different electrolytes on the proton longitudinal
relaxation time ($T_1$, s) of the water population I in RM.

| Electrolyte | Concentration (M) | | |
|---|---|---|---|
| | 1. $10^{-4}$ | 1. $10^{-1}$ | 1. $10^0$ |
| NaCl | 0.37 | 0.40 | 0.44 |
| $NaNO_3$ | 0.44 | 0.51 | 0.48 |
| KCl | 0.46 | 0.42 | 0.40 |
| $KNO_3$ | 0.47 | 0.45 | 0.42 |
| $MgCl_2$ | 0.49 | 0.48 | 0.40 |
| $CdCl_2$ | 0.44 | 0.43 | 0.38 |
| $ZnCl_2$ | 0.38 | 0.30 | – |
| RbCl | 0.47 | 0.44 | – |

CELLS

[1]H NMR study of erythrocytes in essential hypertension.

Human essential hypertension is a disease of social relevance, whose
genesis depends both on genetic and on environmental factors.  Poor discrimination between normotension and essential hypertension can be obtained on
the basis of blood pressure level alone, and any easily measurable parameter, which could discriminate between normality and pathology, would certainly help in the diagnosis.  The optimum would be achieved with a "marker"
of hypertension based on genetic differences since it could be used in pre-
ventive medicine to detect subjects prone to hypertension on genetic basis
before the onset of the pathologic condition.

Spontaneously hypertensive rats are the best, though not ideal, animal
model of human essential hypertension.  Essential hypertension, and genetic
hypertension in rats, are characterized by marked alterations in the membrane transport of several cells, among which are red blood cells.  Therefore, rat erythrocytes have been studied by proton NMR to ask whether the
spectral responses could be used to identify genetically hypertensive individuals, even before the onset of the pressure rise (24).

While no substantial difference can be observed between normotensive
(WKY and MNS) and spontaneously hypertensive (SHR and MHS) strains in the
proton spectra of packed erythrocytes, a distinctly different relaxation
behaviour is detected.  The proton spectra of erythrocytes essentially consist of two broad envelopes of resonances, one (A) to low field and the
other (B) to high field of the water resonance.  For each of the two bands a
longitudinal relaxation time, $T_{1(A)}$ and $T_{1(B)}$, respectively, can be determined by the inversion-recovery pulse sequence, taking the area under the
envelopes as a measure of the magnetization values.  The decay of the magnetization measured in this way can be fitted by a single exponential giving
single values of $T_{1(A)}$ and $T_{1(B)}$ (Fig. 3).

The relaxation time values vary within large limits both for the
normotensive and the hypertensive strains of rats; however, the ratio
$R = T_{1(A)}/T_{1(B)}$ shows an interesting behaviour which is reported in Table 5
(taken from Ref. 24).

This marked difference in the [1]H relaxation behaviour may be related to
a different degree of organization of the intracellular water and/or to a

Table 5. $^1H$ – NMR data of rat erythrocyte suspensions[a] ($B_0$ = 4.7 T, T = 298K).

| | Normotensive | Hypertensive |
|---|---|---|
| Number of rats | 10 | 10 |
| $T_{1(A)}$ (s)[b] | 0.86 ± 0.25 | 0.32 ± 0.08 |
| $T_{1(B)}$ (s)[b] | 0.39 ± 0.15 | 0.35 ± 0.07 |
| R[b] | 2.0 ± 0.6 | 0.9 ± 0.2 |

a)  in 0.9% NaCl in $^2H_2O$; 35% hematocrit.
b)  values are given ± half dispersion.

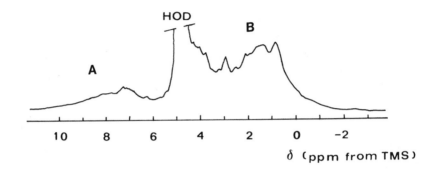

Fig. 3.  $^1H$ NMR spectrum of a suspension of rat
erythrocytes in 0.9% NaCl solution in
$^2H_2O$.  (T = 298 K, $B_0$ = 4.7 T).

different number of exchangeable protons of membrane proteins exposed to the
solvent in the two strains, since the proton relaxation in erythrocytes is
dominated by the water-mediated cross-relaxation.  Both factors may come
into play because, on one side, the erythrocytes of the hypertensive strains
have a smaller volume (25) and thus a larger fraction of membrane bound
water; on the other side different composition or conformation of the membrane proteins (26) may expose a different number of exchangeable protons to
the solvent.  The parameter R seems a good "marker" of genetic hypertension
in rats, because its value changes from approximately 2 in the case of normal subjects to ca. 1 for genetically hypertensive animals.

However, when similar measurements are performed on human erythrocytes
of hypertensive patients and their offsprings and on normotensive subjects
the results are considerably different (27).  Also, in the case of human
erythrocytes, the water-mediated cross-relaxation process is more efficient
for hypertensive specimen than for the normotensive ones, as indicated by
saturation transfer experiments.  At variance with the animal model, however, red blood cells of normotensive people always yield a value of R
larger than 1.5, with a very large variability range, while the value of R
is 1.34 ± 0.06 for all hypertensives, actual or perspective, except four,
for whom a value of R close to unity has been found (as for spontaneously
hypertensive rats).  Several sharp resonances can be extracted from the
broad envelopes of the proton spectra of human erythrocytes by the convolution difference procedure.  A careful inspection of such manipulated spectra
shows marked differences in the low field region (A) for the four hyperten-

sive specimens which also exhibit a distinctly different relaxation behaviour, i.e., R close to unity.

It can be concluded that, in humans:  the parameter R alone cannot be used as a marker for essential hypertension; the combined occurrence of an R value of ca. 1.34 and an efficient saturation transfer mechanism is a strong indication of erythrocyte modifications connected with essential hypertension; an R value close to unity combined with an efficient saturation transfer and a proton NMR spectrum modified in the low field region can be used to identify essential hypertensives.  These hypertensive subjects probably constitute one of the several subgroups of the population of essential hypertensives for which the spontaneously hypertensive rats can be best used as models.

The main lesson to be learned from this study, of considerable importance in clinical application, is that the extrapolation of results obtained from animals to humans is often arbitrary and can lead to gross errors.


TISSUES

NMR studies of regenerating liver of rats.

Regenerating liver is a good model of rapidly dividing tissues and the regenerative process can thus be used as a model of tumoral growth.  Hepatic regeneration is accompanied by metabolic changes and the combined use of high and low resolution NMR appear therefore to be a suitable technical approach to the study of this process.  $^{31}$P-NMR yields information only on a very limited number of metabolites; proton spectra are of such complexity that their interpretation is a formidable if not hopeless task; $^{13}$C therefore appears the nucleus of choice to follow the metabolic changes occurring in the regenerating liver.  The NMR sensitivity of the nucleus, however, is low and fixation of the tissue by suitable means (buffered aqueous formaldehyde) is convenient to allow acquisition of the data over long periods without degradation.

The $^{13}$C spectra of regenerating liver tissue at different times after hepatectomy are reported in Fig. 4.  Dramatic changes are observed in the level of several metabolites (notably triglycerides) indicating that the $^{13}$C-NMR can be used to follow proliferative phenomena of this kind (28). Low resolution NMR has been utilized to measure the proton relaxation times, $T_1$ and $T_2$, of fresh liver tissue in the course of the regeneration (29). The observed variation of $T_2$ with the time after hepatectomy is too small to be meaningful and cannot be used to follow the regenerative process.  Interesting information comes from the measurements of $T_1$:  the data are collected in Table 6 (taken from Ref. 29).

We have examined a large number of specimen (90 samples from non-operated or sham-operated animals and 30 bioptic specimen for each of the chosen times) to verify beyond doubt that the observed modifications were really due to regeneration and not to other phenomena like circadian rhythm (30) or surgical stress and manipulation of the organ (31).

A relationship between $T_1$ changes and the proliferative phenomenon is further supported by the conspicuous metabolic changes consequent to partial hepatectomy observed by $^{13}$C-NMR.  During the first 24 hours after surgery, $T_1$ has been found to increase in parallel with DNA duplication, as determined by autoradiographic data, while in cell cultures the duplication process is accompanied by a faster relaxation (32), suggesting that phenomena other than DNA duplication are responsible for the longer $T_1$ values. Such phenomena might be the expansion of intercellular spaces and the

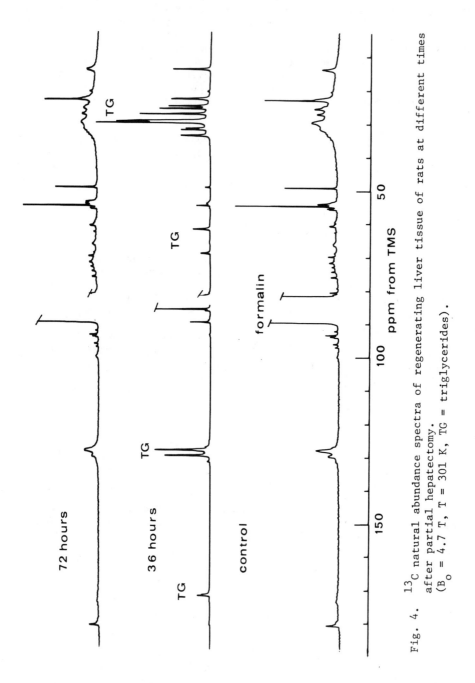

Fig. 4. $^{13}$C natural abundance spectra of regenerating liver tissue of rats at different times after partial hepatectomy.
($B_o$ = 4.7 T, T = 301 K, TG = triglycerides).

Table 6. $^1$H- $T_1$ of regenerating liver tissue of rats as a function of time after partial hepatectomy (T = 310 ± K; $B_O$ = 0.47T). The $T_1$ values are given ± SEM.

| Time (hours) | $T_1$ (s) |
|:---:|:---:|
| 0[a] | 0.215 ± 0.006 |
| 3 | 0.213 ± 0.009 |
| 6 | 0.213 ± 0.005 |
| 12 | 0.233 ± 0.005 |
| 18 | 0.250 ± 0.008 |
| 24 | 0.261 ± 0.004 |
| 30 | 0.258 ± 0.007 |
| 36 | 0.253 ± 0.005 |
| 48 | 0.238 ± 0.006 |
| 60 | 0.231 ± 0.005 |
| 72 | 0.222 ± 0.006 |
| 84 | 0.218 ± 0.005 |
| 108 | 0.215 ± 0.005 |

a) normal and sham-operated rats.

increase of intracellular water, and of its mobility, which are known to accompany the first stages of liver regeneration.

Kinetic equations can be deduced from the relaxation data, which describe the regeneration as the resultant of a proliferation (equation 2) and an inhibition (equation 3) process, whose onset occurs several hours after the partial hepatectomy operation.

$$T_1 = 0.150 + 0.035 \ln t \qquad (2)$$

($T_1$ in s, t in hours; the relationship holds from the 6th hour on)

$$T_1^{inhib.} = 0.232 - 0.072 \ln t \qquad (3)$$

($T_1$ in s, t in hours; the equation holds from the 24th hour on)

Since the $T_1$ value depends upon the fraction X of dividing cells (equation 4, taken from Ref. 29)

$$T_1 = 0.213 + 0.0036 X \qquad (4)$$

the longitudinal relaxation time is an indirect index of the entity of proliferation.

This kind of information could be of interest in the follow-up of the neoplastic growth.

The examples discussed above clearly show that meaningful and successful application of the NMR spectroscopy to living systems can only be achieved with a previous study of complex model systems. Moreover, all the available information from both high and low resolution NMR is required to understand even such models; a constructive approach requires in addition previous knowledge of the systems under study obtained by means of other techniques.

# REFERENCES

1. P. Mansfield and P. G. Morris, "NMR Imaging in Biomedicine," Academic Press, New York (1982).
2. J. H. Battocletti, CRC Critical Revs. Biomed. Engn. 10:1 (1984).
3.a. K. L. Behar, D. L. Rothman, R. G. Shulman, O. A. C. Petroff, and J. W. Prichard, Proc. Natl. Acad. Sci. USA 81:2517 (1984).
   b. P. A. Bottomley, W. A. Edelstein, T. H. Foster, and W. A. Adams, Proc. Natl. Acad. Sci. USA 82:2148 (1985).
4. J. R. Alger, K. L. Behar, D. L. Rothman, and R. G. Shulman, J. Magn. Res. 56:334 (1984).
5. M. Barany, C. Arus, and Y.-C. Chang, Magn. Res. Med. 2:289 (1985).
6. M. L. Martin, J.-J. Delpuech, and G. J. Martin, "Practical NMR Spectroscopy," Heyden & Son Ltd., (1980) Chapter 7.
7. C. A. Boicelli, and A. M. Baldassarri, Practical aspects of in vitro and in vivo $T_1$ and $T_2$ measurements, in "NMR in living systems," Reidel ed., Plenum Publ. Co., in press.
8. P. T. Beall, Magn. Res. Imaging 1:165 (1982).
9. A. Abragam, "Principles of Nuclear Magnetism," Clarendon Press, Oxford (1983) Chapter 3.
10. Proceedings of the EEC Workshop on "Identification and characterization of biological tissues by NMR," Discussion on the effects between various techniques on measurements, Ann. Ist. Super. Sanita 19:57 (1983).
11. J. deGier, M. C. Blok, P. W. M. van Dick, C. Mombers, A. J. Verkley, C. C. M. van der Neut-Kok, and L. L. M. van Deenen, Ann. N.Y. Acad. Sci. 308:85 (1978).
12. M. J. Conrad and S. J. Singer, Biochem. 20:808 (1981).
13. C. A. Boicelli, F. Conti, M. Giomini, and A. M. Giuliani, Chem. Phys. Lett. 89:490 (1982).
14. L. M. Gierasch, J. E. Lacy, K. F. Thompson, A. L. Rockwell, and P. I. Watnick, Biophys. J. 37:275 (1982).
15. C. A. Boicelli, F. Conti, M. Giomini, and A. M. Giuliani, in "Physical methods on biological membranes and their models," F. Conti ed., Plenum Publ. Co., New York (1985) 143.
16. C. A. Boicelli, M. Giomini, and A. M. Giuliani, Appl. Spectry. 38:537 (1984).
17. J. A. Pople, W. G. Schneider and H. J. Bernstein, "High resolution nuclear magnetic resonance," McGraw-Hill, New York (1959) p. 207.
18. R. B. Moon and J. H. Richards, J. Biol. Chem. 248:7276 (1973).
19. C. A. Boicelli, F. Conti, M. Giomini, and A. M. Giuliani, Spectrochim. Acta 38A:299 (1982).
20. C. A. Boicelli, M. Giomini, and A. M. Giuliani, Spectrochim. Acta 37A:559 (1981).
21. C. A. Boicelli, F. Conti, M. Giomini, and A. M. Giuliani, Gazz. Chim. Ital. 113:573 (1983).
22. C. A. Boicelli, G. Giomini, and A. M. Giuliani, in "Future trends in polymer science and technology," Martinus Nijhoff Publ., in press.
23. O. Soderman, G. Arvidson, G. Lindblom, and K. Fontell, Eur. J. Biochem. 134:309 (1983).
24. C. A. Boicelli, M. Giomini, and A. M. Giuliani, It. J. Biochem. 32:161 (1983).
25. S. Sen, G. C. Hoffman, N. T. Stowe, R. R. Smeby, and F. M. Bumpus, J. Clin. Invest. 51:710 (1972).
26.a. Yu. V. Postnov, S. N. Orlov, P. V. Gulak, and A. S. Shevcenko, Pflugers Arch. Ges. Physiol. 365:257 (1976).
   b. M. Canessa, N. Adragna, H. S. Salomon, T. M. Connolly, and D. C. Tosteson, N. Engl. J. Med. 302:772 (1980).
   c. J.-F. Cloix, M.-A. Devynck, E. Derbigny, J.-L. Funck-Brentano, and P. Meyer, Biochem. Biophys. Res. Comm. 105:1577 (1982).

27. C. A. Boicelli, M. Giomini, and A. M. Giuliani, It. J. Biochem. 34:75 (1985).

28. C. A. Boicelli and A. M. Giuliani, Physiol. Chem. Phys. Med. NMR, in press.

29. C. A. Boicelli, B. Baratta, and A. M. Giuliani, Physiol. Chem. Phys. Med. NMR, in press.

30. J. D. de Certaines, J. P. Moulinoux, L. Benoist, A.-M. Bernard, and P. Rivet, Life Sci. 31:505 (1982).

31. P. Fantazzini, L. Lendinara, F. Novello, E. Brosio, and A. DiNola, Biochim. Biophys. Acta 303:250 (1984).

32. P. T. Beall, B. B. Asch, D. C. Chang, D. Median, and C. F. Hazelwood, Biophys. J. 25:238a (1979).

TOWARDS NMR SPECTROSCOPY IN VIVO:   II.   RELATIONSHIP BETWEEN NMR PARAMETERS

AND HISTOLOGY

C. Andrea Boicelli[▲●], Angela M. Baldassarri[▲], Arrigo Bondi[△],
Anna Maria Giuliani[*], and Roberto Toni[●]

[▲]CNR, Instituto San Raffaele, Milano
[●]Instituto di Anatomia Umana Normale, Bologna
[△]Instituto di Anatomia Patologica, Bologna
[*]CNR – ITSE, Area della Ricerca, Montelibretti (Roma)

INTRODUCTION

The future of NMR as an in vivo diagnostic tool, both for imaging techniques and for spectroscopic determinations, requires as a preliminary step
a precise tissue characterization.  In practice, sound relationships should
be established between the histology of a tissue and the relevant NMR parameters.

Ten years ago CT attempted essentially the same correlation exploiting
the Hounsfield numbers, that is the absorption coefficient of the X radiation of the tissues.  The CT achievements, however, have been limited and
uncertain since the results depend on a single parameter and the use of contrast media has been found necessary to increase tissue differentiation,
thus introducing the distribution of the contrast agent as an additional
source of uncertainty.

Several different parameters for each nuclear species are available for
NMR (1) to monitor the specific properties of a tissue.  As a matter of
fact, the quantity monitored in the NMR experiments is always the macroscopic magnetization $\vec{M}$ at the time of sampling.  The characteristic NMR parameters are the modulus of $\vec{M}$ and its spatial distribution (i.e., the nuclear
density), the time constants which describe the evolution of the $\vec{M}$ components along the z axis or in the (x,y) plane (i.e., $T_1$ and $T_2$), the resonance frequency of the nuclear magnetic moments whose resultant is $\vec{M}$ (i.e.,
the chemical shift).

When the NMR parameters are used to attempt a precise tissue characterization, the main problem lies in the heterogeneity of the living matter and
in the histological variability, not easily quantified, of each tissue compartment.  It is intrinsically impossible to evaluate the many components
which contribute to the macroscopic NMR response, and the measured value of
M depends on the physico-chemical properties of each compartment of the
system under examination.  In spite of these difficulties, the NMR technique, compared to the traditional roentgen techniques, has the advantage of
a larger number of measurable parameters, and the probability of success is
thus greater.  Unfortunately, the hope to exploit the NMR response, and in
particular the relaxation parameters, for tissue characterization has not

yet been achieved: relaxation times have indeed proved to be extremely sensitive, but non-specific, parameters (2,3). Nevertheless, the measurement of relaxation times has been particularly useful in establishing the strategy for image sampling suited to study morphological alterations in pathologic conditions (4,5).

The goal of NMR would be to combine the positive results so far obtained with an ability to characterize a tissue. The starting point of such process is obviously the study of in vitro samples. The problems and sources of error in the determination of parameters such as the relaxation times have been discussed elsewhere (6) and in the preceding chapter. Once instrumental difficulties are overcome, one has to verify the possibility of correlating the histological properties of a sample with its NMR responses. Attempts in this direction have been going on for some years (7-9) and several systematic approaches have been tried, but the results are contradictory. This, however, is not as negative as it may appear and there are good reasons to believe that a good NMR characterization of several tissues can be achieved. The experimental examples reported below lend support to this statement.

EXPERIMENTAL

All the relaxation time measurements have been carried out on a Bruker Minispec p20 spectrometer, operating at 20 MHz on protons. The temperature during the experiments has been kept at $37 \pm 1°C$. Great care has been taken with the instrumental setting to reduce the systematic errors to a minimum (6). Standard pulse sequences have been used: inversion-recovery for $T_1$, and spin-echo for $T_2$ determinations. Because of the predictable multicomponent time evolution of the magnetization, a number of data points has been collected large enough (not less than 7 points for each component) to ensure a reliable multicomponent analysis of M as a function of time. The intensity of the signal, proportional to $M(t)$, has been measured 7 μs after the second pulse of the sequence, a time very short compared to the shortest $T_2$, but long enough to avoid interference between transmitter and receiver.

All the specimens have been handled following the same protocol taking all precautions necessary to avoid uncontrollable damage to the tissues (10). The measurements were completed within 45 minutes from surgical ablation. Comparison of the magnetization profile (modulus and bandshape) at the beginning and at the end of the measurements gave no indication of tissue alterations capable of modifying the NMR characteristics of the samples during the time elapsed.

EXAMPLE 1

In the case, previously reported (6), of cardiac hypertrophy induced in rats by administration of isoproterenol, apparently, the use of the NMR to characterize the tissue is problematic, if not hopeless. It is well known that administration of synthetic or natural cathecolamines may induce cardiac hypertrophy or necrosis (11). These are structural alterations of such importance so as to justify the expectation of markedly modified relaxation times. The study of the variations induced on the relaxation times has been carried out on 90 male Wistar rats ($210 \pm 20$ g body weight) treated with two different dosages of isoproterenol (3 and 80 mg/Kg of body weight) injected intraperitoneally twice a day for one week. Untreated animals have been used as controls. The left ventricle with apex has been utilized for the NMR study; a small fraction of the same sample has been subjected to histological analysis. The lesions detected at the histological observation were similar for both treatments with isoproterenol; the typical alterations induced are focal necrosis of myocardial cells, monocyte infiltrates, swelling and proliferation of fibroblasts with the presence of collagen fibers, focal fatty degeneration and interstitial oedema. The NMR results are presented in Table 1, where we report the range of the different relaxation times observed together with the fraction of specimens for which such relaxation behaviors have been measured.

Table 1. Proton NMR $T_1$ and $T_2$ values of rat myocardium and fractions of examined samples presenting the various relaxation behaviors. ($B_0 = 0.47$ T; T = 37 ± 1°C; a: 3 mg/Kg of isoproterenol twice a day; b: 80 mg/Kg of isoproterenol twice a day; c: untreated).

| $T_1$ (s) | a | b | c |
|---|---|---|---|
| 0.30 - 0.45 | 40 | 50 | 10 |
| 0.50 - 0.60 | 75 | 80 | 100 |
| >0.7 | 45 | 55 | 0 |

| $T_2$ (s) | | | |
|---|---|---|---|
| 0.010 - 0.020 | 55 | 10 | 60 |
| 0.040 - 0.045 | 35 | 10 | 100 |
| >0.05 | 85 | 80 | 10 |

It is clear that the histological alterations of the myocardium induce the presence of additional components of the magnetization; very intriguing is the absence of relaxation times associated with histologically intact tissue which has been observed for a certain fraction of samples. This cannot be because at the time of sacrifice all the animals were vital. The apparent disappearance of tissue structures should be ascribed to the superposition of the magnetizations from different phases at the time of sampling; the time evolution of the various components is masked by the intrinsic noise of the method and different behaviors become indistinguishable. In fact, the time evolution of the magnetization reduces the measured signal intensity while the noise contribution remains unchanged and the signal to noise ratio decreases with the time. The deterioration of the signal to noise ratio leads to an overestimation of the measured relaxation times, $T_1$ and $T_2$, independently of the pulse sequence used. It is therefore probable that a tissue component might disappear because of the noise when its magnetization evolves faster than that of another tissue and the ratio of their magnetization values is unfavorable. In general, two tissue components will become indistinguishable for the value of t satisfying equation 1:

$$K n (f_{NO}^A M_0^A - f_{NO}^B M_0^B) + \sum_{m=0}^{n-1} (-1)^m \frac{n!}{(n-m)!} \left( \frac{f_{NO}^A M_0^A}{(T_i^A)^{n-m}} - \frac{f_{NO}^B M_0^B}{(T_i^B)^{n-m}} \right) t^{n-m} \quad (1)$$

In this equation the superscripts A and B identify the two components, $T_i$ represents either $T_1$ or $T_2$, n is the polynomial degree. K is a numerical factor whose value is 0 for the saturation-recovery sequence, -1 for the inversion-recovery sequence, and -2 for the spin-echo, Carr-Purcell and Carr-Purcell-Meiboom-Gill sequences. $M_0$ is the equilibrium magnetization and $f_{NO}$ is a random function representing the rsm noise because of its probabilistic nature; in the actual measurements its contribution to the signal depends on the instantaneous noise value, which may vary between plus or minus its peak value. The apparent relaxation times measured depend on the relative values of the $f_{NO}M_0$ quantity of the various magnetization components. When a saturation—recovery or a progressive saturation sequence are used, the apparent $T_1$ value may deviate from the "true" value by as much as ± 27% if the signal to noise ratio is 25, while the oscillation is only 10% for a signal to noise ratio of 50. The situation becomes rapidly disastrous as the signal to noise ratio decreases. In conclusion, the disappearance of a component of the magnetization can be attributed to an unfavorable signal to noise ratio. Tissue characterization through NMR relaxation times in such conditions is obviously questionable.


EXAMPLE 2

We have examined a different case of heart pathology, which seems instead to lend itself to an NMR description which can be correlated, to a certain extent, with the results of histological examination; it is the case of human papillary muscles from patients suffering from mitral—aortic pathologies (12).

The NMR results are collected in Table 2, together with the observed histological characteristics. Specimens A, B, D, and F are specific of mitral—aortic pathology, E refers to a ventricular aneurysm following infarct, and C to a Fallot tetralogy. $T_1$ increases for the samples with abundant connective tissue and ischemic areas (D, E, and F), while a shorter $T_1$ is measured for samples A, B, and C where hypertrophy of myocardial cells, interstitial oedema and intracellular accumulation of lipoperoxides are the main histological features. Obviously no control data are available. These results show the possibility of a certain gross correlation between histological structure and NMR relaxation data of a tissue.

Table 2.   Proton NMR relaxation times and histological features of human pathological papillary muscle samples.  ($B_o$ = 0.47 T; T = 37 ± 1°C)

| Sample | $T_1$(s) | $T_2$(s) | Histological Features |
|--------|---------|---------|----------------------|
| A | 0.31 0.51 | 0.076 | |
| B | 0.31 0.50 | 0.063 | Hypertrophy of myocardial cells Interstitial oedema Intracellular lipoperoxide accumulation |
| C | 0.34 0.51 | 0.073 | |
| D | 0.48 0.60 | 0.060 | Hypertrophy of myocardial cells Fibroblast proliferation |
| E | 0.80 | 0.017 0.071 | D presents also elastin accumulation E and F present also granulocyte infiltration and areas of necrosis |
| F | 0.67 | 0.077 | |

EXAMPLE 3

Of great interest are the pancreatic endocrine tumors, which are rarely identified because of intrinsic difficulty of diagnosis. Their primary characteristic is to be all histologically similar; therefore, their nature

Table 3. Proton NMR relaxation times of specimens of human endocrine pancreatic tumors. The controls are the fractions of pancreas which appear non-infiltrated by neoplastic cells at the histological analysis. ($B_0$ = 0.47 T, T = 37 ± 1°C).

| Control | | A | | B | | C | | D | |
|---|---|---|---|---|---|---|---|---|---|
| $T_1(s)$ | $T_2(s)$ | $T_1(s)$ | $T_2(s)$ | $T_1(s)$ | $T_2(s)$ | $T_1(s)$ | $T_2(s)$ | $T_1(s)$ | $T_2(s)$ |
| 0.12 | 0.040 | 0.60 | 0.040 | 0.54 | 0.040 | 0.53 | 0.030 | 0.35 | 0.070 |
| 0.18 | | 0.68 | 0.064 | 0.65 | 0.070 | 0.68 | 0.080 | 0.48 | |
| | | | | 0.88 | 0.110 | 0.85 | 0.090 | | |
| | | | | | | 1.04 | 0.110 | | |

A: gastrinoma; B: gastrinoma; C: insulinoma; D: vipoma

183

can only be identified on the basis of immunochemical tests, namely, of their specific reactivity in selected reactions.

Differentiation between normal pancreatic tissue and tissue with neo-plastic infiltrates can be accomplished by means of NMR. The possibility of discrimination is connected with the complete modification of the histolo-gical pattern, because of which the normal pancreatic tissue has values of the relaxation times totally different from the neoplastic pancreatic tissue (Table 3).

Only a limited number of human samples have been examined by NMR (four vipomas, four insulinomas and two gastrinomas), mainly because of the rarity of the pathology and the difficulty of identification. Vipomas and insulin-omas gave internally homogeneous responses, while the two gastrinomas exhi-bited different behavior. It is clear from the results shown in Table 3 that NMR offers a possibility to discriminate between vipoma and insulinoma, while differentiation of gastrinoma B from insulinoma is doubtful. Compari-son of the NMR results with the histological and immunohistochemical charac-teristics of the samples (shown in Table 4) is at this point very instruc-tive and shows that the ultrastructural features do not influence, or more precisely do not explain the NMR behavior of the tissue, while the relative amounts of the gross histological structures can modify the response.

Table 4. Histological features of human endocrine pancreatic tumors. ICA refers to immunochemical tests.

| Histology | A | B | C | D |
|---|---|---|---|---|
| Nucleus + nucleolus | large | large | large | large |
| Chromatin | HS | HS | dense | HS |
| Neoplastic cells | + | ++ | + | + |
| Neo-like cells | NO | NO | ++ | NO |
| Connective fibers | - | -- | - | - |
| APUD-amyloid | - | ++ | ++ | ++ |
| Fat-like tissue | NO | NO | MO | - |
| Necrosis-flogosis | + | + | + | + |
| ICA: gastrin | - | ++ | NO | NO |
| insulin | NO | NO | - | NO |
| VIP | NO | NO | NO | ++ |

A: gastrinoma; B: gastrinoma; C: insulinoma; D: vipoma
HS: highly structured; NO: not observed
--: very low; -: low; +: abundant; ++: very abundant

CONCLUSIONS

The failure of NMR in characterizing tissues can reasonably be ascribed to an incorrect strategy of correlation. Clearly, histologically different structures can give different NMR responses; however, the attempt to correlate the NMR behavior, which is multifactorial in origin, with non-homologous histological structures is logically incorrect: too many competing factors, totally different for each component can justify the NMR results without explaining their origin. Nevertheless, the examples discussed show that, when the histological substrate in its basic structures is comparable in the different terms, some correlation can be attempted between histology and NMR within each series. Unfortunately, the low NMR signal to noise ratio hinders the correlation between NMR behavior and the histological picture. Once this problem is solved, and an appropriate sampling strategy is adopted which is capable of describing completely the evolution of the magnetization of a tissue, then there is hope of correlating NMR parameters with the morphological identification of a pathological state.

# REFERENCES

1.  D. G. Gadian, "Nuclear magnetic resonance and its applications to living systems," Clarendon Press, Oxford (1982), Chapter 6.
2.  P. A. Bottomley, T. H. Foster, R. E. Argensinger, and L. M. Pfeifer, A review of normal tissue hydrogen relaxation times and relaxation mechanisms from 1–100 MHz: dependence on tissue type, NMR frequency, temperature, excision and age. Med. Phys. 11:425 (1984).
3.  P. A. Bottomley, C. J. Hardy, R. E. Argensinger, and G. R. Allen, Relaxation in pathology: are $T_1$'s and $T_2$'s diagnostic? IV Annual Meeting of the Society of Magnetic Resonance in Medicine, Vol. 1, (1985) P. 28.
4.  K. Gersonde, L. Felsberg, T. Tolxdorff, D. Ratzel, and B. Strobel, Analysis of multiple $T_2$ proton relaxation processes in human head and imaging on the basis of selective and assigned $T_2$ values. Magn. Res. Med. 1:463 (1984).
5.  K. Gersonde, M. Staemmler, L. Felsberg, and T. Tolxdorff, Tissue characterization by parameter selective whole-body proton imaging, IV Annual Meeting of the Society of Magnetic Resonance in Medicine, Vol. 1 (1985) P. 50.
6.  C. A. Boicelli and A. M. Baldassarri, Practical aspects of in vitro and in vivo $T_1$ and $T_2$ measurements, in "NMR in living systems," T. Axenrod, Ed., Reidel Publ. Corp., in press.
7.  P. T. Beall and C. F. Hazelwood, Distinction of normal, preneoplastic and neoplastic states by water proton NMR relaxation times, in "NMR imaging," C. L. Partain, A. E. James, Jr., R. D. Rollo, and R. R. Price, Eds., W. B. Saunders Co., Philadelphia (1983), PP. 312-338.
8.  S. S. Ranade, S. Shah, G. V. Talwalker, and S. R. Kasturi, Significance of histopathology in pulsed NMR studies on cancer, in "NMR imaging," C. L. Partain, A. E. James, Jr., F. D. Rollo, and R. R. Price, Eds., W. B. Saunders Co., Philadelphia (1983) PP. 446-452.
9.  S. S. Ranade, S. H. Bharade, G. V. Talwalker, G. K. Sujata, V. T. Shrinivasan, and B. B. Singh, Significance of histopathology in pulsed NMR studies on cancer, Magn. Res. Med. 2:128 (1985).
10. P. T. Bealle, Practical methods for biological NMR sample handling, Magn. Res. Imaging 1:165 (1982).
11. C. I. Chopper, G. Rona, T. Balazs, and R. Gaudry, Comparison of cardiotoxic actions of certain sympathomimetic amines, Can. J. Biochem. 37:35 (1959).
12. R. Toni, C. A. Boicelli, and A. Bondi, Characterization of human pathological papillary muscles by [1]H-NMR spectroscopic and histologic analysis, Int. J. Cardiol., in press.

# THEORY OF NMR IMAGING

E. R. Andrew

Departments of Physics, Radiology and
Nuclear Engineering Sciences
University of Florida
Gainesville, Florida   32611, U.S.A.

## INTRODUCTION

In conventional nuclear magnetic resonance (NMR) it is customary to place a small homogeneous specimen, typically less than 1 ml, of pure liquid or solid in a very uniform magnetic field, often uniform to a part in $10^9$, and NMR spectra and relaxation times are recorded and interpreted.  In contrast with conventional NMR spectroscopy, NMR imaging is concerned with applications to heterogeneous specimens, for example parts of the human body, which are not small, and furthermore they are placed in a deliberately non-uniform magnetic field.

The purpose of the non-uniform field is to label or encode different parts of the specimen with recognizably different NMR frequencies, enabling the structure and internal processes of the specimen to be derived and displayed.  The use of field gradients in NMR to encode spatial information goes back to the work of Hahn,[1] Gabillard[2,3] and Carr and Purcell.[4]  They have been used in the study of phase separations,[5] information storage,[6,7] and in the investigation of periodic structures by the NMR diffraction method.[8]

In writing this article it has been assumed that the reader is familiar with the fundamentals of conventional NMR.  Notwithstanding the differences between conventional NMR and NMR imaging, the basic NMR phenomena remain the same in both applications and a formal description of the NMR equipment reads much the same for both.  The object of interest is placed in the field of a magnet and is surrounded by a radiofrequency coil that is supplied from a radiofrequency generator.

The NMR signal is picked up in a receiver coil, which may be the same
coil as the transmitter coil and after amplification the signal is
recorded and displayed. A dedicated computer instructs the whole
system, gathers and records the data and performs all necessary
calculations. The main differences in equipment are the much larger
aperture magnets that are required for examining human subjects and the
addition of coils to generate field gradients and facilities for
manipulating the gradients.

When imaging the human body and other living systems, the proton
($^1$H) is by far the most commonly used nucleus. Hydrogen is the most
abundant chemical element in the body, it is isotopically almost 100%
abundant, and it has the highest magnetic moment among stable nuclei.
Oxygen has no convenient isotope. For carbon the isotope $^{13}$C is 1.1%
abundant with a low magnetic moment. The principal isotope of nitrogen
is $^{14}$N with a low magnetic moment and also a quadrupole moment while $^{15}$N
has a low abundance. Phosphorus is of considerable interest on account
of the important metabolites which contain it. $^{31}$P is 100% abundant and
it has a reasonable magnetic moment; phosphorus is however rather dilute
in living systems. Summarizing, protons are by far the best nuclei for
human imaging; $^{31}$P nuclei are of substantial interest and after that are
one may mention $^{13}$C, $^{14}$N, $^{15}$N, $^{19}$F, $^{13}$Na.


IMAGING TECHNIQUES

Many different techniques have been described for NMR imaging[9-12],
and a basic classification has been described by Brunner and Ernst.[13]
First we may arrange to isolate a small volume and collect the NMR
signal from it. This elemental volume may then be traversed through a
plane in the object of interest enabling us to build an NMR image of the
plane. This is the sequential point method and it is inevitably slow.

Next we may arrange to gather the NMR signal from a whole line or
column of n elements simultaneously by a Fourier transform procedure,
which is n times faster. This is line scanning.

Then we might gather the NMR signal from a whole plane of $n^2$
elements simultaneously and process the data in such a way that we get
an image of the plane. This is planar imaging. It may not necessarily
be faster than line scanning, but since NMR signals are being gathered
from the whole plane all the time it will certainly give a much better
signal/noise ratio in the image.

Finally we might gather the NMR signal from the whole three-dimensional (3D) object simultaneously and process the data in such a way as to characterize all $n^3$ volume elements.  This is 3D imaging.

The first two methods (sequential point and line scanning) were important in the early days of NMR imaging, but have now been superseded by the third (planar imaging) except for special purposes; almost all medical imaging is now done by planar imaging.  3D imaging is available on many instruments but takes longer, typically 20 minutes or more, and gives more information than is usually needed.  On the other hand, a single slice or several adjacent slices, may be imaged in a few minutes.

In order to pursue planar imaging it is first necessary to define the slice to be imaged.  This is usually done by the selective excitation method.[14,15]  A field gradient is applied along say the Z direction and the object is irradiated with a 90° pulse having a narrow spectral width, corresponding to a narrow range of magnetic field values.  Only those nuclei in a slice of the object perpendicular to Z which experience this narrow range of field values will be excited.  In this way we have selectively excited the nuclei in this slice with a 90° pulse, and the remainder of the object remains untouched.

We now switch the field gradient into the defined slice (XY plane) and let the NMR free induction decay (FID) evolve.  This may be recorded and Fourier transformed on-line by computer to give the NMR spectrum of that slice.  The intrinsic response of the proton NMR signal in pure water is extremely sharp, of order 0.1 Hz.  In human tissues the intrinsic response of soft tissues is somewhat broader, of order 5 Hz, but still quite sharp.  Consequently in a field gradient of say 1G/cm ($10^{-2}$ T/m), different parts of the specimen experience different field strengths, and the NMR spectrum is a one-dimensional (1D) projection of proton density along the direction of the gradient.[16]  Such 1D projections yield some structural information, but in order to obtain a 2D image or picture of proton density it is necessary to manipulate this 1D structural probe, and there are several ways in which this may be done.

One procedure consists in applying the gradient in a number of successive directions in the defined plane, obtaining n 1D projections, each read to n data points.  The situation is now formally similar to that in CT X-ray scanning which also produces a series of equiangular 1D projections.  As in CT scanning using back projection or other methods a proton density image may be reconstructed by computer.  This was the method employed by Lauterbur[1] in his pioneering paper in Nature in 1973, in which he first realized proton NMR images in two tubes of water. This 2D projection-reconstruction method of planar imaging was later used in some commercial NMR scanners, but has nowadays largely given way to an alternative procedure called 2D Fourier imaging. Whereas the 2D projection-reconstruction method is based on a radial system of coordinates, the 2D Fourier imaging method is based on cartesian coordinates which is more straightforward to handle; moreover it is more free from artifacts and is readily extended to 3D and 4D.

In the 2D Fourier imaging method, devised by Kumar, Welti and Ernst[17], a slice is again defined in the XY plane by selective excitation. A field gradient $G_x$ is then applied along the X direction for a time $t_x$, after which a gradient $G_y$ is applied along the Y direction for a time $t_y$. The NMR signal is read as a function $t_y$ to n data points. The process is repeated for a different time $t_x$, indeed for n different times $t_x$, yielding an array of $n^2$ data points on which a 2D Fourier transform can be performed, giving an image of n × n pixels (picture elements).

Since this procedure is central to the practical generation of NMR images we now analyze the process in detail. Let the proton density at any point $(x,y)$ in the defined slice be $\rho(x,y)$. Then, neglecting relaxation effects, the NMR signal from an element of area dxdy at $(x,y)$ in the slice will be proportional to

$$\rho\ dxdy\ \exp(i\gamma Bt) \tag{1}$$

where $\gamma$ is the nuclear gyromagnetic ratio and B is the magnetic induction field at $(x,y)$. During the time $t_x$

$$B = B_0 + xG_x\ , \tag{2}$$

where $B_0$ is the value of B at $(0,0)$. During the subsequent time $t_y$

$$B = B_0 + yG_y\ . \tag{3}$$

After substituting (2) and (3) in (1) and detecting the NMR signal at angular frequency $\omega_0 = \gamma B_0$ , the NMR signal from the element is proportional to

$$\rho\ dxdy\ \exp\left[i\gamma(xG_x t_x + yG_y t_y)\right]. \tag{4}$$

For the whole slice the NMR signal is therefore

$$S(t_x, t_y) = \iint \rho(x,y) \exp[i\gamma(xG_x t_x + yG_y t_y)] \, dx \, dy \qquad (5)$$

$$= A \iint \rho(\omega_x, \omega_y) \exp[i(\omega_x t_x + \omega_y t_y)] \, d\omega_x \, d\omega_y \qquad (6)$$

where $\quad \omega_x = x\gamma G_x, \quad \omega_y = y\gamma G_y, \quad A = (\gamma^2 G_x G_y)^{-1}. \qquad (7)$

From (6) we see that the NMR signal $S(t_x, t_y)$ is the 2D Fourier transform of the proton density in the slice $\rho$. From the reciprocal property of Fourier transforms it therefore follows that $\rho(x,y)$, which is the quantity we want in order to construct the image, is just the 2D Fourier transform of $S(t_x, t_y)$, which we measure, for an array of values $t_x$ and $t_y$.

We see from (5) and (6) that in the analysis $t_x$ always appears multiplied by $G_x$. So instead of incrementing $t_x$ through n successive values we can equally well hold $t_x$ constant and successively increment $G_x$ through n values, which has practical advantages. This is the Spin-warp variation of 2D Fourier imaging.[18]

The imaging of a single slice, or of several adjacent slices, may give sufficient information for clinical purposes. If however a complete NMR measurement of all $n^3$ voxels (volume elements) characterizing the 3D object is desired, a planar imaging method may take a long time with $n \sim 100$. In this situation simultaneous or true 3D imaging methods have their attractions.

In a true 3D imaging method NMR signals are gathered from the whole 3D object in every measurement; they are collected and processed in such a way that the NMR signal from all $n^3$ volume elements is determined. The NMR image of any selected slice of arbitrary orientation may then be displayed. The 3D image of the whole object may be displayed as a series of n 2D images of coplanar slices, each with n × n pixels.

One procedure is to extend the 2D Fourier imaging method to 3D. There is no need to select a slice. We apply a gradient $G_x$ along X for a time $t_x$, then $G_y$ along Y for the time $t_y$ and finally $G_z$ along Z for time $t_z$. The NMR F1D is recorded to n data points during $t_z$. The procedure is repeated for n values of $t_y$ and for each of these for n values of $t_x$. Following the previous argument we see that the NMR signal from the whole object is

$$S(t_x, t_y, t_z) = A \iiint \rho(\omega_x, \omega_y, \omega_z) \exp[i(\omega_x t_x + \omega_y t_y + \omega_z t_z)] \, d\omega_x \, d\omega_y \, d\omega_z \qquad (8)$$

where     $\omega_x = xYG_x$,     $\omega_y = yYG_y$,     $\omega_z = zYG_z$,     $A = (Y^3G_xG_yG_z)$ . (9)

From (8) we observe that the NMR signal $S(t_x,t_y,t_z)$ is the 3D Fourier transform of the proton density $\rho$.   It therefore follows that $\rho(x,y,z)$,  which characterizes the nuclear density throughout the 3D object, is just the 3D Fourier transform of $S(t_x,t_y,t_z)$, which we measure.

For convenience in the foregoing discussion it has been assumed that the object is divided up into n × n × n volume elements.  We may simply extend the argument to a subdivision into $n_x$ × $n_y$ × $n_z$ volume elements and obtain unequal resolution in the three spatial dimensions.

If we take a specimen of any organic liquid, apply a 90° pulse, observe the F1D and then Fourier transform it, we get the high-resolution NMR spectrum of that liquid.  Now let us take a structured specimen containing a variety of materials, and apply a gradient $G_x$ along X for a time $t_x$, and then after $t_x$ remove the gradient and record the F1D as a function of t without the gradient; then repeat the procedure for n values of $G_x$.  After 2D Fourier transformation we obtain a series of n high-resolution NMR spectra for n successive planes normal to X.  Now let us extend the procedure and apply a gradient $G_x$ along X for time $t_x$, then $G_y$ along Y for time $t_y$ and then record the NMR signal to n data points in absence of a gradient.  Now after 3D Fourier transformation we obtain a series of high-resolution NMR spectra for all $n^2$ pixels in the XY plane.  Finally this may be extended to 4D, three spatial dimensions and one spectroscopic dimension.  We may apply gradients $G_x$, $G_y$, $G_z$ along X,Y,Z respectively for times $t_x$, $t_y$, $t_z$ respectively and then record the NMR signal as a function of time t in absence of any gradient.  After 4D Fourier transformation we obtain a series of high-resolution NMR spectra from all $n^3$ voxels constituting the object in 3D.  To do all this would be very time consuming. Nevertheless by convolution with suitable window functions it may be used to select particular volumes for in vivo NMR spectroscopy[19], and is of particular value for in vivo $^{31}$P NMR spectroscopy.  Alternatively we may obtain a 2D or 3D image for each NMR spectral line.

PULSE SEQUENCES AND TISSUE CONTRAST

Living tissues vary widely in their relaxation properties.  Values of $T_1$ from various tissues typically range from 200 to 1000 ms; values of $T_2$ are typically five to ten times shorter than $T_1$.  Moreover as Damadian[20] first demonstrated in 1971 with in vitro samples, cancerous tissues have significantly longer values of $T_1$ and $T_2$ than the corresponding normal tissues. Tissue contrast may be obtained by exploiting these differences in $T_1$ and $T_2$.

Tissue contrast may be enhanced by administration of paramagnetic contrast agents such as solutions of chelates of gadolinium, which induce shorter relaxation times in the tissues they enter. Such contrast agents must have unpaired electrons, and experimental work has been carreid out on a variety of transition and rare earth compounds, on stable free radicals and spin labels, and using molecular oxygen.

The inversion recovery sequence is valuable for displaying $T_1$ contrast. This sequence consists of an initial 180° pulse which inverts the nuclear magnetization, followed after a time TI by a 90° pulse which generates the FID. After the 180° pulse protons in the various tissues undergo longitudinal relaxation, recovering in an approximately exponential manner, each with its own particular value of $T_1$. If the value of TI is made equal to the time at which the magnetization crosses zero for the longer relaxation components, no NMR signal will result from these tissues. On the other hand the shortest relaxation time components will be almost back to their full values, and will give a strong signal; for intermediate relaxation times there will be a dispersion of responses. In this way a $T_1$-weighted image is obtained in which short $T_1$ components appear brighter.

$T_1$-weighted images may also be obtained with a saturation-recovery sequence, namely a series of 90° pulses whose spacing TR is comparable with the shorter $T_1$ values. These shorter $T_1$ tissues relax fairly completely between pulses and give strong signals after each pulse. Long $T_1$ tissues relax rather little between pulses and give weak signals, with a dispersion of responses for intermediate values of $T_1$.

$T_2$-weighted images may be obtained with a 90°-$\tau$-180° spin-echo sequence. If the time interval TE between the 90° pulse and the echo (TE = $2\tau$) is comparable with the shorter $T_2$ values, the echo FID from these components will have substantially decayed whereas those from the longer $T_2$ components will not and will give stronger signals. In an image generated from these echo FID's longer $T_2$ components will appear brighter and we have a $T_2$-weighted image.

ECONOMICAL USE OF TIME

In the 2D Fourier transform method of imaging we apply a series of n 90° selective pulses each followed by different combinations of field gradient values as described earlier. After each pulse we read the FID which may last 10 ms depending on the gradient values. We then wait say 2000 ms for the nuclear magnetization to relax longitudinally before applying the next pulse. If n is 128, an image is obtained in about 4 minutes. However we have only made NMR measurements in 10 ms out of every 2000 ms, an efficiency of only 0.5%. A very large amount of time is wasted between the end of the FID and the next pulse, just waiting for longitudinal relaxation to take place. We now consider ways of improving this efficiency.

First we can insert a series of 180° pulses after each 90° pulse giving spin echoes at for example 50, 100, 150, 200 ms and we can reconstruct images from each set of echoes. The echoes decay with time $T_2$, varying from one tissue to another. Tissues with longer values of $T_2$, particularly cancerous tissue,[20] will progressively stand out in later echo images.

This useful multi-echo procedure still uses only about 200 ms of the 2000 ms available, and has increased the efficiency in the use of time to 10%. The next step is to attack an adjacent virgin slice by selecting a second slice and repeating the whole procedure. Then we may move to a third slice and so on. With the parameters given we could examine ten slices before returning to the first slice, which will by then have fully relaxed. This is the multi-echo/multi-slice procedure, which fully utilizes all the available time. In this example a total of 40 images are gathered in 4 minutes, which is 6s per image, competitive with CT X-ray scans.

The fastest method of obtaining an NMR image is by the echo planar imaging method devised by Mansfield.[21] A field gradient is applied to the specimen and is reversed cyclically. This generates a series of echoes which when Fourier transformed have a periodicity imposed in frequency space, and this of course corresponds to real space. The NMR response therefore is concentrated in rows perpendicular to the gradient direction. If a small gradient is added at right angles one observes the rows obliquely and can read every pixel in the defined slice separately and get a complete image in one NMR excitation. This image from one shot may not have a good signal/noise ratio and for a normal still picture would need averaging a number of times. However the importance is that it allows moving pictures to be obtained in real time, where the quality of an individual frame is not important and the eye performs the necessary integration over a series of frames.[22]

## MAGNETS

The central component of any NMR imaging system is the magnet. First generation NMR imaging systems for human whole-body imaging used resistive magnets generating a magnetic field up to 0.15 T. Such magnets consist of four or six discrete water-cooled coils. In most systems the field is horizontal and the patient lies on a couch which is slid inside the magnet until the section of anatomical interest is in the center of the magnet. In one system[23] the field is vertical and the patient is placed horizontally between the coils. This configuration allows a simpler radiofrequency coil to be constructed with its axis perpendicular to the magnetic field.

Currently the trend is to work at higher field strengths using superconducting magnets. These magnets generate very stable fields in a 1m diameter bore. The optimum field strength for NMR proton imaging is a matter of much current interest and controversy. Although systems are available up to 2T a common range of field strengths in use is 0.3 to 0.6T. An increase of field strength to within this range does yield improvements in image quality without significant complications. Superconducting magnets are however substantially more expensive than resistive magnets. Superconductive systems have been mounted in trailers for mobile operation. At each hospital visited the field is run up to its operating value and after use is run down to zero before departure to the next clinical site.

Large permanent magnets are also sometimes used for NMR imaging. In one system[24] the field is vertical between plane parallel polefaces and the patient is slid horizontally into this gap. Permanent magnets require no electrical power or refrigerants and have no running costs; they also have smaller stray fields. They are however extremely heavy.

## REFERENCES

1. E. L. Hahn, Spin echoes, Phys. Rev. 94: 630(1950).
2. R. Gabillard, Resonance nucleaire mesure du temps de relaxation $T_2$ en presence d'une inhomogeneite de champ magnetique superieure a la largeur de raie, C. R. Acad. Sci. Paris 232: 1551 (1951).
3. R. Gabillard, A steady state transient technique in nuclear resonance, Phys. Rev. 85: 694 (1952).
4. H. Y. Carr and E. M. Purcell, Effects of diffusion on free precession in nuclear magnetic resonance experiments, Phys. Rev. 96: 630 (1954).

5. G. K. Walters and W. M. Fairbank, Phase separation in He$^3$-He$^4$ solutions, Phys. Rev. 103: 262 (1956).

6. A. G. Anderson, R. L. Garvin, E. L. Hahn et al, J. Appl. Phys. 26: 1324 (1955).

7. E. R. Andrew, A. Finney and P. Mansfield, Information storage by NMR, Royal Radar Establishment Report PD/24/026/AT (1970).

8. P. Mansfield and P. K. Grannell, NMR diffraction in solids, J. Phys. C: Solid St. Phys. 6: L422 (1973).

9. E. R. Andrew, NMR Imaging, Acc. Chem. Res. 16: 114 (1983).

10. E. R. Andrew, NMR Imaging of intact biological systems, Phil. Trans. Roy. Soc. B 289: 471 (1980).

11. E. R. Andrew, NMR imaging in medicine: physical principles, Phil. Trans. Roy. Soc. B in press (1985).

12. P. Mansfield and P. G. Morris, NMR Imaging in Biomedicine, Academic Press, New York (1982).

13. P. Brunner and R. R. Ernst, Sensitivity and performance time in NMR imaging, J. Mag. Res. 33: 83 (1979).

14. A. N. Garroway, P. K. Grannell and P. Mansfield, Image formation in NMR by a selective irradiative process, J. Phys. C: Solid St. Phys. 7: L 457 (1974).

15. P. C. Lauterbur, C. S. Dulcey, C. M. Lai, et al, Magnetic Resonance Zeugmatography, Proc. 18th Ampere Congress, Nottingham 27 (1974).

16. P. C. Lauterbur, Image formation by induced local interactions: examples employing nuclear magnetic resonance, Nature 262: 190 (1973).

17. A. Kumar, D. Welti and R. R. Ernst, NMR Fourier zeugmatography, J. Mag. Res. 18: 69 (1975).

18. W. Edelstein, J.M.S. Hutchison, G. Johnson and T. Redpath, Spin warp NMR imaging and applications to human whole-body imaging, Phys. Med. Biol. 25: 751 (1980).

19. T. H. Mareci and R. H. Brooker, High-resolution magnetic resonance spectra from a sensitive region defined with pulsed field gradients, J. Mag. Res. 57: 157 (1984).

20. R. Damadian, Tumor detection by nuclear magnetic resonance, Science 171: 1151 (1971).

21. P. Mansfield and I. L. Pykett, Biological and Medical imaging by NMR, J. Mag. Res. 29: 355 (1978).

22. Rzedzian, R., Mansfield, P. et al., Real time NMR clinical imaging in paediatrics, Lancet 1983 ii, 1281.

23. Mallard, J., Hutchison, J.M.S. et al.  In vivo NMR imaging in
    medicine: the Aberdeen approach, Phil. Trans. Roy. Soc. B 289: 519
    (1980).

24. Fonar, Melville, New York (1983).

SOME OBSERVATIONS ON NMR IMAGING PARTICULARLY

IN LOWER FIELDS

I. R. Young[+] & G. M. Bydder[*]

[+]GEC Research Laboratories, East Lane, Wembley, Middx
[*]NMR Unit, Hammersmith Hospital, Ducane Road, London W12

ABSTRACT

MR Imaging is a complex technique and the simple working rules necessary to begin with may not be valid when extrapolated outside their original
context.

Increasing experience also may lead to modification of clinical practice. An active process of reassessment of the explicit and implicit working rules current in MRI is a necessary process and in this paper effects of
magnetic field strength, the comparative value of spin and field echo, and
aspects of sequence comparison are discussed.

KEYWORDS

NMR Imaging, Imaging Field, Inversion Recovery, Field Echo.

INTRODUCTION

Magnetic Resonance Imaging is a subtle and complex process, and it is
both easy and dangerous to trivialize, by seeking to define a few very simple rules by which to encompass it. Though it is not practicable to examine
all its variations and problems in a manageable paper, an attempt is made
here to highlight some of the important, though, with one exception, neglected factors that should be considered.

Three key simplifications to understanding MRI which have been made are
that high field, preferably using surface coils, is automatically better
than low, that spin echo based data acquisition is all that is needed and
that a range of different sequences including inversion recovery are not
necessary. All three are more or less flawed, and the propositions underlying them need much greater study. This paper recounts some of the evidence that justifies this re-evaluation.

It is reasonable to suggest that these concepts owe their existence to
a lack of knowledge about the parameters of the tissues being studied, and
an increasing number of clinical results is sufficient justification to
probe further. For example, many tumours do not have values of T2 that
differ significantly from those of the normal tissue around them as might be
expected[1] so that the use of spin echo (SE) sequences which are primarily T2

199

dependent may be unproductive, and the relatively small changes in T1 that often occur at the same time mean that the maximum sensitivity to that parameter is needed - so that inversion recovery (IR) is to be preferred.

In general, tissue parameters are so variable, even in the normal population, that it is unwise to guess that any given imaging procedure will ensure the contrast that is expected. In particular, the possibility of there being multiple components in the relaxation behaviour of tissue which may or may not be properly detected make it unwise to try and conjecture what an image would have looked like if only it had been taken using the appropriate procedure, rather than another.

Another example of an aspect of MRI that is regarded with a measure of optimism which is hard to defend is the use of surface coils[2,3]. However, the majority of lesions which cannot be better studied with other modalities are deep seated, and these coils are not a quick and easy answer to examining them. Indeed, superficial pathology in most parts of the body except the brain is much more easily and effectively examined by biopsy than RM imaging. Further, the starting point of a clinical analysis is comparison between the two sides of the body whenever symmetry permits so that an image of a complete section of the body is frequently more desirable than one showing one limited region on one side.

The paper examines the risks of maintaining too dogmatic a view of imaging methods by considering a few specific instances where clear features of clinical performance call into question the wisdom of persisting with a single strategy.

CHOICE OF FIELD LEVEL

Though the decision to consider one field rather than another is usually presented as being one of sensitivity only, other factors do enter. Contrast is more important than signal in detecting lesions - and its balance changes with field in quite subtle ways, which affect the strategy of imaging, and its effectiveness. Further, the changes in T1 with field and the presence of chemical shift means that the level of artifact in images alters.

The argument about the changes in signal-to-noise ratio has been rehearsed extensively in the past[4,5] so that the conclusion reached by Gadian[6] (derived from Hoult and Lauterbur[7]) in a system in which the probe is fully loaded by a spherical conducting object makes a suitable starting point. This develops the relationship

$$\psi \quad B_0 \, g^{1/2} \sigma^{-1/2} \tag{1}$$

where g is the radius of the object being scanned and $\sigma$ is its conductivity (which increases with frequency, and in the range of interest approximately doubles for a frequency change of 10 (or a dependancy of $\omega^{0.3}$))[8]. It is necessary to set this relation in the context of an imaging experiment. For example, equation (1) assumes a constant bandwidth, which is not realistic in two respects.

a)  T1 increases with field[9] meaning that with constant sequence repetition time there is less signal recovery.
b)  the frequency difference between pixels is proportional to field.

This latter statement has been reviewed more extensively elsewhere[10] and the effect can be summarized as bieng due to one of:

i)    tissue T2 which seems to be only weakly dependent on field, if at all,[9]

ii)    apparent relative displacement of tissues due to chemical shift,

iii)    field inhomogeneity (primarily in the slice selection direction, as the largest dimension in a voxel),

v)    body susceptibility effects, which are relatively unimportant in the head though may be significant in the abdomen.

Which factor is of most importance depends on the use to which the machine is put, and to its general quality. The chemical shift artifact is, in practice, the most important of the three, and techniques which recognize it and can be used to eliminate it are attractive, even though they add to imaging time by requiring two sets of data[11]. However, Figs. 1a and 1b illustrate a clinically important situation in which no simple correction procedure is possible - for it depends on both lipid and water component signals being present, and having roughly the same magnitude. Fig. 1a shows a typical spin echo image with tR = 544 msec and tE = 44 msec, while Fig. 1b is an image of the same subject acquired using partial saturation with tR = 500 msec, and with a delay (tA) of 22.5 msec between the centre of the 90 degree pulse and the field echo. This delay is chosen so that the lipid and water spins, initially aligned but with a frequency difference of around 3.5 ppm, are 180 degrees out of phase at the echo peak, and, as shown, largely cancel. The short time to acquisition means that the annulus fibrosa (the rim round the disc which has a relatively short T2) is well seen, which is clinically important as it is this which bears on the cord and nerve roots producing the symptoms of much disc disease. (All images were acquired using the Picker prototype cryogenic imager at Hammersmith Hospital which operates at 0.15T[12] with matrices and slice width as given in the figure legends).

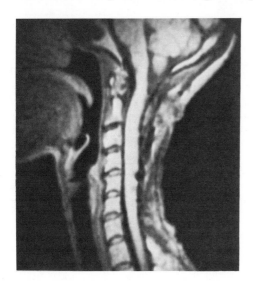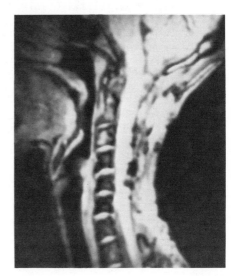

Figure 1.
Images of the cervical spine of a patient with a tumour of the cord, acquired using 512 projections on a 256 x 256 matrix with a slice thickness of 3.5mm. Fig. 1a was acquired using SE544/44 sequence; Fig. 1b using a PS500 sequence with a field echo at 22.5 msec after the exciting 90 degree pulse. At this time the lipid and water signals are out of phase and cancel, giving the appearance of Fig. 1b. The short time to the echo means that the annulus fibrosa round the discs is well seen, without the high level signal from the bone marrow to mark it.

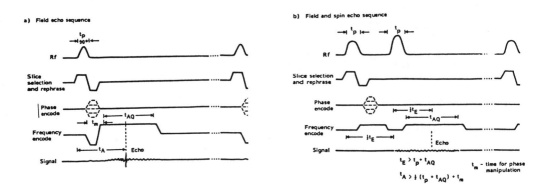

Figure 2.

Diagram of the form of spin echo and field echo data acquisitions which shows that, for constant direction of data collection, the echo in the latter will always form at an earlier time than with the former, meaning that the signal will be greater particularly from tissue with shorter T2.

In order that there shall be no confusion between artifacts and annulus, it is necessary that the chemical shift artifact be kept below, at most, 0.5 pixel. Techniques which attempt to identify what is artifact and what is genuine fail in examples such as that above including those in which phase encoding is done in non-preferred directions, such as along the body. In this case, provision must be made to avoid aliasing and these tend to take too long to avoid losing signals from tissues with short T2 values. As a result the bandwidth needed to acquire data is determined by the need to ensure that the frequency difference between pixels is greater than $7 \times 10^{-6} \gamma B_0$. The technique illustrated in Fig. 1, which is applicable to many other orthopaedic applications, particularly as cartilage is another tissue with a short T2, is an example where the strict proportionality of f (the bandwidth) and field must be maintained as the latter is changed if clinical capability is to be retained.

For completeness, two other factors which are field dependent need to be considered. The first of these reflects the time between excitation and data acquisition. In spin echo experiments this is established by the value of tE needed, but in IR direct acquisition by field echo[13] is an option that minimizes the development of T2 based contrast to oppose that derived from T1 and partial saturation (PS) and saturation recovery (SR) sequences, by definition, use that form of acquisition. For any given duration of data acquisition (as Fig. 2 indicates) tA (in a field echo) will always be less than tE. Dephasing due to field errors and eddy currents begins at the time of excitation and continues uncompensated until data acquisition is completed, so that (in Fig. 2) a phase error of $\gamma \delta B_0 t$ (where t is the time from excitation to the end of data acquisition – Fig. 2) ultimately develops. The corresponding error in a symmetrical spin echo is $\delta B \gamma ts/2$ where ts is the data sampling period. $\delta B$ contains components due to field errors ($\delta B_0$) and eddy currents (which include time dependent field errors ($\delta B(t)$). Since it is the absolute magnitude of $\delta B$ which matters, which increases with field with magnets of constant quality, field echo techniques are easier in low fields. Finally, the filling factor of a low field receiver coil designed to image a complete section is better than that for probes suitable at greater field levels. This arises since there are two requirements in such a coil:

a)  homogeneity
b)  sensitivity

The latter is (by reciprocity) a function of the ratio of the volume of a voxcel to that of the coil. Thus, the smaller the probe the better for any given study, and the greater the need for coils which are homogeneous over the greatest possible fraction of their volume. Particularly in the head quasi-spherical geometry coils[14,15] have been shown to have these attributes. However, amongst the requirements for good homogeneity are a significant number of turns, which form coils which become harder to tune as the field increases. Capacitive and inductive coupling are also less troublesome at low field. Thus, the complete signal-to-noise ratio relationship can be written as:

$$k \ (\omega) \ B_0 \ g^{1/2} \ \sigma^{-1/2} \ f^{-1/2} \ \exp(-t_A/T2) \ (1-\exp(-t_R/T1)) \qquad (2)$$

for a partial saturation (PS) experiment, where $k(\omega)$ is a term expressing the relative efficiency of the probe design with field, but which generally reduces with field and f is the bandwidth. Assuming a fixed imaging matrix (constant value of g) and slice width, all the terms in this expression with the exception of the field itself show a tendency to diminish with field.

The actual relationship is a function of the experiment being performed. As Bottomley et al.[9] have pointed out the T1 values of many tissues show dependencies on field which fall in a range around $B_0^{0.35}$. In very fast repeated sequences (tR small), the field dependence of $(1-\exp(-t_R/T1))$ is significant, though in slow multi-slice procedures the term may change little.

All in all, it is reasonable to say that the improvement in signal-to-noise ratio with field is likely to be less than as $B_0^{0.35}$, and, more generally, lie between $B_0^{0.15}$ and $B_0^{0.3}$.

CONTRAST TO NOISE RATIO

The available data about the dependence of T1 on field relates almost completely to normal tissue[9], and the spread of tissue parameters in pathological tissue is so wide that it may continue to be difficult to draw useful conclusions from examples where the same tissue is not studied in different fields. However, as is now documented (principally by Bottomley et al.[9], but also for example, by Mansfield and Morris[16]), the field dependence of many tissues can usefully be represented by a relationship of the form:

$$T1 = a \ \omega^b \qquad (3)$$

where a and b are values characteristic of each tissue, b is usually in the region of 0.3 to 0.4 for normal tissues. CSF, however, which is relatively pure water shows much less change in the range of fields of interest[17].

Taken together these restrictions mean a contraction in the range of brain T1 values as the field increases with the signals from typical lesions being sandwiched between those from grey matter and CSF. As is discussed further in Section 7, the signal from CSF tends to become dominant as tR is increased in order to allow additional slices to be interleaved, and there is difficulty in detecting periventricular lesions as their signals lie between those of normal brain and CSF. Fig. 3 illustrates the variations in signal for various tissues at various fields, using values for b from Bottomley et al.[9] where available, values from our own observations for CSF, and assuming a value of b = 0.3 for the lesion (assumed to be edema or infarction, with values of T1 of 650 msec and T2 of 150 msec, as measured at 0.15T). Fig. 3 was plotted for an SE1000/60 sequence, but the general pattern shown tends to exist in useful SE

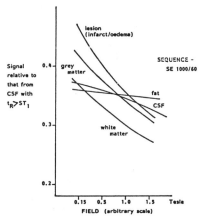

COMPUTED SIGNAL VARIATIONS WITH FIELD(LESION BEHAVIOUR
WITH FIELD SPECULATIVE)

Values computed from Bottomly et al Med Phys 11 425 (1984)
except lesion coeff. assumed 0.3 start 650 ms,0.15T
various measurements July-Sept 1984

Figure 3.

Plot of the relative signal for an SE1000/60 sequence at different fields using as starting values for tissue parameters those
measured at 0.15T on the Hammersmith machine. The function used
is that given in eq. (3) and the powers are those found by
Bottomley et al.[9]. The lesion variations were calculated using a
value of b (eq. (3)) of 0.3, and the starting values at 0.15T are
T1 = 650 msec, T2 = 150 msec. The model used for the sequence is

$$S \approx S_0 \ (1-\exp(^{-t}R/T1))\exp(^{-t}E/T2)$$

($S_0$ is available signal at $t_R > 5T1$)

sequences where in lower fields CSF signals are lower than those from brain
though pathological signals exceed them. T2 is assumed to be constant at
all field levels and tissue parameters at 0.15T are those given in Table 1.

FAST OPERATION

Contrast is also affected by other consequences of changing field which
then arise from the change in T1. As has been discussed elsewhere, slice
shape in any system which involves no non-selective inverting pulses after
the 90 degree pulse in a function of the ratios tR/T1 and tR/T2[18]. The
signal behaviour is such that the contrast is reduced below what might be
expected for simple models, as is illustrated in Fig. 4 (at 0.15T) for the
tissue pairs white matter/lesion and lesion/CSF. The parameters for the
lesion are typical of those of a multiple sclerosis plaque. The sequence
used is PS, but the argument is similar for other circumstances except
where a non-interleaved SE or IR scan is used. The degradation increases
with a reduction in tR (at fixed T1 and T2) so that as the field in which
the examination is made is increased (i.e., T1 increases) there is a relative loss of contrast if the value of tR used is not adjusted appro-
priately.

Though one of the advantages that has been advanced for operating at
high field is a reduction in scanning time, it seems quite unlikely that
much of the gain proposed is realizable only with difficulty. The one case
when the slice shape artifact does not reduce contrast beyond what might be

Table 1
Parameters of Various Tissues at 0.15T

| Tissue | Relative Proton Density | T1 (msec) | T2 (msec) | T1/T2 |
|---|---|---|---|---|
| Adult White Matter | 0.9 | 380 | 85 | 4.5 |
| Adult Gray Matter | 1 | 520 | 95 | 5.5 |
| Neonate Brain | | | | |
| Gray Matter | 1.1 | 1100 | 250 | 4.4 |
| White Matter | 1.2 | 1300 | 250 | 5.2 |
| Infarct | 1.2 | 1400 | 250 | 5.6 |
| Fat | 0.8 | 170 | 80 | 1.4 |
| Brain Infarction/Edema | 1 | 650 | 120-180 | 3.6-5.4* |
| MS Plaque | | | | typically |
| Brain Tumour | 1 | 700-1200 | 120-130 | 3.3-5.0** |
| (typical metastasis of abdominal tumour) | | | | |
| CSF | 1.2 | 1500 | 1000 | 1.5 |
| Meningioma | 1 | 600 | 100 | 5.0 |
| Liver | 1 | 250 | 50 | 5.6 |
| Muscle | 1 | 250 | 50 | 5.0 |
| Spleen | 1 | 600 | 100 | 4.0 |

\* – Values used for calculation: T1 650 msec  T2 150 msec
\*\* – Values used for calculation: T1 800 msec  T2 200 msec

Values of typical tissue parameters at 0.15T as measured at various times at Hammersmith. Sequences used have been variously SR, IR and SE all with $t_R$ of 1500 msec. and $t_I$ of 500 msec in IR. For SE various values of $t_E$ were used. The results were obtained during normal clinical imaging and were not acquired specially. All are the means of widely spread values.

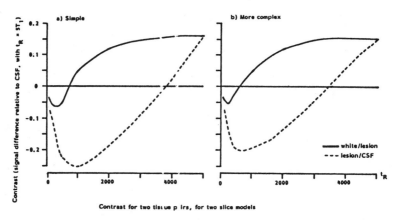

Figure 4.

Plot of the theoretical contrast differences in partial saturation
at various repetition rates using the simple model

$$S = S_0 \ (1-\exp(^{-t}R/T1))\exp(^{-t}A/T2)$$

and the more refined model

$$S = \frac{S_0 \ (1-\exp(^{-t}R/T1))\exp(^{-t}A/T2)}{1-\cos\alpha \ (\exp(^{-t}R/T1) + \exp(^{t}R/T2))+\exp(^{-t}R/T1)\exp(^{-t}R/T2)}$$

(in Fig. 4b) ( $\alpha$ is the magnetisation precession angle in excitation) for tissue pairs white matter/lesion and lesion/CSF. Tissue
parameters are given in Table 1, $t_A$ is the time to the peak of the
echo in the data acquisition.


expected is in the case of non-interleaved SE sequence when the 180 degree
pulse can be non-selective. Unfortunately, the gain here too is less than
satisfactory, as, particularly in rapidly repeated sequences, contrast differences due to T1 and T2 tend to be in opposition[19].

SCANNING PERFORMANCE

It has been argued also that rapidly repeated sequences give a better
contrast-to-noise ratio than slower ones, and that specifically, inversion
recovery (IR) is inferior to PS[20] in this respect, though the work referred
to used simple models for the sequences, and made no allowance for the
exploitation of intervals in the sequences. Further, it is clearly a simplification to suggest a performance criterion for a complex clinical situation based on only one pair of tissues. The idea of a figure of merit has
been developed elsewhere[10], based on three tissue pairs, and the results
from various sequences compared with those from an IR sequence. Scanning
efficiencies (specified below) were used as the basis of the study. Then:

$$\text{Figure of Merit (FOM)} = \frac{(E_A + E_B + E_C)_X}{(E_A + E_B + E_C)\text{IR REF}} \qquad (4)$$

for three tissue pairs A, B, C and a sequence X compared with the IR reference sequence.

206

The efficiencies were given by:

$$E = m^{3/2} n\, p^{1/2} \sum_{S=1}^{P} \quad CAS$$

Where CAS is the contrast developed in the sth echo of a sequence with repetition time t. Where the individual images are not needed, they can be added to improve the efficiency (which is allowed for in the eq. (4) up to p echoes) - though as Reference 10 points out, this procedure is not by any means universally beneficial. It is assumed that if t is less than tREF (the repetition time of the reference IR1500/500 sequence) then any extra repetitions in the same time permit a wide slice to be subdivided into m (= tREF/t ). n is the number of slices that can be interleaved.

Examination of a variety of sequences suggests that while it is certainly true that PS is an effective sequence, it is not significantly more so than IR, and both are markedly superior to many SE sequences, particularly those with short tR and short tE. Table 2, using typical tissue parameters given in Table 1, examines the same issue rather further, in that it looks at the relative figures of merit for two clinical situations, showing that the slightly simplistic view that equal weight can be given to each image of a multiple echo sequence has a major impact on what is otherwise a not terribly encouraging performance. (In body studies the need for gating complicates assessment, though techniques such as respiratory ordered phase encoding (ROPE)[21] which do not change scan times can be directly compared with other non-gated procedures).

While it is still true that SE sequences are not as productive as is often considered, what emerges are the differences between performances in the various situations. This emphasizes the weakness of the case that suggests that there is a sequence which is the answer to all clinical circumstances.

FIELD ECHO (FE) AND SPIN ECHO (SE) DATA ACQUISITION METHODS

As has been mentioned before, the echo in FE will always occur earlier than that in SE for data acquisitions of the same bandwidth (data acquisition duration for a constant sized matrix). Thus, there will be reduction in the signal (as represented by the exp (-tA/T2) term in eq. (2)), by an amount which tends to increase the longer the data acquisition period becomes because of the extra time needed before the inverting pulse in SE. The use of an asymmetric spin echo is possible, but this is in practice much more nearly a form of field echo than it is a spin echo. Table 3, using the timing given in Fig. 2, illustrates the point. The relative gain to be obtained with field echo in the body is apparent. The differences between head and body imaging are most marked when discussing spin echo methods, for not only are the T2 values of body tissues less, but the effect of motion is greater the longer the delay between excitation and data collection. This is because, even if the data collection period is locked by the gating so that the moving tissue is always in the same place, there will be some loss of accuracy in the formation of the echo as motion during the tE period will not be precisely matched before and after the inverting pulse. The benefits of multiple echoes are also much less obvious in the body, and their general utility needs assessment - in particular how to judge their efficiency and relate their performance to the other figures of merit. In Table 2 the figure of merit of the individual echoes were added, which is, as is discussed below, probably an overstatement.

Assessing the additional clinical information in a series of echoes is, however, more difficult, though this ought to be allowed for in the

Table 2

| Sequence | Clinical Situation | | Notes and Effective No. of Slices |
|---|---|---|---|
| | A | B | |
| PS200 (with 20 msec data acq.) | 1.49 | 1.44 | 15 |
| PS1000 (with 20 msec data acq.) | .44 | .20 | 15 |
| IR 1500/500 (with 20 msec FE data acq.) | 1 | 1 | 10 |
| SE 200/40 (20 msec data acq.) | .84 | .67 | 15 |
| SE 1500/80 (50 msec data acq.) | 1.29 | 1.49 | 10 (data acq. finished after 105 msec) |
| SE 1000 with 4 echoes (40,80,120,160) (all 20 msec data acq.) | 2.24 | 2.51 | 7 individual FOM added |

All referred to the result for IR 1500/500 with FE
acquisition in the same situation.

Figures of merit of a number of sequences calculated using equation (4) from the parameters given in Table 1.  The two situations are:

A.   Lesion such as an MS plaque between white matter and CSF.

B.   Tumour in the mid brain surrounded by edema.  Contrast is relevant between tumour and edema and edema and gray and white matter.

Sequence choice is intended to display the different strengths and weaknesses of typical choices.

Table 3

| Tissues | 20 msec acquisition FE echo at 15 msec SE at 30 msec | 40 msec acquisition FE at 30 msec SE at 50 msec |
|---|---|---|
| White Matter | 1.19 | 1.27 |
| Tumour | 1.08 | 1.11 |
| Liver | 1.34 | 1.49 |
| Muscle | 1.34 | 1.49 |
| Fat | 1.21 | 1.28 |
| | Ratios of FE/SE | |

Relative amplitudes of signals from various
tissues using Field Echo and Spin Echo Data
Collections.

Relative signals calculated using the parameters in Table 1 for a
number of tissues using FE and SE data acquisitions. Two acquisition times (20 msec and 40 msec) are used in each case, with the
times to the echo peaks being those which would be considered
necessary at Hammersmith.

figure of merit. Multiple echoes where the dependence is genuinely due to
T2 are barely possible with field echo data acquisition, and, though multi-
echo spin-echo data acquisition can be used with inversion recovery
sequences, the reduction in T1 contrast that follows seems unjustified
unless the aim is to obtain a numerical value.

Fig. 5a and 5b show the contrast obtained with multiple echoes from a
number of tissue pairs of clinical relevance with two significantly different sequences. Since even with 6 or 8 echoes the accuracy of a T2 measurement is not much improved as diffusion effects may still be significant[22] and multiple exponents inadequately resolved, the additional clinical information to be gained from extra echoes is confined to contrast
which is ambiguous in one image being resolved in another. From Fig. 5 it
is clear that the intermediate echoes contribute only limited additional
information to that from the two extreme images (remembering that, in
effect, two clinical situations are shown). In assessing the figure of
merit, therefore, for a multiple echo sequence, it is reasonable to add
those for two echoes of a set, to produce a composite result, regarding any
other echoes as being means of improving the noise level, even if the contrast may be impaired.

On the other hand, as observed in Section 2, field echoes are more
effective in visualizing important tissues such as cartilage and disk
walls. It is not possible to quantify the benefit that field echoes convey
in this way - since the absence of these tissues will be quite acceptable
in some examinations though essential in others. Discounting this feature
implies that the merit of spin echo based sequences will be overstated
relative to field echo ones, but even ignoring this factor spin echo acquisition is not (as Table 2 indicates) particularly impressive.

Other factors such as the different appearances of flow are as difficult to quantify. However, the enhanced signal from flow with partial
saturation[23] images which can be obtained quickly (as tR is short) and is a
useful marker in various clinical situations is an additional bonus. While
spin echo methods offer a more accurate method of quantifying flow[24] the
appearance is often ambiguous, and usually the signal intensity is less.
The following illustration is of a result which cannot be obtained simply

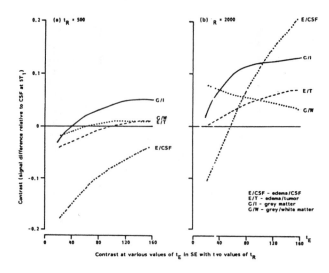

Figure 5.

Curves showing the behaviour of the contrast between a number of
tissue pairs at various spin echo tE times for two basic repetition times (500 msec and 2000 msec). The tissue pairs are:

A.  White and gray matter
B.  Gray matter and an infarcted region
C.  Edema and tumour
D.  Edema and CSF.


using SE, but which lacks accuracy when compared with what can be done with
that sequence.  Fig. 6 shows a pair of images in which Fig. 6a was acquired
using a saturation recovery sequence with tR = 200 msec, field echo data
acquisition (tA = 225 msec) and Fig. 6b was acquired using a partial saturation with the same tR and tA.  The saturation method used was a 90 degree
pulse followed by multiple spoiler gradient pulses.  These sequences result
in images which are quick to acquire (around 1.7 minutes each), but have
good signal-to-noise ratio.  The PS sequence, however, because of slice
shape artifact[18] is not readily quantifiable - since the measurements taken
are so dependent on tissue time constants.  The pair of images does indicate the presence of flow well - as the brighter CSF in the PS image shows
(at the arrows) - but flow is not readily quantifiable.

The accurate measurement of flow is best done using SE methods with the
pulsed gradients and phase measurements proposed by Stejsdal and Tanner[25]
and examined by Packer[26].  The method used is a differential one - comparing phases in images taken with different gradient amplitudes or intervals,
and so is slower.  However, detailed mapping of flow in vessels has proved
possible as described in Reference 24.

INVERSION RECOVERY

The sensitivity of IR to small changes in T1 is greater than that of
other sequences (as the usual relationship for the sequence suggests, particularly if the repetition time is substantially greater than T1).  The
problem that accompanies this is that signal levels are low, and the level
of background signal may appear noticeably in the image.  As observed previously, this arises due to the signal range being 1, and the image appearance is determined by the method of reconstruction[27].  One practical virtue
of the sensitivity of IR sequences is that they give better performance
with contrast agents such as Gadolinium-DTPA[28].  Another is the selectivity

210

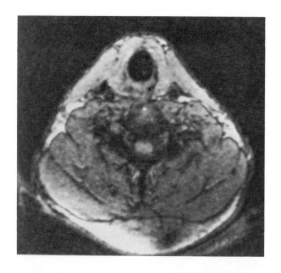

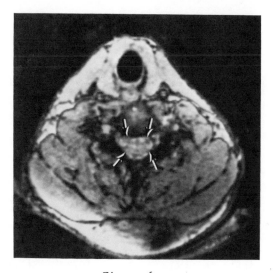

Figure 6.
Pairs of images both acquired with tR of 200 msec, matrix of 256
x 256 and slice thickness of 5mm of the neck of a patient. Fig.
6a was acquired using SR and Fig. 6b using PS. The SR sequence
used a single 90 degree pulse followed by burst of spoiler pulses
(4 of 6 msec each). Note (at the arrows) the CSF signal which
suggests movement.


with which the signals from tissue with known values of Tl can be eliminated. The values of tI needed to produce cancellation of a tissue is:

$$tI = \frac{TI}{\ln(0.5(1-\exp(-tR/T1)))}$$

As described elsewhere[29] this has clinical applications in eliminating
the peripheral fat in abdominal images which is responsible, to a significant degree, for the motion artifact which has resulted in generally disap-

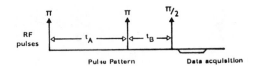

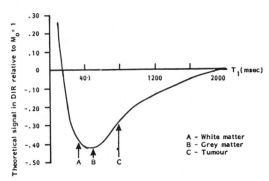

Double Inversion Recovery (DIR) Sequence Characteristics

Figure 7.
Diagram of the characteristics of the double inversion recovery
sequence for a number of tissues – including fat and CSF which
are the tissues the signals from which are suppressed in Fig. 8b.

pointing abdominal results. The high contrast obtainable with magnitude
reconstruction in this imaging method has given improved clinical performance.

Signal levels are only substantial well away from the crossover point
(where the signal is zero), and this is even more true of double inversion
recovery sequences, in which two 180 pulses are used – with the sequence
shown in Fig. 7. The signal relationship is

$$S = S_0 \, (1 - 2E_B \, (1 - E_A) - E_R)$$

where $E_A = \exp(-t_A/T1)$, $Eg = \exp(tB/T1)$ $E_R = \exp(t_R/T1)$ and the cancellation
values are obtained numerically.

This sequence, as is shown in Fig. 8a and b, goes some way towards cor-
recting the contrast problems discussed earlier, particularly as field
levels increase. In Fig. 8a, which shows an SE1500/80 image where the
signal from CSF is similar to that from the brain and possible edema, contrast is confused though the double inversion recovery image (Fig. 8b)
which is designed to cancel both CSF and fat signals results in much more
contrast. Though the images look of comparable quality, numerical analysis
would suggest that Fig. 8a has a better figure of merit than Fig. 8b –
though clearly the former lacks information available in the latter. This
arises because the cancellations in the double inversion recovery sequence
are achieved at the expense of signal – whereas, inevitably, calculation
places a premium on it.

While IR sequences acquired with a field echo have a minimum of contrast ambiguity in the case of sequences with larger tI values, SE acquisition is often employed, and multiple echoes can be obtained in order to
derive T2 information. A sequence with a value of tI which is short is the
sole instance of a case when T1 and T2 contrast values add though, even in
this case, unless tR is very long complex contrast ambiguities can arise.

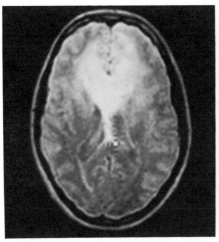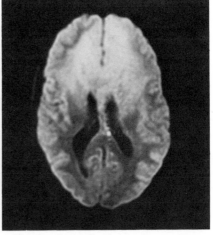

Figure 8.
Images both acquired with a matrix of 256 x 256 and slice thickness
of 5mm in which Fig. 8a is a conventional SE image (with tR of 1500
msec and tE of 80 msec) while Fig. 8b in a double inversion recovery
image with tIA of 900 msec tIB of 120 msec and tE of 80 msec.  tR
was 2000 msec.


CONCLUSION

An analysis of NMR imaging based on any one criterion will be challenged under most circumstances since the complexities of the topic are
such that it is generally feasible to find an anomaly.  Thus, the figure of
merit discussed earlier can be challenged on its ability to allow for the
subtlety of an appropriate double inversion recovery image.  However, the
approach does suggest that it is an oversimplification to suggest that
there are single sequences which are universally better than others.  The
differences between field and spin echo are perhaps the dominant factor in
altering the relative figures of merit of the sequences, particularly in
the body.  These, in turn, enter the argument about the variations of performance with change in field level, for it is relatively easier to work
with field echoes in lower field systems than it is in higher ones.  Particularly in the body, again, this reduces the predicted gain in performance
with increasing field to a very moderate figure.

ACKNOWLEDGEMENTS

We are grateful to the DHSS, and particularly to Mr. G. R. Higson and
Mr. J. L. Williams, for the help and support throughout the program from
which this work is derived.

REFERENCES

1.  I. M. Mackay, G. M. Bydder, I. R. Young, Magnetic Resonance Imaging of
    Central Nervous System Tumors Which do Not Display Evidence of an
    Increase in Tl or T2, J. Comp. Asst. Tomog. (in press).
2.  J. J. H. Ackerman, T. H. Grove, G. C. Wong, D. G. Gadian, G. K. Radda,
    Mapping of Metabolites in Whole Animals by 31P NMR using Surface
    Coils, Nature (London) 283:167 (1980).
3.  J. L. Evelhoch, M. G. Crowley, J. J. H. Ackerman, The Effect of Sur-
    face Coil B1 Inhomogeneity on Spatial Localization and T1 Measure-
    ments, J. Mag. Res. Med. (ABS) 1(2):150-151 (1984).

4.  I. R. Young, Signal and Contrast in NMR Imaging, <u>Brit</u>. <u>Med</u>. <u>Bull</u>. 40(2):139-147 (1984).

5.  C-N Chen, V. J. Sank, D. I. Hoult, Probing Image Frequency Dependence, Proc. 3rd. Ann. Mtg. Soc. Mag. Res. Med., New York City, NY 148 (1984).

6.  D. G. Gadian, Nuclear Magnetic Resonancer and Its Applications to Living Systems, Clarendon Press, Oxford, p. 161 et seq. (1982).

7.  D. I. Hoult, P. C. Lauterbur, The Sensitivity of the Zeugmatographic Experiment Involving Human Samples, <u>J</u>. <u>Mag</u>. <u>Res</u>. 34:425-453 (1979).

8.  E. H. Grant, Interaction of Radio Waves and Microwaves with Biological Material, <u>Br</u>. <u>J</u>. <u>Cancer</u>, 45 Suppl. V 1 (1982).

9.  P. A. Bottomley, T. H. Foster, R. E. Argersinger, L. M. Pfeifer, A Review of Normal Tissue Hydrogen NMR Relaxation Times and Relaxation Mechanisms from 1-100MHz Dependence on Tissue Type, <u>Med</u>. <u>Phys</u>. 11:425 (1984).

10. I. R. Young, M. Burl, G. M. Bydder, A Study of the Comparative Efficiencies of Different Pulse Sequences in Magnetic Resonance Imaging (submitted to <u>J</u>. <u>Comp</u>. <u>Asst</u>. <u>Tomog</u>.)

11. D. Kunz, W. Vollman, W. Mehnhard, Separation of Fat and Water in: "MR Imaging, Magnetic Resonance Imaging and Spectroscopy," M. A. Hopf, G. M. Bydder, eds., <u>Eur</u>. <u>Soc</u>. <u>Mag</u>. <u>Res</u>. <u>Med</u>. <u>Biol</u>., Geneva, Swi., pp 36-41 (1985).

12. I. R. Young, D. R. Bailes, M. Burl, A. G. Collins, D. T. Smith, M. J. McDonnell, J. S. Orr, L. M. Banks, G. M. Bydder, R. H. Greenspan, R. E. Steiner, Initial Clinical Evaluation of a Whole Body, NMR Tomograph, <u>J</u>. <u>Comp</u>. <u>Asst</u>. <u>Tomog</u>, 6:1-18 (1982).

13. R. J. Sutherland, J. M. S. Hutchison, Three Dimension NMR Imaging Using Selective Excitation, <u>J</u>. <u>Phys</u>. <u>E</u>. <u>Sci</u>. <u>Instrum</u>, 11:79 (1978).

14. P. C. Butson, I. R. Young, G. M. Bydder, Closely Coupled Receiver Coils as a Means of Improving the Signal-to-Noise Ratio in: "Magnetic Resonance Imaging of the Brain, Magnetic Resonance Imaging and Spectroscopy," M. A. Hopf, G. M. Bydder, eds., <u>Eur</u>. <u>Soc</u>. <u>Mag</u>. <u>Res</u>. <u>Med</u>. <u>Biol</u>., Geneva, Swi., pp 307-313 (1985).

15. G. M. Bydder, P. C. Butson, R. R. Harman, D. J. Gilderdale, I. R. Young, Use of Spherical Receiver Coils in MR Imaging of the Brain, <u>J</u>. <u>Comp</u>. <u>Asst</u>. <u>Tomog</u>. 9(2):413-414 (1985).

16. P. Mansfield, P. G. Morris, NMR Imaging in: "Biomedicine," Academic Press, NY, pp. 15-30 (1982).

17. D. G. Gadian, J. R. Griffiths, M. A. Foster, Private Communications, Sept. (1984).

18. I. R. Young, D. J. Bryant, J. A. Payne, Variations in Slice Shape and Absorption as Artifacts in the Determination of Tissue Parameters in NMR Imaging, <u>Mag</u>. <u>Res</u>. <u>Med</u>. (in press).

19. I. R. Young, G. M. Bydder, Some Factors Involving Slice Shape Which Affect Contrast in Nuclear Magnetic Resonance (NMR) Imaging, <u>Ann</u>. <u>de</u> <u>Radiologie</u> 28(2):112-118 (1985).

20. W. A. Edelstein, P. A. Bottomley, H. R. Hart, L. S. Smith, Signal Noise and Contrast in Nuclear Magnetic Resonance (NMR) Imaging, <u>J</u>. <u>Comp</u>. <u>Asst</u>. <u>Tomog</u>. 7:391 (1983).

21. D. R. Bailes, D. J. Gilderdale, G. M. Bydder, A. G. Collins, D. N. Firmin, Respiratory Ordered Phase Encoding (ROPE), a Method for Reducing Respiratory Motion Artifact in Magnetic Resonance Imaging, <u>J</u>. <u>Comp</u>. <u>Asst</u>. <u>Tomog</u>. (in press).

22. H. Y. Carr, E. M. Purcell, Effects of Diffusion on Free Precession in Nuclear Magnetic Resonance Experiments, <u>Phys</u>. <u>Rev</u>. 94:630-638 (1958).

23. I. R. Young, D. R. Bailes, A. G. Collins, D. J. Gilderdale, Image Options in NMR, in "NMR Imaging," R. L. Witcofski, N. Karsteadt, C. L. Partain, eds., Bowman Gray School of Medicine, Winston Salem, NC, 15-23 (1982).

24.  D. J. Bryant, J. A. Payne, D. N. Firmin, D. B. Longmore, Measurement Flow with NMR Imaging Using a Gradient Pulse and Phase Difference Technique, J. Comp. Asst. Tomog. 8(4):588 (1984).

25.  E. O. Stejskal, J. E. Tanner, Spin Diffusion Measurements. Spin Echoes in the Presence of a Time-Dependent Field Gradient, J. Chem. Phys. 42:288-292 (1965).

26.  K. J. Packer, The Study of Slow Coherent Molecular Motion by Pulsed Nuclear Magnetic Resonance, Mol. Phys. 17:355 (1969).

27.  I. R. Young, D. R. Bailes, G. M. Bydder, Apparent Changes of Appearance of Inversion Recovery Images, Mag. Res. Med. 2:81-85 (1985).

28.  D. G. Gadian, J. A. Payne, D. J. Bryant, I. R. Young, D. H. Carr, G. M. Bydder, Gadolinium DTPA as a Contrast Agent in MR Imaging Theoretical Projections and Practical Observations, J. Comp. Asst. Tomog. 9(2):242-251 (1985).

29.  G. M. Bydder, I. R. Young, MRI Clinical Use of the Inversion Recovery Sequence, J. Comp. Asst. Tomog. (in press).

# SIGNAL, NOISE AND R. F. POWER IN MAGNETIC RESONANCE IMAGING

D. I. Hoult

Biomedical Engineering and Instrumentation Branch,
Division of Research Services, Building 13, Room 3W13
National Institutes of Health, Bethesda, M.D. 20205, U.S.A.

## ABSTRACT

The influences on magnetic resonance imaging of probe design, relaxation times, chemical shift and power deposition are considered in the light of the controversy surrounding the notion of an optimal imaging field strength. It is shown that the noise in the experiment originates in the patient, and that in consequence, the signal-to-noise ratio (S/N) increases, at the most, linearly with field. The removal of chemical shift artifacts is discussed, and the use of a Carr-Purcell sequence recommended as a way of maintaining signal-to-noise ratio while eliminating artifacts. The concept of desired image S/N is then introduced, and it is shown that there exists a vaguely defined field strength at which that ratio is attained in the minimum time. Finally, the dangers of excessive power deposition in a patient are highlighted, and the use of a field in the range 0.5 to 1 Tesla advocated as giving good signal-to-noise ratio and versatility while not exceeding recommended power limits.

## INTRODUCTION

It is well known in traditional NMR studies that probe design has a considerable bearing on spectrum signal-to-noise ratio,[1] as of course, do $T_1$, $T_2$ and sample concentration. The same factors affect the quality of a proton image, but for very different reasons, and the aim of this writing is to outline in broad terms the workings of the factors, while also considering the influences of chemical shift and r.f. power on the imaging experiment. To begin, we examine the origins of the signal and noise. On the assumption that the imaging experiment is functioning correctly, we need not consider the signal from the entire sample (a human,) but rather, can concentrate upon the signal from the elementary volume (voxel) which gives rise to the brightness of a single picture element (pixel) – i.e. to the numerical content of one element of the data matrix.[2] The f.i.d. (which may be in the form of an echo) from the voxel of choice is generated by its precessing nuclear magnetization's inducing in the receiving coil a small voltage which is amplified and recorded in the usual way. However, the noise associated with the signal does not arise from the voxel, nor, for the most part, from the probe. Rather, its origins are in the Brownian motion of the electrolytes in the human body.[3] The rotational component of this motion induces magnetically a random voltage in the receiving coil, and the strength of this voltage is powerfully dependent on the size of the sample (approximately 5/2 power of linear dimension,) and the square root of its electrical conductivity, for motion of electrolytes is, of course, associated with electrical conduction,- a factor of some consequence when a $B_1$ field is applied, for heat is generated.[3,4] Unfortunately, no way has been found of removing this noise, which like the NMR signal itself, increases with frequency, and so, for constant conductivity, the f.i.d. signal-to-noise ratio (S/N) only increases linearly with frequency. To make matters worse, the conductivity of the human body tends to increase with frequency too, and so while from the head, f.i.d. S/N does tend to vary linearly with Larmor frequency $\nu_0$ our measurements[5] indicate that from the body the dependence is only as $\nu_0^{0.8}$. As both the signal and the noise originate from the sample, it follows that, in a very real sense, the sample dictates its own S/N, and the only way to improve matters is to reduce the volume of sample which the receiving coil "sees," (to write loosely,) thereby reducing substantially the induced noise. The ultimate in this process is, of course, a surface coil,[6] whose active volume is so small that the induced noise is now negligible in comparison to the noise generated by the probe's resistance. However, the price paid is loss of field of view.

## FROM F.I.D. TO PROJECTION

With most imaging strategies which collect an appreciable number of f.i.d.s. (so as to obtain full spatial information,) the step following data collection is, as in spectroscopy, Fourier transformation. However, the aim of the transformation is to take advantage of the relationship between spatial distance and frequency created by the imposition of a field gradient. With the use of a linear gradient, distance and frequency become synonymous - they are yoked (ζευγμα) together; hence Lauterbur's coinage of the term "zeugmatography".[7] However, transverse relaxation $T_2$ and chemical shift $\delta$ spoil the relationship. A decrease in $T_2$ causes a spread of frequency, while a chemical shift causes a change of frequency. These effects are translated, because of the assumption that the synonymy is accurate, into, respectively, a blurring of, and an erroneous shift of perceived image spatial position.[8] Further, a decrease of $T_2$ also results in a decrease of amplitude in the transform - a dependency which may or may not be desirable.

The simplest way of eliminating the image artifacts these effects cause is to reduce the length of time $\Delta t$ for which an f.i.d. is digitized, so that the inequalities

$$\Delta t \ll T_2 \quad ; \quad \Delta t \ll 1/\nu_0 \delta \qquad\qquad 1$$

are satisfied (Here $\delta$ is the chemical shift range in p.p.m., and $\nu_0$ is the Larmor frequency in MHz.) However, once these inequalities are satisfied, the S/N in the transform becomes proportional to $\sqrt{\Delta t}$, and so a compromise between S/N and artifacts is needed. Given a proton chemical shift range of over 4 p.p.m.[9], it is clear that at high field strengths (e.g. 2 Tesla) $\Delta t$ is becoming small ($\ll 3$ ms,) while the gradient strengths needed to maintain high spatial resolution are becoming large ($\gg 10^{-2}$ T/m). Thus a compromise value of $\Delta t \sim 1/\delta\nu_0$ can produce images with little or no artifact, but this value is well below the compromise ($\Delta t \sim 30$ ms) necessary to render $T_2$ effects negligible, and thus we must ask if there is any way of maintaining image fidelity while recovering the S/N lost when $\Delta t$ is grossly restricted.

Three approaches are possible. The first is that the above arguments are invalid if there is negligible chemical shift in the sample. Thus, for example, the normal head contains little fat, so there is little evidence of artifact in a high field image, even when $\Delta t = 30$ ms. The signal-to-noise ratio is, of course, excellent in such images, for full advantage can then be taken of the linear dependence of S/N upon frequency. (However, with an abnormal head, or the torso, the situation may be very different.) The second approach is to regard the chemical shift as a blessing rather than a curse, in that it contains extra information which may be of clinical use. Thus the technique of chemical shift imaging,[10] which produces separate images of, say water and fat, has recently become popular. However, it should be noticed that with the exception of echo-planar methods,[11] the production of a chemical shift image takes appreciably longer than that of a "composite" image - a point of some significance in a typical radiology department. Further, while the extra time taken to collect the additional data does result in improved S/N in any particular image, (e.g. the water image,) integration of the chemical shift spectrum associated with each voxel, in order to reestablish a composite image, negates the improvement. Thus chemical shift imaging is no real solution to the problem of chemical shift artifacts; rather it is a technique for obtaining spectral information, and at the moment, it is not clear what clinical value such information holds. The third approach utilizes an echo train - the familiar Carr-Purcell sequence. Using $180^{\circ}$ echo pulses, the data lasting a time $\Delta t$ are repeatedly regenerated for as long ($\sim T_2$) as is desired. By co-addition of the images formed from each echo, the full S/N can be recovered, and as an added bonus, $T_2$ information can easily be extracted. However, it is not easy to put such a scheme into practice, for a variety of technical reasons, and further the many $180^{\circ}$ pulses generate considerable heating of the patient - a point to be considered in more detail later. Thus considerable research is in progress on the problem of selective, minimum energy $180^{\circ}$ refocusing pulses. The importance of this research may be seen from the fact that in a body image, transform S/N varies only as $\nu_0^{0.3}$ when $\Delta t$ is restricted,[5] whereas if, by image co-addition, the full effective value of $\Delta t \sim T_2$ can be used, S/N varies as $\nu_0^{0.8}$, giving far more credence to the use of higher field systems.

## FROM PROJECTION TO IMAGE

It takes, in most circumstances, far more than 1 f.i.d. to make an image. Two factors govern the actual number of f.i.d.s needed. The first is the S/N required from our voxel of interest (an n-fold increase in the number of f.i.d.s gathered results, as usual, in a $\sqrt{n}$-fold increase in S/N,) and the second is the minimum number required for the image reconstruction protocol to work (typically 256.) At low fields, say 0.1T, it may be necessary to average several sets of data, but as we increase field strength and f.i.d. S/N improves, there will come a point when the minimum number of f.i.d.s is sufficient to produce good images. At what frequency this subjectively assessed point is reached is obviously debatable, for one viewer may require a S/N of 20:1 while another may insist on 60:1. However, if the multiple echo method may be employed, a good argument may be made that sufficient S/N is available in a body image in the region of 0.7T. This being the case, we must examine how long it takes to obtain an image at higher fields. No matter what protocol may be employed, the "gold standard" by which f.i.d. repetition rate is judged is the longitudinal relaxation time $T_1$, and for all body tissues, this increases with frequency.[12,13] Thus the penalty paid for pushing the field strength beyond the minimum necessary is an increase in imaging time - the same penalty we pay for using a field which is too low. It follows that if we are interested in the "best" field for imaging, we must be careful in establishing our criteria. If we want the ultimate in S/N ratio and care but little for the time taken to obtain it, then clearly the highest field is called for. However, if we wish to have good image quality in the minimum time, then there exists a vaguely defined optimum in the mid-field range. It might be thought that a complicating factor in this argument is the use of the lengthened $T_1$ value (as compared to $T_2$, which varies but little with field) to obtain more slices in a multi-slice experiment. However, this is not so. The factor govering the repetition rate of f.i.d.s from differing slices is not saturation ($T_1$), it is $T_2$, and thus the minimum time taken to obtain a given number of slices is almost independent of field strength, once averaging of images is no longer required. Finally, it is worth pointing out that there is not too much that can be accomplished with excess S/N. The slice thickness may be reduced to the point where it is comparable to the basic resolution of the image, but the latter may only be improved by increasing the number of "views" (i.e. the number of f.i.d.s needed to form the image) and thus, once again more time is required, a waste if motion of one sort or another is blurring the image anyway.

## POWER DEPOSITION

We have already seen that the application of a $B_1$ transmitting field to a human deposits energy because the body is a conductor. There naturally arises therefore, the questions of how much heating is necessary, and whether or not it is dangerous. Neither question is easy to answer. While a healthy person can lie on a beach under the full summer sun and absorb of the order of 1 kW for some time, a patient with thermoregulatory, vasodilatory and cardiovascular problems may be able to handle far less stress. Further, that ability will be influenced by the humidity of the imaging suite, the air flow over the patient and his or her nervous state. Ultimately, it may be necessary for the physician to make an assessment (based on research not yet performed) of what the patient can tolerate. Meanwhile the various governmental bodies responsible for regulation of such matters have recommended limits based on, and comparable to, a person's resting metabolic rate[14,15]($\sim$1.2 W/kg). Turning to the question of how much heat is dissipated in the imaging experiment, the answer is, of course, totally dependent on the protocol employed. However, while it is possible in theory to produce images without the use of 180° echo pulses, in practice, for reasons concerned with field homogeneity and chemical shift, they are inevitably used in current imaging systems, and constitute the main offender in terms of patient heating, especially if multiple echoes are used.[16] We must therefore ask what determines the strength of the $B_1$ field used in an imaging experiment. The criterion must be that the field affects uniformly all magnetization within its designated orb of influence, and while, in practice, magnetic field inhomogeneity may affect the issue, the fundamental governing factor is once again the chemical shift range. If the selective 90° pulse which determines the width and location of the slice of interest does not cover a frequency range much greater than that of the chemical shift, an image may comprise water signal from one section and fat from an adjacent section – an artifact difficult to detect. Once the slice has been selected, any refocusing pulse must cover satisfactorily the chosen frequency range. Thus $B_1$ must satisfy the inequalities

$$B_1 \gg 2\pi/\gamma T_2 \; ; \; B_1 \gg 2\pi\delta\nu_0/\gamma \qquad\qquad 2$$

Now during the pulse, the instantaneous power deposition is governed by the proportionality[3]

$$W \propto \nu_0^2 \, B_1^2 \, \sigma \qquad\qquad 3$$

where $\sigma$ is the electrical conductivity of the body. We therefore see that as we increase in field strength, and the chemical shift becomes an important factor in determing $B_1$'s intensity, the energy deposited by a 180° pulse becomes proportional to at least the cubic power of frequency $\nu_0$ (180° pulse length is dependent on $1/B_1$, and $\sigma$ may increase with increasing frequency.) Now we have seen that to obtain the maximum signal-to-noise ratio from a slice, the use of multiple echoes is essential if artifacts are to be avoided. However, inequality 1 shows that the time aperture $\Delta t$ various inversely with Larmor frequency, and thus, in a highly efficient multi-echo, multi-slice experiment, the rate at which 180° pulses are applied is proportional to frequency. It follows that for this rather efficient experiment, power deposition in the person increases as at least the fourth power of frequency, and not withstanding any questions as to what constitutes satisfactory fulfillment of In. 2 , a reasonably accurate assessment of the frequency at which the power deposition safety limit is reached can be made. For example, if the power deposited in the torso is given by the experimentally determined equation

$$W = 3 \times 10^{-7} \, \nu_1^2 \, \nu_0^{2.4} \; \stackrel{x}{\div} 3 \qquad\qquad 4$$

where $\nu_1$ is the Larmor frequency in the rotating frame, and if

$$\nu_1 = 3 \, \nu_0 \, \delta \qquad\qquad 5$$

then for rectangular 180° pulses repeated at a rate of one every $1/\delta\nu_0$ seconds, the deposition is given by

$$W = 4.5 \times 10^{-7} \, \delta^2 \, \nu_0^{4.4} \qquad\qquad 6$$

and, for example, 30 watts are deposited at 32 MHz. Clearly, the assumptions made in the above calculation can be challenged and the coefficient in Eq. 6 debated. The important point is that the order of magnitude of the result is comparable to the body's resting metabolic rate, and further because of the powerful dependency on Larmor frequency, even considerable changes in permitted power, or the coefficient, do not have a great effect on the frequency at which the power deposition is appreciable. We may therefore conclude that such deposition in the body is of serious concern as we increase in frequency, and that it places restrictions on the efficiency of data gathering so long as 180° echo pulses are essential for faithful and rapid imaging.

# CONCLUSION

Clearly, there is much room for research concerning the removal of chemical shift effects and the minimization of power deposition. Indeed it may well be that by the time this paper is published, the arguments it contains will be outdated. However, at the time of writing, they do appear to indicate that, along with questions of installation costs and the volume of influence of the magnet's fringe field, a medium field instrument (0.5 to 1T) represents the best compromise for the radiology department concerned with routine diagnosis rather than research. Such an instrument can produce high quality images in a versatile manner while not consuming excessive time, and as its technology is not quite so experimental, it is probably also a little more reliable. Meanwhile, it is hoped that the present writing will help underline the fact that it is not sufficient to judge performance purely on the basis of a manufacturer's carefully selected best images. There is more to a pretty picture than meets the eye!

# REFERENCES

1.  D. I. Hoult and R. E. Richards, J. Magn. Reson. 24:71 (1976).
2.  D. I. Hoult, Brit. Med. Bull. 40:132 (1984).
3.  D. I. Hoult and P. C. Lauterbur, J. Magn. Reson. 34:425 (1979).
4.  P. A. Bottomley and E. R. Andrew, Phys. Med. Biol. 23:630 (1978).
5.  D. I. Hoult, C. -N. Chen, and V. J. Sank, submitted to Magn. Res. Med.
6.  J. J. H. Ackerman, T. H. Grove, G. G. Wong, D. Gadian, and G. K. Radda, Nature 283:167 (1980).
7.  P. C. Lauterbur, Nature 242:190 (1973).
8.  A. J. Dwyer, R. H. Knop, and D. I. Hoult, J. Comp. Ass. Tomog. 9:16 (1985).
9.  R. E. Gordon, P. E. Hanley, and D. Shaw, Prog. NMR Spec. 15:1 (1982).
10. B. R. Rosen, I. L. Pykett, and T. J. Brady, Nuclear Magnetic Resonance Chemical Shift Imaging, in "Biomedical Magnetic Resonance," T. L. James and A. R. Margulis, eds., Radiology Research Education Foundation, San Francisco (1984).
11. P. Mansfield, Magn. Res. Med. 1:370 (1984).
12. P. T. Beall, S. R. Amtey, and S. R. Kasturi, "NMR Data Handbook for Biomedical Applications," Pergamon Press, New York (1984).
13. P. A. Bottomley, T. H. Foster, R. E. Argersinger, and L. M. Pfeifer, General Electric Company Technical Information Series, Report No. 84CRD072, Schenectady, New York (1984).
14. Office of Radiological Health "Guidelines for Evaluating Electromagnetic Risk for Trials of Clinical NMR Systems," Communications of February 25th and December 28, Food and Drug Administration, Rockville, MD (1982).
15. National Radiological Protection Board, Brit. J. Radiol. 56:974 (1983).
16. P. A. Bottomley, R. W. Redington, W. A. Edelstein, and J. F. Schenck, Magn. Res. Med., In press.

# HIGH FIELD NMR IMAGING AND SPECTROSCOPY

Paul A. Bottomley

General Electric Corporate Research
and Development Center, PO Box 8
Schenectady, New York 12301

## INTRODUCTION

The combination of proton ($^1$H) NMR imaging and phosphorus ($^{31}$P), carbon ($^{13}$C) and $^1$H NMR chemical shift spectroscopy techniques for clinical applications has been a major goal of our research program. It is hoped that such a combination could provide a comprehensive dossier of the bodies' anatomical and biochemical function to serve in the monitoring of disease states and their response to therapy and recovery. It was our perception that the major problems involved in combining the two technologies were initially instrumental and not due to any insurmountable physical obstacles. Thus the stringent requirements of chemical shift spectroscopy in the body necessitated the introduction of highly homogeneous, high field, large bore superconducting magnets. The relatively high NMR frequencies demanded of the NMR coils used in these magnet systems necessitated the development of new RF coil designs for $^1$H NMR imaging. The application of strong gradient magnetic fields to achieve spatial localization in NMR imaging is usually incompatible with the high magnetic field homogeneity required for resolution of chemical shift information. Hence new techniques for obtaining spatially localized spectra were required.

We have constructed a whole-body NMR research system based on a 1.5 T, 1 m bore magnet with homogeneity of the order 0.5 ppm across the head. This system has been used to produce $^1$H head, body, and high-resolution surface-coil NMR images, as well as spatially localized $^{31}$P, $^{13}$C, and $^1$H spectra of the head and body, and $^1$H images of different chemically shifted species of the head and limbs. An overview of these imaging and spectroscopy techniques and results is presented here. Two other magnetic field dependent parameters important to clinical high-field imaging, the RF power deposited by NMR pulses, and the NMR relaxation times, are also discussed.

## NMR IMAGING

### Imaging Sequences

NMR images can be generated from a sample placed in the magnet by application of a complex sequence of gradient and RF magnetic field pulses. A typical sequence for generating transaxial images is exemplified in Fig. 1[1]. The sequence commences with the selective excitation of nuclei in a thin slice of desired thickness lying perpendicular to the z-axis by application of a selective excitation RF pulse during interval $q_1$ in the presence of a z-gradient. This is followed by an inverting RF pulse in interval $q_3$ to generate an NMR signal during intervals $q_4$ and $q_5$. The NMR signal is observed in the presence of an x-gradient so that its NMR frequency spectrum is a one-dimensional projection of the slice along the x-axis. The projection is obtained by Fourier transformation of the NMR signal. Spatial information in the y-direction within the plane results from application of variable amplitude y-gradient pulses during interval $q_2$ in subsequent repetitions of the imaging sequence. A second Fourier transformation with respect to the y-gradient amplitude yields the complete planar image of the selected slice. In practice, signals are often averaged several times prior to advancing the y-gradient in order to improve the signal-to-noise ratio. The sequence is repeated with $n_y$ different y-gradient values and the NMR signal sampled at $n_x$ equally spaced points in the time-domain to yield an $n_x$ by $n_y$ point image upon reconstruction.

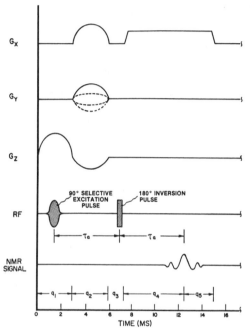

**Fig. 1.** Typical gradient/RF pulse sequence used for performing an NMR imaging experiment. The z-axis is coincident with the cylindrical axis of the sample-tube and the magnet, with the x-axis horizontal and orthogonal to z. $G_x = \partial Bo/\partial x$, $G_y = \partial Bo/\partial y$ and $G_z = \partial B_o/\partial z$ are the linear x-, y-, and z- imaging gradients in the main magnetic field $B_o$. $\tau_a$ is the period between selective and inversion RF pulses. The selective excitation pulse consists of sinc-function modulated RF.

## RF Coils

The RF coil used for excitation and detection of NMR signals from the head at 1.5 T (64 MHz) was initially a 25 cm diameter slotted-tube resonator[2,3]. The resonator consisted of a 30 cm long cylinder of copper sheet with two 20 cm long windows cut on opposite sides, each window opening subtending a $100^o$ angle at the axis (Fig. 2). The key to the high-frequency performance of this structure is the use of distributed rather than lumped tuning capcitances symmetrically located at 4 breaks in the copper at the ends of the cylinder adjacent to the windows.

Distributing the capacitance in this manner results in a four-fold reduction in the voltage and electric field between adjacent conductor, decreasing the self-capacitance of the structure and raising its self-resonance frequency. The use of capacitively-coupled copper guard-rings at RF ground on the inside of the coil-former minimizes capacitive coupling to the sample. This coil proved suitable for NMR experiments on the head at frequencies well-above 70 MHz, whereas use of the conventional "half-turn" saddle geometry[4] was precluded above about 50 MHz on a comparably-sized structure due to its self-resonance properties[2]. The use of distributed impedance networks in NMR coil designs has recently been extended to 16 or more elements in the "bird-cage" resonator design[5]. Such multi-element strategies can provide improved RF field uniformities.

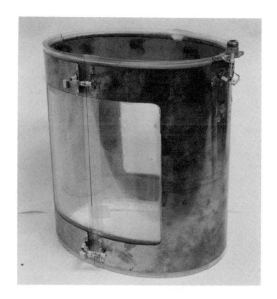

Fig. 2 A slotted tube resonator NMR coil used for head imaging at 64 MHz (1.5 T). The RF field is directed through the centre of the windows.

## Images and Contrast

Examples of transaxial $^1$H NMR images through the head and body obtained by application of the imaging sequence shown in Fig. 1, are presented in Fig. 3A, B[2,6]. Fig. 3C, D show higher resolution images through the eye and the knee-joint respectively. These images were detected using a 10 cm diameter single turn circular NMR coil located on the surface of the body adjacent to the respective anatomy[7,8]. Surface coils of relatively small radii provide the best signal-to-noise ratio ($\psi$) for imaging tissues close to the surface because their restricted spatial sensitivity significantly reduces the detected noise from the sample, and because the region of interest is close to the coil, generating a relatively large signal. It is this improvement in $\psi$ which permits the reduction of the image point size, and the consequent improvement in spatial resolution. In surface coil imaging a conventional whole-body or head transmitter coil is usually employed for excitation, so that the RF excitation field is uniform across the region of interest.

The NMR image intensity in a selected (transaxial) plane in the sample is approximately given by

$$S(x,y) \propto \rho(x,y) \left[1 - \exp\left(\frac{\tau}{T_1(x,y)}\right)\right] \qquad (1)$$

where $\tau$ is the repetition period of the sequence of Fig. 1, $\rho(x,y)$ is the proton nuclear spin density at $(x,y)$, $T_1$ is the spin-lattice relaxation time at $(x,y)$, and the spin-spin relaxation time $T_2 \ll \tau$. Thus tissue $T_1$'s are a major consideration in determining the image signal strength, and also affect the image scan time via the choice of the $\tau$ parameter. It can be shown that optimum contrast and signal-to-noise ratio results from a choice of $\tau \sim T_1$ with this sequence. Differences amongst tissue relaxation times also provides the major mechanism for image contrast and the discrimination of disease.

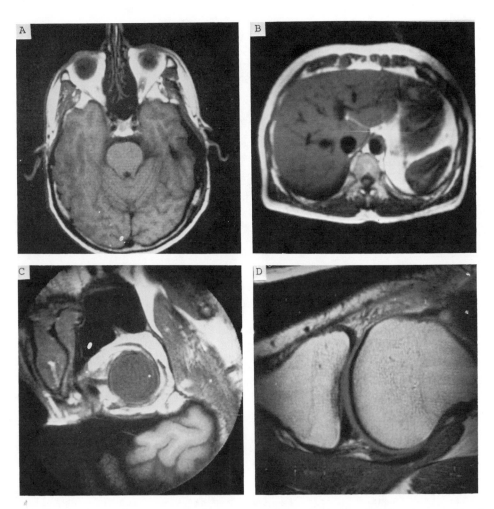

**Fig. 3.** 1.5 T NMR images recorded through (A) the head at eye-level (scan time, 102 s; resolution, 1x1x4 mm per picture point), (B) the body through the liver (scan time, 5 min; resolution, 2x2x5 mm per picture point), (C) through the eye in a coronal plane and (D) the knee in a sagittal plane using a 10 cm diameter surface coil (scan time, 3.4 min; resolution, 0.5x0.5x3 mm per picture point). Image array sizes were 256x256 throughout.

## NMR Relaxation

Recently, we reviewed the published $^1$H NMR $T_1$'s and $T_2$'s of normal tissue as a function of NMR frequency ($\nu$), tissue type, species, temperature, excision, and age.[10] Tissue type and NMR frequency were observed to be the main factors affecting $T_1$ and it was found that the frequency dispersions of all tissues could be fitted to the expression $T_1 = A\nu^B$ in the range 1-100 MHz, with A and B ($\sim 1/3$) tissue-dependent constants. $T_2$ was found to be essentially constant with NMR frequency, and often multicomponent. The results are tabulated in Table 1: the $T_1$ dispersion for liver is depicted in Fig. 4. Typically, tissue $T_1$'s change by only about 25% from 25 MHz (0.5 T) to 64 MHz (1.5 T). As the NMR signal-to-noise ratio $\psi \propto \nu^\alpha$ with $1 \leq \alpha \leq 7/4$, depending on whether the dominant noise source is the sample or the NMR coil,[11] this elongation in $T_1$ does not override the inherent $\psi$ advantage of the higher operating field.

Table 1

MEAN $^1$H TISSUE $T_1$ and $T_2$ RELAXATION TIMES

| Tissue | $T_1^1$ | | | $T_2^2$ | |
|---|---|---|---|---|---|
| | A | B | SD (%) | $T_2$ (ms) | SD (ms) |
| Muscle | | | | | |
| skeletal | .000455 | .4203 | 18 | 47 | 13 |
| heart | .00130 | .3618 | 16 | 57 | 16 |
| Liver | .000534 | .3799 | 22 | 43 | 14 |
| Kidney$^3$ | .00745 | .2488 | 27 | 58 | 24 |
| Spleen | .00200 | .3321 | 19 | 62 | 27 |
| Adipose | .0113 | .1743 | 28 | 84 | 36 |
| Brain | | | | | |
| grey matter | .00362 | .3082 | 17 | 101 | 13 |
| white matter | .00152 | .3477 | 17 | 92 | 22 |
| unspecified | .00232 | .3307 | 19 | 76 | 21 |
| Lung | .00407 | .2958 | 19 | 79 | 29 |
| Marrow$^4$ | | | | 59 | 24 |
| Breast$^5$ | | | | 49 | 16 |

1. $T_1 = A\nu^B \pm$ SD %, where $\nu = ^1$H NMR frequency in Hz, SD = standard deviation expressed as a percentage of $T_1$, $T_1$ in sec.

2. Assumes $T_2$ is independent of frequency. Multicomponent data is omitted from the computations. $T_2$ is in ms. SD = standard deviation in ms.

3. Averages medulla and cortex.

4. Insufficient data for a $T_1$ fit.

5. Use skeletal muscle and/or adipose $T_1$ fits.

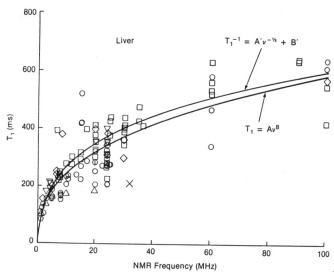

Fig. 4. $T_1$ dispersion data for liver fitted to $T_1 = A\nu^B$ with A = 0.000534, B = 0.3799 and standard deviation from the curve of 22% using a method of least squares. The mean cited standard deviation for each point expressed as a percentage of the $T_1$ value is about (9±5)%. Different symbols denote different species: human samples are represented by diamonds.

### RF Power Deposition

An additional consideration for clinical high-field imaging is the power deposited in the body by the RF pulses[12-14]. Power deposition is usually expressed as the specific absorption rate P in W/kg. In a cylinder of tissue, a θ radian NMR pulse of duration T deposits power

$$P(r) \sim (1.5 \times 10^{-19}) \nu^2 r^2 \theta^2 / \tau T \tag{2}$$

at radius r.[14] At 64 MHz, imaging sequences applied to the whole body can approach levels comparable to the average body basal metabolic rate of ~ 1 W/kg.

Average power deposition in an NMR imaging sequence can also be measured directly by monitoring the power input to the NMR coil, and substracting the coil losses by measuring the coil quality factors (Q) with and without the subject present. The average power deposited is

$$P^* = \frac{\tau}{mT} w_t \left[ 1 - \frac{Q(\text{loaded})}{Q(\text{empty})} \right] \tag{3}$$

where m is the subject's mass and $w_t$ is the measured pulse power corrected for cable losses.[14] The average power deposition measured at 64 MHz during a whole-body imaging experiment is plotted as a function of mass in Fig. 5 assuming the Fig. 1 imaging sequence with τ=0.2s, T = 0.7 s, and θ=π. The power deposited by the selective π/2 pulse is generally egligible in comparison to the π pulse because of the $\theta^2$ dependence of P n equation (2), and because selective excitation pulses are inherently f longer duration T which is inversely proportional to P (equations (2), 3)). The measured power deposition levels in this example are about /10 the average resting body metabolic rate.

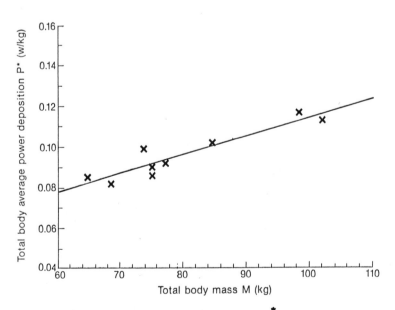

**Fig. 5.** Total body average power deposition $P^*$ (W/kg) as a function of total body mass in adult males using the imaging sequence of Fig. 1 at 64 MHz (τ=0.2s, T = 0.7 ms, and θ=π)[14].

## Spatial Localization

Initial human [31]P and [13]C spectroscopy studies benefitted from both the sensitivity advantage and the spatial selectivity provided by surface coils[2]. When used for both excitation and detection of the NMR signal, the surface coil sensitivity is approximately confined to a hemisphere subtended by the coil circumference and extending about one radius deep. A serious problem encountered when using surface coils for spatial localization in this manner, is undesirable signal contributions to the spectra from surface tissues in deep organ studies[15] (Fig. 6A). To eliminate surface tissue contributions and to provide accurately controlled depth-resolved surface-coil spectra (DRESS) we developed a localization technique employing a selective excitation pulse applied in the presence of a pulsed gradient magnetic field directed parallel to the surface-coil axis[16] (Fig. 7). This sequence results in localization of the NMR signal to a disk lying at the intersection of the selectively excited plane parallel to the surface coil, and the surface coil sensitivity profile.

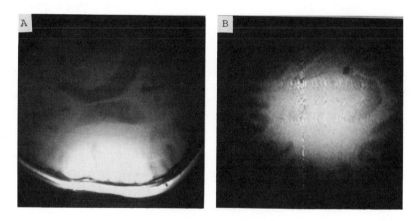

Fig. 6(A). Transaxial [1]H NMR image recorded at 64 MHz using a 6.5 cm surface detection coil located above the temple (array size, 256x256; $\tau=1.0$s; slice thickness, 4 mm). The hemispherical surface coil sensitivity profile is evident as the bright region lower centre. Up to about 50% of the [1]H signal derives from surface tissue. (B) Sagittal [1]H NMR image of a sensitive disk localized by the DRESS method[16] with similar coil location as in (A) (depth, 3.5 cm).

A conventional [1]H image of such a disk 3.5 cm deep in the brain is shown in Fig. 6B, recorded using a 6.5 cm diameter surface coil. [31]P spectra from the head as a function of depth are shown in Fig. 8.[16] These were also detected using a 6.5 cm diameter surface coil. The depth of the sensitive disk is varied simply by offsetting the frequency of the NMR pulses in a single side-band transmitter. The spectrum at 35 mm deep in Fig. 8 corresponds to brain, as characterized by a large phosphodiester (PD) to adenosine triphosphate (ATP) ratio, and a reduced phosphocreatine (PCr) to ATP ratio compared to the surface muscle spectrum. We find the application of [1]H surface-coil imaging immediately prior to acquisition of the spectroscopic information, invaluable for determining the precise location and identity of the tissue undergoing spectroscopic examination.[15]

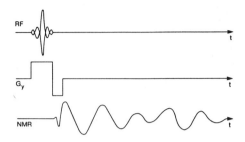

Fig. 7. DRESS pulse sequence.[16] A sinc function-modulated 90° RF pulse selects a plane parallel to the surface coil when applied in conjunction with a magnetic field gradient ($G_y$) directed coaxial to the coil. Data is acquired (NMR) as soon as the nuclei are rephased by the negative $G_y$ lobe.

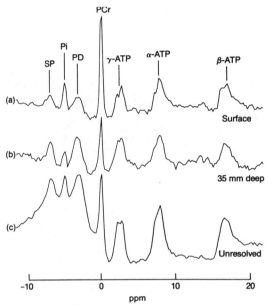

Fig. 8. [16] $^{31}$P DRESS from the surface of the human head (a), and 35 mm deep (b). The surface coil was located above the temple. (c) is a spatially unresolved spectrum recorded with the gradient turned off. The averaging times were 10, 20 and 5 min, respectively ($\tau=1s$). Chemical shifts are relative to PCr. A 3 Hz line-broadening exponential filter was applied to each spectrum, but no baseline flattening was attempted. The spectrometer gains are in the ratio 2:4:1 for (a), (b), and (c), respectively. (SP, sugar phosphates and phosphomonoesters; $P_i$ inorganic phosphate and blood sugar phosphate; PD, phosphodiesters; $\alpha-$, $\beta-$, $\gamma$-ATP, $\alpha-$, $\beta-$, $\gamma$-phosphates of ATP; $\gamma$-ATP and $\alpha$-ATP may contain contributions from adenosine diphosphate.)

## $H_2O$ Suppression

When the DRESS sequence is applied to the $^1$H resonance in the head, only a single $H_2O$ resonance is observed in the brain whilst surface tissue also exhibits a lipid ($-CH_2-$) resonance[16] (Fig. 9). It has been shown that if the $H_2O$ resonance in brain is suppressed, then other biologically important metabolites, such as lactate can be observed at mM-levels[17]. The amplitude of the lactate resonance appears as sensitive to hypoxia and ischemia as the Pi resonance in $^{31}$P spectra and the resonance at 1.3 pm in the spectrum contains 3-fold as many nuclei. Given the 15-fold sensitivity advantage inherent in $^1$H NMR compared to $^{31}$P NMR at the same field, in vivo $H_2O$ suppressed spectroscopy could provide spectacular sensitivity/scan time advantages over $^{31}$P for some metabolic studies and clinical applications.

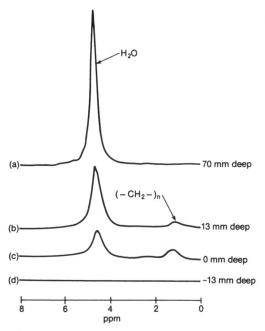

**Fig. 9.** A series of $^1$H DRESS[16] as a function of depth recorded from the human head above the temple (slice thickness, 5 mm; $\tau$=4.5 s; acquisition time, 9.0 s per spectrum; no exponential filtering). The spectrometer gain is the same for each spectrum. (a) was recorded at a depth of 70 mm below the surface of the skin, (b) was recorded with the sensitive plane at the surface, and (d) was obtained from 13 mm outside the head.

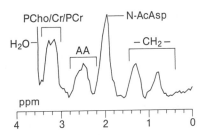

**Fig. 10.** Localized $^1$H spectrum form the human head recorded at a depth of 5 cm using $H_2O$-suppressed DRESS[18] with a 3-cm diameter surface coil located above the temple (acquisition time, 1.0 s; slice thickness, 5 mm; PCho/PCr/Cr, phosphocholine and total creatine pool; AA, amino acids; $-CH_2-$, lipid resonances from scalp tissue where DRESS slice intersects the surface).

We recently obtained metabolite-level [1]H spectra from the human brain at 1.5 T in an acquisition period of 2s (c.f. Fig. 8) using the DRESS technique modified for $H_2O$-suppression[18] (Fig. 10). The modification consisted of adding a long 100 ms duration sinc function modulated $\pi/2$ NMR pulse applied in the absence of imaging gradients immediately prior to the DRESS sequence in Fig. 7. This long pulse is precisely tuned to the $H_2O$ resonance so that its effect when combined with the $\pi/2$ slice-selective pulse is to invert the $H_2O$ resonance, thereby removing it from the spectrum.[18] In practice the $H_2O$ resonance is attenuated about 30-fold, which is sufficient to avoid receiver saturation and enable detection of mM-level metabolites. The N-acetylaspartate (N-AcAsp) resonance in Fig. 10 is at approximately a 10 mM concentration. Lactate is not identifiable in this spectrum of a normal volunteer.

### Chemical Shift Imaging

This method of $H_2O$-suppression by selective irradiation can also be incorporated in the conventional high-field imaging sequence depicted in Fig. 1. If the chemical shift spectrum of a sample is relatively simple, then the contributions of various preselected resonances in the spectrum can be removed from the image simply by applying the long chemical-selective irradiation pulse to the undesired resonance immediately prior to performing the conventional imaging sequence.[19,20] For example, in the body where the dominant resonances are from $H_2O$ and $-CH_2-$, chemical shift images can be obtained by respectively pre-irradiating the $-CH_2-$ and $H_2O$ resonances. The application of the technique to the head is illustrated in Fig. 11. Note that the $-CH_2-$ image contain negligible contributions from the brain consistant with Fig. 9. The likely cause of this lack of NMR-visible lipid in the brain is that brain lipids are rigidly bound and exhibit short $T_2$'s ($<3$ ms). Therefore they do not contribute to the spectra or images on the time-scale of these NMR experiments.

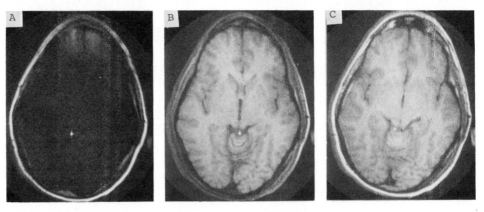

**Fig. 11.** [1]H transaxial NMR images representing the $-CH_2-$ (A) and $H_2O$ (B), distribution in the head obtained by chemical-selective irradiation[19,20]. (C) is a conventional image recorded with the chemical-selective irradiation pulse turned off. (Array size, 256x256; resolution 1x1x4 mm per picture point; image scan time, 5 min; $\tau = 0.2$s; duration of chemical selective irradiation pulse, 40 ms).

For heterogeneous objects where the chemical shift spectra contain more than two peaks it is possible to obtain chemical shift images of each species by using a 3-dimensional (3-D) or 4-dimensional (4-D) chemical shift imaging sequence in which one dimension is the chemical shift axis.[21,22] The 3-D sequence is identical to that shown in Fig. 1 except that the $G_x$-gradient is turned off during data acquisition intervals $q_4$ and $q_5$, and instead, the amplitude of the $G_x$-lobe during $q_2$ is varied in a similar fashion to the $G_y$-lobe (but linearly independent of the $G_y$ amplitude) in subsequent applications of the sequence. The spatial dependence of chemical shift spectra from the sample is determined from a 3-D Fourier transformation with respect to time, and the $G_x$ and $G_y$ amplitudes. Results are shown in Fig. 12 using an 8x8 point spatial array of spectra containing 128 points, and a whole-volume head imaging NMR coils. The $^1H$ image in Fig. 12A shows 2 bottles containing the characteristic spectrum of ethanol: Fig. 12B is a $^{31}P$ spectroscopic image of the whole human head recorded in about 1/2 hr. The lack of discernible spectra in Fig. 12B compared to Fig. 8 confirms the substantial signal-to-noise ratio advantage of surface coils relative to whole volume coils alluded to earlier.

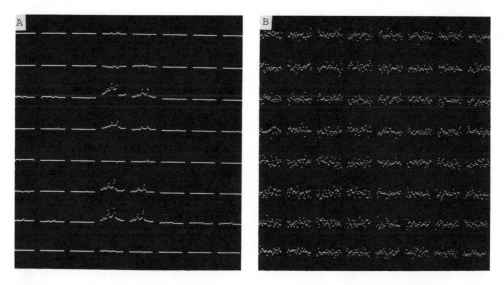

Fig. 12. (a) Transaxial $^1H$ 3-D chemical shift image of 2 bottles of ethanol located near the centre (array size, 8x8x128; spatial resolution 3x3x3 cm. (B) Transaxial $^{31}P$ 3-D chemical shift image through the human head above the temple (same spatial parameters; scan time ~ 1/2 hr.)

CONCLUSIONS

High quality, high resolution $^1H$ NMR images can be obtained from the human body at 1.5 T. The images show excellent contrast due to differences in tissue NMR relaxation times, and RF power levels typically do not substantially exceed basal metabolic levels. Imaging and spectroscopy techniques can be combined to yield spatially localized $^1H$ and $^{31}P$ spectra from the human body in clinically viable acquisition times of 2.0s to 20 min. Such spectra, acquired noninvasively, can provide a profile of key metabolites that reflect the state of health of the examined tissue.

Presently, in vivo applications of the DRESS technique for obtaining localized $^{31}P$ NMR include the detection of spectra from the normal human heart[23], and the noninvasive detection of regional myocardial ischemia in dogs.[24] We have also improved the DRESS method to enable acquisition of $^{31}P$ spectra from multiple depths in essentially the same time as required for single spectral acquisition.[25] Such advances render clinical applications of $^{31}P$ spectroscopy technically viable. Although the diagnostic value of the information thereby obtained awaits longer-term evaluation, initial indications are most promising.

REFERENCES

1. P. A. Bottomley, W. A. Edelstein, W. M. Leue, H. R. Hart, J. F. Schenck, and R. W. Redington, Magn. Reson. Med. 1:69 (1982).
2. P. A. Bottomley, H. R. Hart, W. A. Edelstein, J. F. Schenck, W. M. Leue, O. M. Mueller, and R. W. Redington, Radiol. 150:441 (1984).
3. D. W. Alderman and D. M. Grant, J. Magn. Reson. 36:447 (1979).
4. P. A. Bottomley, in: "NMR Imaging Proc. Internatl. Symp. on NMR Imaging: Winston-Salem, NC, Oct. 1-3, 1984," R. L. Witcofski, N. Karstaedt, and C. L. Partain, eds. Bowman Gray School of Medicine, Winston-Salem, NC:25 (1982).
5. C. E. Hayes, W. A. Edelstein, J. F. Schenck, O. M. Mueller, and M. Eash, J. Magn. Res. (in press 1985).
6. W. A. Edelstein, O. M. Mueller, P. A. Bottomley, J. F. Schenck, L. S. Smith, M. O'Donnell, W. M. Leue, and R. W. Redington, Magn. Reson. Med. 1:113 (1984).
7. W. A. Edelstein, J. F. Schenck, H. R. Hart, C. J. Hardy, T. H. Foster, and P. A. Bottomley, J. Am. Med. Assoc. 253:828 (1985).
8. J. F. Schenck, H. R. Hart, T. H. Foster, W. A. Edelstein, P. A. Bottomley, R. W. Redington, C. J. Hardy, R. A. Zimmerman, and L. T. Bilaniuk, Am. J. Neuroradiol. 6:193 (1985).
9. W. A. Edelstein, P. A. Bottomley, H. R. Hart, and L. S. Smith, J. Comp. Assist. Tomogr. 7:391 (1983).

10. P. A. Bottomley, T. H. Foster, r. E. Argersinger, and L. M. Pfeifer, Med. Phys. 11:245 (1984).

11. D. I. Hoult and P. C. Lauterbur, J. Magn. Reson. 34:425 (1979).
12. P. A. Bottomley and E. R. Andrew, Phys. Med. Biol. 23:630 (1978).
13. P. A. Bottomley and W. A. Edelstein, Med. Phys. 8:510 (1981).
14. P. A. Bottomley, R. W. Redington, W. A. Edelstein, and J. F. Schenck, Magn. Reson. Med. 2:336 (1985).
15. P. A. Bottomley, W. A. Edelstein, H. R. Hart, J. F. Schenck, and L. S. Smith, Magn. Reson. Med. 1:410 (1984).
16. P. A. Bottomley, T. H. Foster, and R. D. Darrow, J. Magn. Reson 59:338 (1984).
17. K. L. Behar, J. A. den Hollander, M. E. Stromski, T. Ogino, R. Shulman, O. A. C. Petroff, and J. W. Prichard, Proc. Natl. Acad. Sci. USA 80:4945 (1983).
18. P. A. Bottomley, W. A. Edelstein, T. H. Foster, and W. A. Adams, Proc. Natl. Acad. Sci. USA 82:2148 (1985).
19. P. A. Bottomley, T. H. Foster, and W. M. Leue, Lancet i:1120 (1984).
20. P. A. Bottomley, T. H. Foster, and W. M. Leue, Proc. Natl. Acad. Sci. USA 81:6856 (1984).
21. P. A. Bottomley, L. S. Smith, W. A. Edelstein, H. R. Hart, O. M. Mueller, W. M. Leue, R. Darrow, and R. W. Redington , Magn. Reson. Med. 1:111 (1984).
22. P. A. Bottomley and W. A. Edelstein, US Patent 4506223 (1985).
23. P. A. Bottomley, Science (in press, 1986).
24. P. A. Bottomley, R. J. Herfkens, L. S. Smith, S. Brazzamano, R. Blinder, L. W. Hedlund, J. L. Swain, and R. W. Redington (submitted for publication, 1985).
25. P. A. Bottomley, L. S. Smith, W. M. Leue, and C. Charles, J. Magn. Reson. (in press, 1985).